# Hysterical Men

# Hysterical Men

## THE HIDDEN HISTORY OF MALE NERVOUS ILLNESS

**Mark S. Micale**

HARVARD UNIVERSITY PRESS
Cambridge, Massachusetts
London, England
2008

Printed in the United States of America

*Library of Congress Cataloging-in-Publication Data*
Micale, Mark S., 1957–
    Hysterical men : the hidden history of male nervous illness /
Mark S. Micale.
        p. ; cm.
    Includes bibliographical references and index.
    ISBN 978-0-674-03166-1 (alk. paper)
    1. Hysteria—History.    2. Men—Mental health—History.
I. Title.    [DNLM: 1. Hysteria—history.    2. Gender Identity.
3. History, Modern 1601–.    4. Men—psychology.
WM 11.1 M6192h    2008]
RC532.M533    2008
616.85′240081—dc22            2008026043

*In memory of Janet Oppenheim and Roy Porter*

# CONTENTS

# ILLUSTRATIONS

# Acknowledgments

In the course of writing this book, I have incurred many debts. For material support over the years, I am grateful to the Harvard Society of Fellows, the Morse Fellowship Program at Yale University, the London Unit of the Wellcome Institute for the History of Medicine, the National Institutes of Health, the Manchester University Department of History, the British Academy, the University of Illinois Center for Advanced Study, and the UIUC Humanities Research Board.

On the research front, I want to acknowledge assistance from the staffs of the four great libraries where I conducted the bulk of my research: the Countway Library of Medicine in Boston, the National Library of Medicine in Bethesda, Maryland, the Wellcome Library for the History of Medicine in London, and the Bibliothèque de la Faculté de Médecine in Paris.

While my encounter with books was central to the evolution of this project, its main ideas have been honed by contact and controversy with scholars at other institutions and events. In particular, I recall lively and illuminating discussions with audiences at the Congress on Freud's Pre-Psychoanalytic Writings in Ghent, Belgium; the Harvard University Center for Cultural and Literary Studies; the Deutsch-Amerikanisches Institut at the University of Freiburg; and the "Men and Madness" symposium at Manchester Metropolitan University, organized by Berthold Schoene-Harwood.

As I reflect back on the decisive reading experiences underpinning this study, none seems more important than *The Inward Gaze: Masculinity and Subjectivity in Modern Culture* (1992), written by the British literary historian Peter Middleton. My book is in some sense an extrapolation of Middleton's analysis of literary and popular-cultural sources to the field of the history of medicine. Discovering Susan Bordo's work on the masculinization of Western philosophy since Descartes proved to be another epiphany. I first realized that I had to end my book with a chapter on Freud after listening in 1993 to a brilliant lecture on bisexuality in the psychoanalytic corpus delivered by Elisabeth Young-Bruehl to Yale's Muriel Gardiner Group in Psychoanalysis and the Humanities. For some time now, too, my thinking about male hysteria has dovetailed with Juliet Mitchell's work derived from clinical psychoanalysis, a fact from which I draw inspiration. More than any other scholar, the French historian of psychology Jacqueline Carroy has highlighted the interplay of medical, psychological, and literary languages in nineteenth-century culture; her precedent led me to explore this connection in my own historical story.

A book that attempts to cover a broad range of time periods and cultures is necessarily beholden to the work of many scholarly specialists. Most important, my first chapter, which is the farthest from my own areas of expertise, relies heavily on the voluminous and invaluable scholarship of Roy Porter and George Rousseau. Janet Oppenheim's *"Shattered Nerves": Doctors, Patients, and Depression in Victorian England* (1991) has provided a model of exacting scholarship, and her fifth chapter on "Manly Nerves" was a welcome revelation. I also want to salute the pioneering research of Robert Nye and John Tosh on, respectively, the history of French and British masculinities in the nineteenth century.

Other intellectual debts are more particular. Many years ago, Guenter Risse first brought to my attention the Georgian-era treatise on the nervous distempers as a medical genre. Elaine Showalter, a major voice in the historiography of hysteria, once sagely counseled me to make more of Charcot's many memorable case histories in my discussion of his work. At a critical moment, Robert Nye provided a superbly perceptive assessment of this project that kept me on track and sharpened my thinking on key points. In a conversation at an AAHM meeting long ago, Nancy Tomes casually conjured up the term "male malady" and then donated it to me. Fernando Vidal introduced me to the Huston/Sartre film *Freud: The Secret Passion,* and David Areford helped me to track down Francis Bacon's collection of French medical photographs in Dublin. Jim Gilbert and I worked side by side on our books about masculinity, sharing many conversations as well as a mutual dissatisfaction with the "crisis paradigm" in masculinity studies. Finally, over the past twenty-five years, Peter Gay has read nearly all of my scholarly work in progress, to my immeasurable benefit. At the University of Illinois in Urbana-Champaign, my colleagues have been wholly supportive—without, however, inquiring too closely into the nature of my passion for male hysteria. I wish to thank all of these individuals.

In the later stages of this project, my principal debt has been to Joyce Seltzer of Harvard University Press. In addition to her patience and fine editorial work, she has played an important role in shaping the book intellectually.

I dedicate this book to Janet Oppenheim and Roy Porter, two gifted practitioners of the historian's craft. I wish they were here to receive copies of it.

# NOTE ON USAGE

Defining one's subject matter is an essential requirement of all historical inquiry, but this preliminary task proved maddeningly difficult in the case of hysteria. Medical observers through the ages have characterized what they diagnosed as hysteria in exceedingly various, even contradictory, ways. The past models of the disorder analyzed in this book were derived from many different patient populations, institutional settings, disease paradigms, medical specialties, and social environments. Given the highly diverse disease formulations under study, it is likely that many different morbid phenomena were involved.

Given the limitations of the historical sources, it is impossible to rediagnose retrospectively with any reasonable degree of accuracy and consistency what past hysteria patients "really had." In the pages that follow, therefore, I conceptualize "the history of hysteria" as an evolving textual tradition whose subject is the diverse and diffuse behaviors designated as hysterical by physicians. The fact that today's medicine might interpret differently what earlier hysteria doctors declared to be the subject of their discourse is irrelevant to my story. It is physicians and their diagnostic behavior, rather than patients and what ailed them, that remain center stage in my account. Likewise, when I use the words "disease," "disorder," "sickness," and "hysteria," I am not making a judgment about the clinical identity or pathological status of the cases under discussion. I intend these terms in a neutral, descriptive sense, and, if it were not so cumbersome visually, I would cite them in quotation marks throughout.

IV7

:dge—and

;—how

? . . . We

lves.

# Hysteria: The Male Malady

IN JOHN HUSTON'S 1962 film *Freud: The Secret Passion,*
with a screenplay by Jean Paul Sartre, the young Sigmund Freud
(played by Montgomery Clift) appears in Paris during the middle
of the 1880s. In a dramatic scene near the beginning of the film,
Freud is observing Jean-Martin Charcot, then the most celebrated
physician in France, as Charcot demonstrates his new theories of
hysteria and hypnosis. Viewers sense at once that Huston has modeled his scene on one of the best-known representations of European science in the nineteenth century, André Brouillet's colossal
painting *A Clinical Lesson at the Salpêtrière,* which hung in the Paris
Salon of 1887.[1] The action is set in a lecture hall at the Salpêtrière
hospital in Paris, and the central figure of the master-physician
Charcot is surrounded by a clutch of attentive and adoring medical
students, including Freud, who has journeyed to Paris from Vienna
where he felt stifled by the hidebound medical instruction.

In the scene, an attendant wheels a female patient into the amphitheater for public demonstration. Her name is Jeanne; she appears young and fragile, with her chemise pulled provocatively

1

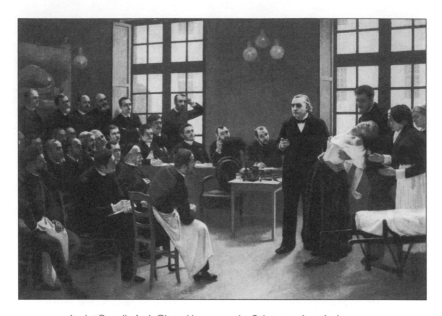

André Brouillet's *A Clinical Lesson at the Salpêtrière* (1886), the most famous icon in the history of hysteria. All the figures in the painting—including the patient and nurses—have been identified.

down around her arms. She suffers from a severe paraplegia that developed, Charcot tells us, following a railroad accident. A male medical student places Jeanne in a deep hypnotic trance by having her stare at a burning candle. Charcot then takes over: using suggestive hypnotics, he conjures away the patient's paralysis and commands her to walk again, thereby melodramatically demonstrating the "non-organic" or hysterical nature of the malady.[2] It is a familiar historical image—a legendary medical showman, a hysterical woman rather luridly placed on public display in the name of high science.

In Brouillet's painting, the gendered division of the canvas could not be more striking: sober, active, authoritative male science, bearded and clad formally in black, on one side of the image, and passive, vulnerable, but voluptuous femininity, highlighted with crimson lipstick, on the other side. But Huston's film, created in America during the age of Freud, includes another feature, one not found in Brouillet's painting seventy-five years earlier. In the movie, a second hysterical patient, an adult male, is brought before the audience after Jeanne. Charcot introduces the man as Servais. Servais's case appears to be one of paralysis agitans, or Parkinson's disease, a progressive degenerative neurological disorder marked by a rhythmic tremor of the extremities. Charcot explains that the patient, a woodcutter by occupation, had been chopping wood a year ago when he was nearly struck by lightning during a thunderstorm. Since then, despite no sign of organic injury, the patient's hands and legs have shaken uncontrollably, which prevents him from earning his living. After placing Servais in a somnambulic trance, Charcot with an autocratic clap of the hands instructs the patient to stop quivering. Again, the hysterical symptom vanishes quasi-miraculously.

At this point, the two hysterical patients—one male and one female—stand side by side in the lecture hall, deeply entranced and symptom-free. (Rumor has it that the two actors were real hospital patients, undergoing actual hypnosis for the film in the presence of their doctors on the studio set.) Charcot then proceeds to re-induce their distinguishing symptoms by means of hypnosis, but this time he ingeniously exchanges symptoms between the two patients: he commands Jeanne to shake nervously in the Parkinsonian manner and Servais to suffer a paralyzed leg. The patients' psyches comply, and the two symptoms magically reappear, but embodied in the patient of the opposite sex: Jeanne begins to tremble, while Servais collapses to the floor. "Gentlemen," Charcot intones in a thick French accent to the rapt audience, "you ave zhust witnessed za birth of an isterical symptom." The musical score swells, Freud's eyes widen in astonishment, and viewers are swept back to Vienna

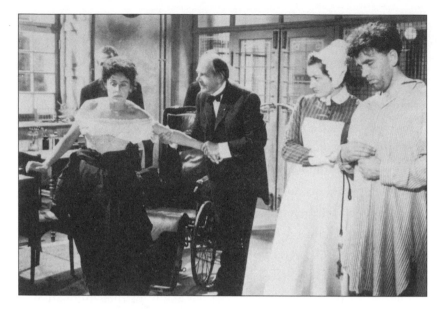

A scene from the film *Freud: The Secret Passion* (1962), directed by
John Huston. Charcot demonstrates on a hypnotized male and
female hysterical patient.

for the next segment of Freud's early career, including historic encounters with his own cast of famously neurotic patients.[3]

The action in this film scene is so fast that it is easy to pass over
the episode. But the scene deserves our close attention. Huston's
film set was an impressively faithful reconstruction, based on detailed knowledge of nineteenth-century medical publications, lith-
ographs, and photographs.[4] This accounts for our familiarity with
its main visual and narrative elements—with the striking exception
of the figure of Servais. What on earth is a *male* patient doing on
stage as the chosen clinical subject of the most renowned hysteria
doctor in history? How are we to understand the difference between the artistic rendition of hysteria in Brouillet's Victorian-era
painting and Huston's cinematic representation informed by mid-
twentieth-century psychoanalysis and existentialism? What are the

implications of ascribing a classically "female" disorder to an adult member of the opposite sex? And why are psychopathologies gendered at all in Western medicine?

THE DISEASE CATEGORY "hysteria" is as old as man—or, rather, as woman. Hysteria is among the oldest described disorders in the history of medicine, and among the most gendered. Facts commonly known about the subject are that the term *hysteria* traces etymologically to the Greek and Sanskrit words for uterus or womb, and that hysteria served for millennia of medical history as a male-authored commentary, often blatant in its misogyny, on women. In Greco-Roman medical writing, hysteria was believed to develop when the female reproductive system was inactive or ungratified over time. In Plato's *Timaeus* and certain Hippocratic texts, we find graphic descriptions of the uterus as a restless animal, rampaging its way through the female body as a result of unnatural prolonged abstinence and giving rise to a bizarre battery of symptoms, including a sensation of suffocation, heart palpitations, and loss of voice. Prescribed treatments for the malady through the ages included massage of the pelvic area, ovarian pressure, the application of scented drugs to entice the uterus back into place, and, most to the point, immediate marriage.

On first glance, the more recent medical era seems an extension of the view that hysteria is a pathological phenomenon exclusive to women. Pampered eighteenth-century salon ladies fainted from hysterical vapors. In Victorian Europe, a gallery of middle-class invalids—Charlotte Perkins Gilman, Alice James, and Eleanor Marx are only the best-known examples—recorded their nervous sufferings in memorable fictional and autobiographical accounts. And at the end of the 1800s, Freud's fabled collection of hysterical female patients helped launch the new psychology of psychoanalysis.

Like the scene in Brouillet's painting, these associations are powerfully engraved in our historical imagination. They do not, however, represent the entire story. Hysteria, it turns out, has operated
within past social and intellectual cultures that did not have as their
sole purpose the definition and oppression of women. Renaissance
treatises on "hypochondriacal melancholia" in fact discoursed on
the effects of the "black bile" on men's minds and bodies more than
on women's. In Georgian England and Scotland, high-society physicians produced dozens of treatises on the "nervous distempers" in
both sexes, while their counterparts in the arts wrote extensively
about their personal nervous symptoms. A distinguished cast of figures in nineteenth-century Europe and America, including Charles
Darwin, John Ruskin, John Addington Symonds, Francis Galton,
George Beard, James Sully, Edmund Gosse, Joseph Lister, Louis
Agassiz, and William James, were plagued by debilitating nervous
ailments.[5] In Paris, Charcot demonstrated his theories on scores of
male patients, just like Servais in *Freud: The Secret Passion.* Hysteria
in modern times has also been a *male* malady.[6]

The full historical story of the male nervous maladies, however,
has yet to be told, and the reasons for this cultivated silence are
themselves highly instructive. Since ancient times, physicians, philosophers, and natural scientists closely observed and extravagantly
theorized female weakness, emotionality, and madness. What this
long procession of male experts signally failed to see, to acknowledge, and to ponder was the existence of masculine nervous and
mental illness among all social classes and in diverse guises. They
did so despite rampant counter-evidence in the clinic and the laboratory, on the streets and the battlefields. The information we do
have about this subject comes to us almost exclusively from letters,
diaries, memoirs, novels, and autobiographies, which is to say from
nonmedical sources. Furthermore, the well-known individual cases

listed above were either handled very privately at the time or were formally diagnosed with non-derogatory diagnoses, such as "nerve exhaustion" and "neurasthenia." The reasons for suppressing male neurosis from the official discourses of science and medicine as well as from popular view range from the personal and psychological to the professional and the political. They constitute a chapter in Western medical history that is marked not by the steady, rational accumulation of knowledge, but by anxiety, ambivalence, and selective amnesia. In a real sense, this is a book about something that did not happen in history, a thought experiment resisted over the generations, a reality of human behavior that was rarely observed by the observational science par excellence. Today, we have in many ways moved beyond the ideas and attitudes chronicled in the following chapters. The story, however, has had some enduring consequences, and the greatly altered circumstances of the early twenty-first century make it possible, and important, to recover that hidden history.

# CHAPTER 1

# Hysterick Women and Hypochondriack Men

AN EGYPTIAN MEDICAL PAPYRUS dating from around 1900 B.C., one of the oldest surviving documents known to medical history, records a series of curious behavioral disturbances in adult women. As the ancient Egyptians interpreted it, the cause of these abnormalities was the movement of the uterus, which they believed to be an autonomous, free-floating organism that could move upward from its normal pelvic position. Such a dislocation, they reasoned, applied pressure on the diaphragm and gave rise to a battery of bizarre physical and mental symptoms. Egyptian doctors developed an array of medications to entice the errant womb back down into its correct position. Foremost among their measures were the placement of aromatic substances on the vulva to draw the womb downward, and the swallowing of foul-tasting substances to repel the uterus away from the upper parts.

This ancient Middle Eastern source furnished the basis for classical Greek medical and philosophical theories of hysteria. The ancient Greeks adopted the notion of the migratory uterus and embroidered upon the connections, only implicit in the Egyptian text, between hysteria and sexual dissatisfaction. In an often-cited passage in the *Timaeus,* Plato in the fourth century B.C. discoursed colorfully about the vagaries of female reproductive physiology: "The animal within them [women] is desirous of procreating children, and when remaining unfruitful long beyond its proper time, gets discontented and angry, and wandering in every direction through the body, closes up the passages of the breath, and by obstructing respiration, drives them to extremity, causing all varieties of disease."[1] Various texts of the school of Hippocrates from the fifth century B.C. onward explain similarly that a mature woman's deprivation of sexual relations causes a restless womb to move upward in search of gratification. As the female reproductive parts move or function irregularly—ascending or descending, convulsing or prolapsing—they can cause dizziness, motor paralyses, sensory losses, and respiratory distress (including *globus hystericus,* the sensation of a ball lodged in the throat), as well as extravagant emotional behaviors. Ancient Greek therapies included uterine fumigations, the application of tight abdominal bandages, and a regular regimen of marital sexual intercourse.[2]

With the growth of anatomical knowledge, the hypothesis of the morbidly wandering womb became increasingly untenable. Nevertheless, ancient Roman physicians continued to associate hysteria exclusively with the female generative system. The principal causes of hysterical disorders, they conjectured, were "diseases of the womb" and disruptions of female reproductive processes, including amenorrhea, miscarriage, premature births, and menopause. Galen of Pergamon, in the second century C.E., formulated a particularly popular theory tracing the origins of the malady to the retention of excessive menstrual blood. Not surprisingly, Roman physicians identified cases of hysteria most often in virgins, widows, and spinsters. Engraved in the *Corpus Hippocraticum* and the Galenic writings, these hypotheses formed a medical ideology that remained influential for millennia of medical history. The descriptive and theoretical details evolved, but the basic doctrine of gynecological determinism endured until remarkably late into the modern medical period.[3] Males, according to these age-old theories, were definitionally excluded from the disease.

The coming of Christian civilization in the Latin West initiated the first paradigm shift in the history of hysteria. From the fifth to the thirteenth centuries, naturalistic pagan views were increasingly displaced by supernatural formulations. In the writings of St. Augustine, human suffering, including organic and mental illness, was perceived to be a manifestation of innate evil consequent upon original sin. Hysteria in particular, with its erratic symptoms, was viewed as a sign of possession by the devil. The hysterical female was now interpreted alternately as a victim of bewitchment to be pitied, or as the devil's soul mate to be despised. No less powerful than the classical image of the disease, the demonological model envisioned hysterical anesthesias, mutisms, and convulsions as *stigmati diaboli* or marks of the devil.

This sea change in thinking about the disorder brought with it changes in treatment. The elaborate pharmacopoeia of ancient times was replaced during this long period by supernatural invocations—prayers, incantations, amulets, and exorcisms. Furthermore, with the demonization of hysteria came widespread persecution of the afflicted. During the late medieval and renaissance periods, the scene of interrogation of the female hysteric shifted from the hospital to the church and courtroom, which became the loci of spectacular interrogations. Official manuals for the detection of witches, often virulently misogynistic, supplied instructions for the detection, torture, and at times execution of the witch/hysteric. As exclusively as classical medicine, demonological theories conceptualized hysteria as archetypically female. There were no male witches.

## Hysteria Demystified

The first medical discourse on hysteria in the male population appeared during the later Renaissance period.[4] An idea of hysteria conceived naturalistically first emerged as an ailment of the human mind and body, possessing the status of an integrated disease entity, and designated with language derivative of the modern English noun "hysteria."

Physicians during the 1500s and 1600s increasingly took the position that disease should be placed wholly within the province of medical explanation and ministration, rather than religion. With the emergence of a modern, secular world view, what was once regarded as a divinely created soul in spiritual distress came more and more to be construed as a naturalistic mind, psyche, or personality that suffered emotionally or psychologically. In the work of Paracelsus in Switzerland, Johannes Weyer in the Netherlands, and Ambroise Paré in France, hysteria ceased to be viewed as a demonic visitation and instead became a medical malady. By the middle of the seventeenth century, the disorder had effectively been renaturalized as part of the larger demystification of mental life occurring across western and central Europe.[5]

During the following century and a half, the British Isles generated the richest and most voluminous commentary on this freshly demystified hysteria. England's early representative of the new secularizing movement was Edward Jorden (1569?–1633). In 1603 Jorden, a prominent member of the London College of Physicians, authored *A Briefe Discourse of a Disease Called the Suffocation of the Mother*.[6] The work was occasioned by a controversial case of witchcraft involving the fourteen-year-old daughter of a city alderman who had suddenly been smitten by a bizarre array of nervous symptoms, including convulsions, loss of sight and speech, and a lack of sensation on the left side of her body.[7] Jorden's *Discourse* runs to only 55 compact pages, and its full title indicates its aim: *A briefe discourse of a disease called the suffocation of the Mother. Written uppon occasion which hath beene of late taken thereby, to suspect possession of an evill spirit, or some such like supernaturall power. Wherein is declared that divers strange actions and passions of the body of man, which in the common opinion, are imputed to the Divell, have their true natural causes, and do accompanie this disease.* Published in the midst of the witch-craft craze, Jorden's pamphlet, which he wrote in the English vernacular for the public's enlightenment, is a forceful and clear-headed defense of the naturalness of hysterical phenomena.

Jorden boldly re-medicalized the disorder by going back twenty centuries to Hippocratic and Galenic ideas, which he embraced uncritically. Jordenian hysteria occurs when the womb, deprived of health-giving moisture derived from sexual intercourse, worms its way upward in the body cavity in search of nourishment. Throughout his exposition, Jorden, who lards his discussion with classical textual citations, labels the disorder "suffocation of the Mother," a colloquialism for "suffocation of the womb." All the cases he cites involve women. Despite its progressive ideological and humanitarian goals, Jorden's late Elizabethan tract is a conservative document that rehabilitated the uterine hypothesis within British medical thought for the next three-quarters of a century.

Nearly two decades after Jorden's essay, Robert Burton's sprawling and eccentric masterpiece, *The Anatomy of Melancholy*, appeared.[8] Burton (1577–1640) passed the bulk of his adulthood in the cloistered splendor of Renaissance Oxford. There, as a lifelong fellow of Christ Church College, he taught theology, medicine, and the classics. Written under the pseudonym of Democritus Junior, his tome appeared in 1621 and was an immediate success, with five editions published during the author's lifetime. Burton's subject is the human mind in all of its kaleidoscopic moods and manifestations. In the tradition of the Renaissance treatise on humanity, the book draws on nearly the whole of human knowledge, including psychology, medicine, literature, philosophy, philology, history, astrology, art, and travel. Burton had read comprehensively in the book culture of his time, and his erudite work is chock-full of excerpts from and allusions to classical, medieval, and contemporary texts.[9] Burtonian melancholy embraces an enormous range of behaviors, from fatigue and insomnia to stuttering and digestive disorders. From today's clinical perspective, it is a hodgepodge of neurotic and psychotic reactions, including obsessions, phobias, anxiety states, and hallucinations.

Listed among the forms and symptoms of the affliction is "Maids', Nuns', and Widows' Melancholy," commonly considered the Burtonian version of hysteria. Burton regards this malady as a species of "hypochondriacal melancholy" and cites Hippocrates and Aretaeus of Cappadocia among its early observers. In the classical manner, he traces the disorder partly to venereal starvation. Not surprisingly, in the opinion of this solitary scholar, "the best and surest" among the repertoire of remedies "is to see them [the victims] well placed and married to good husbands in due time." Burton's recital of hysterical symptoms fills three pages, ranging from "a vexation of the mind" and "much solitariness, weeping, and distraction" to "fits of the mother" and "great pains in their heads . . . hearts and hypochondries." His account grows increasingly engaged autobiographically, until the author catches himself querulously: "But where am I? Into what subject have I rushed? What have I to do with nuns, maids, virgins, widows? I am a bachelor myself, and lead a monastic life in a college; *nae ego sane ineptus qui haec dixerim* [it is certainly very foolish of me to speak thus]."[10]

Into what subject indeed? Tracing his own "bachelor's melancholy" to the monastic celibacy then required of college dons, Bur-

ton's wandering narrative is replete with personal asides. Throughout his more than one thousand pages, he draws his ideas and
insights about the human mind and condition equally from his
reading, his knowledge of other people, and self-observation. Burton's early seventeenth-century textbook of abnormal psychology
looks both backward and forward. Unremarkably, Burton attributes
hysteria to a mishmash of classical humoral and gynecological factors and interprets mental aberrations as the work of God, sin, and
the devil. Burton formally limits "maids', nuns', and virgins' melancholy" to one sex, yet his omnibus concept of melancholy is not
gender-specific—a fact that enables the author to discuss melancholy men, including the intricacies and intimacies of their interior
lives, far more than he discusses melancholy women. Burton's great
book of 1621 thus initiated a tradition of male psychological self-
portraiture that exerted a strong influence on medical and literary
intellectuals in Britain for the following 150 years.[11]

William Harvey's *Anatomical Exercises on the Generation of Animals*
was published in 1651, thirty years after Burton's *Anatomy* and fifty
years after Jorden's *Briefe Discourse*. Harvey's earlier work, *De Motu
Cordis* (1628), announced to the world the circulation of the blood
and is ranked among the premier classics of the history of medicine. Harvey (1578–1657) is deservedly less renowned for his later
forays into reproductive biology. Creative, observationally oriented,
and free from past precedents in other areas of his scientific thought,
Harvey adhered conservatively to a uterine theory of hysteria, leaving no doubt about his beliefs: in his *Anatomical Exercises* he asserts
that "the uterus is a most important organ, and brings the whole
body to sympathize with it." He goes on to add:

> No one of the least experience can be ignorant what grievous
> symptoms arise when the uterus either rises up or falls down,

or is in any way put out of place, or is seized with spasms—how dreadful, then, are the mental aberrations, the delirium, the melancholy, the paroxysms of frenzy, as if the affected person were under the dominion of spells, and all arising from unnatural states of the uterus.[12]

Jorden, Burton, and Harvey are representative of English renaissance medical thought about the "hysterical passions," as they were then commonly called. Despite the modern qualities of these writings, hysteria throughout this period remained an exclusively female condition. Popular synonyms in late sixteenth- and early seventeenth-century English medicine included *uteri adscensus, suffocatio uterina,* and *strangulatio vulvae.* The modernity of Jorden, Burton, and Harvey rests in the re-medicalization of supernatural hysteria and the initiation of a tradition of keen psychological observation; but late Tudor and early Stuart medical writers did not question the inherited wisdom regarding hysteria's gender identity.

There is one exception to this rule, however, which came not from a scientific but a literary figure of the late Elizabethan and early Jacobean periods. In Act Two, Scene 4 of *King Lear,* published in 1606, Shakespeare has Lear register for the first time his personal and political disintegration. After expressing anguish over his rejection by his daughters Goneril and Regan, and the sight of his servant in their stocks, Lear cries out:

O, how this mother swells up toward my heart!
*Hysterica passio!* down, thou climbing sorrow,
Thy element's below.

There seems to be no precedent in medical history for Shakespeare's image of the pathogenic and peripatetic womb rising through the body cavity to the throat, either as a literal physical event in the male body or as a metaphor for emotional and existential anxiety in men.[13]

## The Revolutionary Period

This situation changed dramatically during the last quarter of the 1600s. The transformation of human understanding known as the scientific revolution introduced new methods of inquiry, like the empirical experimentalism of Francis Bacon and the analytical rationalism of René Descartes. The discoveries in physics and astronomy of Copernicus, Brahe, Kepler, Galileo, and Huygens, and the reordering of the cosmos that resulted from them, were achieved through a willingness to question inherited scientific authorities and to revise, if not reject, classical teachings. In medicine, Andreas Vesalius and his successors introduced new and more accurate pictures of the interior of the human body, while Harvey challenged Galenic authority in the field of cardiovascular physiology.

One effect of these changes was to begin to pry loose the age-old association of hysteria with female reproductive anatomy and physiology. European doctors now began to conduct autopsies on patients believed to have suffered from hysteria, and time and again they found no postmortem uterine pathology. In place of the waning gynecological explanations, new ideas about causation, centering on the brain and nervous system, appeared during the 1670s and 1680s. A neurological phase in the history of hysteria took form and provided the theoretical framework for the first medical speculations about the disorder in males.

Two celebrated English physicians put forth critiques of the ancient womb theory during the closing decades of the seventeenth century. Thomas Willis (1621–1675) was professor of natural philosophy at Oxford with a thriving private medical practice in London. In his *Cerebri Anatome* [*Anatomy of the Brain*] of 1664, Willis provided the most complete and accurate account of the human nervous system up to that time.[14] Willis was convinced that the brain and spinal cord played a much larger role than previously realized in the genesis of many illnesses, including hysteria. In his *Practice of Physick* of 1684, he rejected as errant nonsense the notion that the uterus, held in place by an intricate network of ligaments, could detach itself and move through a space densely occupied by bodily organs.[15] Willis instead proposed the cerebral origin and seat of hysteria: "The Distemper named from the Womb is chiefly and primarily Convulsive, and chiefly depends on the Brain and the nervous stock [system] being affected."[16] Elsewhere, Willis demonstrated beyond doubt on the autopsy table that patients who had been diagnosed with hysteria in every case disclosed no structural uterine abnormalities.

Thomas Sydenham agreed. A founder of modern clinical medicine and epistemology, Sydenham (1624–1689) was among the first physicians to emphasize the maintenance of detailed medical records and the unbiased observation of patients. Like his contemporary Willis, Sydenham maintained an elite urban practice that included private clients with all manner of nervous complaints. Sydenham's comments on hysteria are scattered in two relatively unknown works, his *Epistolary Dissertation* of 1681–82 and the posthumously published *Processus Integri* of 1693. When it came to hysteria, Sydenham, the "English Hippocrates," was expressly anti-Hippocratic. He had no truck whatsoever with the old gynecological explanations; in their place he formulated a kind of neuropsychological model of the disease. Sydenham believed that the condition he observed was produced by the irregular distribution of "animal spirits" between body and mind. This maldistribution, he hypothesized, was caused most often by sudden and violent emotions, including anger, fear, love, and grief. Sydenham judged hysteria to be infinitely more common than was previously believed; he stressed the clinical fluidity of the disorder, and he highlighted its extraordinary capacity to morph symptomatologically into other disease forms. It is surely no coincidence that the first medical intellectuals explicitly to reject the womb theory also defended the possibility—in fact the undeniability—of hysterical breakdown in men.

In the 1670s and 1680s, Willis and Sydenham specifically introduced the notion of a masculine variant of the disease through the creation of a novel diagnostic entity, "hystero-hypochondriasis." Up to that time, the familiar term "hypochondriasis" denoted a somatic disorder centered on the hypochondrium, or the area below the rib cage, that was accompanied by a mystifying multiplicity of symptoms. In the ancient system of humoral medicine, these symptoms were imagined to arise from an excess of black bile secreted by the hypochondrium into the body. In Burton's time, hypochondria and hysteria were grouped under the diagnostic umbrella of melancholia. Willis, Sydenham, and their medical contemporaries, however, separated out the symptom cluster of hypochondriasis from Burton's encyclopedic melancholia and granted it status as an independent diagnostic entity.[17] Freed of its association with the more severe psychopathologies encompassed by melancholy, hypochondriasis was now paired with hysteria. Both hysteria and hypochondria designated disorders of the abdominal viscera with an erratic array of mental and physical symptoms released upward in the body cavity. The main difference between the two, according to Willis and Sydenham, was that hysteria afflicted women and hypochondriasis men.

For Willis, hysteria and hypochondriasis were kindred clinical categories, sibling syndromes with similar symptomatologies that traced to the nervous system.[18] In the tenth chapter of *An Essay on the Pathology of the Brain and Nervous Stock in which Convulsive Diseases are Treated of* (1667), Willis applies the diagnosis of hysteria democratically: "Women of all ages and conditions are obnoxious to these kind of Distempers, in the rich and poor, in Virgins, Wives, and Widows; yea, sometimes the same kind of Passions infest Men."[19] In his efforts to discredit the entrenched womb theory, Willis later strategically cites the presence of hysteria in three groups previously excluded from the diagnosis: prepubertal females, postmenopausal women, and adult men. Earlier in the same work, he obligingly illustrates the last contention by relating the story of a forty-year-old man seized with convulsive movements preceded by depression. The patient also suffered from dizziness and choking, with the sensation of a large object moving from his stomach up to his heart. This sensation, Willis reports, was followed by epileptiform attacks, each lasting about fifteen minutes and of such violence that it required four men to restrain the patient.[20] Written in 1667, Willis's passage may well record the first rudimentary "case history" of a male hysteric.

In the 1680s, Sydenham pushed Willis's diagnostic rapprochement of female hysteria and male hypochondriasis a step further. For Willis, female hysteria was an affliction that resembled male hypochondriasis; that is, the two disorders were descriptively and clinically analogous phenomena. Sydenham, however, maintained that hysteria and hypochondriasis were for all intents and purposes the identical disorder—he claimed explicitly that what he observed in his male and female patients was the same pathological entity, which previously had been labeled differently only because of linguistic tradition. In Sydenham's view, men and women could suffer equally from either hysteria or hypochondriasis, just as they might fall prey to gout, malaria, or melancholy.

Late in 1681, the Worcester physician William Cole wrote to Sydenham asking him to set down on paper his beliefs regarding "the hysterical passions." His own health failing, Sydenham responded with an extended letter to his colleague known as the *Epistolary Dissertation to Dr. Cole* (1681–1682), in which he dismisses impatiently the classical explanations of hysteria and declares flatly that men too can be victims:

> Of all chronic diseases, hysteria—unless I err—is the commonest; since just as fevers . . . equal two thirds of the number of all chronic diseases taken together, so do hysterical complaints (or complaints so called) make one half of the remaining third. As to females, if we except those who lead a hard and hardy life, there is rarely one who is wholly free from them—and females, be it remembered, form one half of the adults of the world. Then, again, such male subjects as lead a sedentary or studious life, and grow pale over their books and papers, are similarly afflicted; since, however much antiquity may have laid the blame of hysteria upon the uterus, hypochondriasis (which we impute to some obstruction of the spleen or viscera) is as like it, as one egg is to another.[21]

A debate about the precise clinical relation between hysteria and hypochondriasis—and by extension between female and male neurosis—ran through late seventeenth- and eighteenth-century European medicine. A few physicians, like the German Friedrich Hoffmann, argued that the two disorders were falsely conflated and sought to restore the traditional place of the uterus in the pathogenesis of hysteria.[22] But for the next hundred years Willis's and Sydenham's interpretations prevailed, and British physicians in particular embraced the mixed hystero-hypochondriasis concept. To be sure, Willis's and Sydenham's innovations were only partial: they still reveal traces of humoral thinking; both men continued to employ different terminology for the nervous disorders in the two sexes; and both imagined a higher rate of occurrence in women, resulting from an alleged fragility of the female nervous system. Nonetheless, the sense of a decisive departure from past medical thinking is unmistakable.

What led Willis and Sydenham to apply a diagnostic category previously limited strictly to the members of one sex to the opposite sex? Doubtless a number of factors were involved. The new philosophical empiricism of the seventeenth century encouraged medical elites to see and record the nervous disorders in their male patients in a way they previously had not done. It is likely more than happenstance that Willis was renowned for basing his ideas not on speculative theories but on anatomical observations and pathological studies, whereas Sydenham was fabled for his unprejudiced observational powers. Furthermore, the new scientific attention to the nervous system that characterized the final third of the 1600s provided a key precondition for Willis's and Sydenham's work. While both men continued to perceive women as more vulnerable to nervous afflictions, they also regarded both sexes as possessing the same basic nervous anatomy and physiology, a statement that could not be made about the male and female reproductive systems. The new nerve-centered theories of neurosis, in other words, were much less gendered than the preceding (or succeeding) disease models.

Willis and Sydenham wrote during a period of widespread innovation and creativity in many areas of British life, thought, and society. In the political, intellectual, and scientific culture of the time, no less than in the history of hysteria, the 1670s and 1680s were a revolutionary age in England. Following a decade of escalating confrontation between the crown and parliament, the "Glorious Revolution" of 1688 discarded the overweening Catholic Stuart royal line and ushered in a new system of Protestant Hanoverian government that balanced monarchical and legislative authority. Two years later, the philosopher (and physician) John Locke, a parliamentary sympathizer writing in political exile in Holland, published his *Two Treatises of Civil Government*. Locke's classic of political theory provided the definitive critique of royal absolutism and political patriarchalism, and enshrined the new principles of political liberalism and individualism. The year before the revolution Isaac Newton had published his *Principia,* the culminating synthesis of the scientific revolution, which marked a permanent break from the static, classical world picture. It is clear retrospectively that these diverse but contemporaneous developments were all predicated on a critical questioning, at times a subversion, of traditional, inherited sources of authority, and that each one initiated paradigmatic change in its field. In one small corner of late Stuart culture, the rejection of Hippocratic and Galenic teachings about hysteria, including a new and more liberal application of the diagnosis to both sexes, was part of the revolutionary atmosphere of the age.

## The Nervous Culture of Georgian Britain

The ideas of Willis and Sydenham worked themselves out across the eighteenth century in England and Scotland. In the long and colorful history of hysteria, before Paris and Vienna came London, Edinburgh, Oxford, and Cambridge, where a kind of "nervous culture" formed during the 1700s.[23] That culture fully and comfortably featured both men and women.

A concatenation of circumstances fostered the flowering of Georgian medical culture.[24] The scientific revolution of the previous hundred and fifty years, and the deeper processes of secularization subtending it, released enormous intellectual energies in Europe. In the face of declining theological explanations, the possibility of new, naturalistic domains of inquiry, including sciences of the body and mind, took shape. The new theories of human nature, extending to ideas of health, illness, and disease, that formed at this time centered specifically on the nervous system. This was due in part to the increased knowledge of neuroanatomy and neurophysiology, and in part to Lockean psychology and epistemology with its emphasis on human beings as malleable, sensate creatures. Physicians came to conceptualize the human body as a brain and spinal column with an infinity of neural pathways radiating outward from this cerebrospinal axis. The role of the central nervous system was to convey and coordinate sensory messages throughout the body; all thought, perception, and sensation were mediated through it.[25] Exactly how the nerves organized sensation and motion remained unknown—eighteenth-century scientists speculated extravagantly about nervous organization as a network of fibers, string, pipes, and cords that operated mechanically, hydraulically, electrically, and so forth.[26] Whatever the model was thought to be, the nervous system's role was all-important to Georgian thinkers, and when it failed or malfunctioned, nervous breakdown ensued. Reflecting the new pathological centrality of the nerves, the medical Scotsman Robert Whytt observed in 1765 that "all diseases may, in some sense, be called affections of the nervous system, because, in almost every disease, the nerves are more or less hurt."[27]

The concept of "the nervous distempers," which had gained currency by the 1730s, reflected these new beliefs. The notion of the distempers traces back to the classical doctrine of the temperaments, in which an imbalance of one of the body's four main humors—blood, phlegm, black bile, and yellow bile—was believed to produce disease. Distempered, the human nervous system could

wreak devastating havoc on body and mind. From today's perspective, eighteenth-century nervous disorders embraced an inchoate
combination of mental and physical complaints that would most
likely now be labeled as psychosomatic and psychoneurotic.[28] The
main varieties of the distempers were hysteria, hypochondria, the
spleen, and the vapors, with little clear demarcation among them,
although doctors separated these from more severe pathologies
such as mania, frenzy, delirium, and madness.

Developments in imaginative literature, social theory, and moral
philosophy buttressed the neurocentrism of eighteenth-century
medicine. The 1700s, especially the decades between 1730 and
1790, brought a number of overlapping cults of sensibility. Physicians emphasized sensibility as a property of the nervous system.
Analogously, mid-century Scottish moralists and philosophers like
Francis Hutcheson, David Hume, and Adam Smith dwelled on the
passions and sentiments, rather than the Cartesian faculty of ratio-
cination, as key constituent parts of human nature. Reinforcing this
trend were developments in theology. From the Restoration onward, Anglican clergymen and theologians of Latitudinarian persuasion, reacting against both the emotional severity of Puritan-
ism and the materialist rationalism of Hobbes, sermonized on
certain human sentiments—pity, benevolence, empathy, humani-
tarianism—as forces of moral virtue.[29]

Above all, this was the "age of sensibility." Prose fiction, poetry, and drama during the second half of the eighteenth century
abounded in "sentimental" characters whose emotionality was featured in one work after another.[30] A reaction against the preceding
century's preoccupation with philosophical rationalism and Hobbes's theory of the innate selfishness of man, the new philosophy of
feeling encouraged displays of sentiment that were lavish, spontaneous, and public. Later generations found it easy to parody sen-

sibility as sentimentality. The important point for our purposes is that the eighteenth-century doctrine of sensibility in British culture extended notably to both sexes. The treatises of Hume and Smith theorize about human nature generically, while novelists of sensibility populated their stories with affected heroes and heroines alike.

Henry MacKenzie's *The Man of Feeling* (1771) is the emblematic text of this culture.[31] Born and raised in mid-Enlightenment Edinburgh and the son of a well-to-do doctor, MacKenzie (1745–1831) followed in the literary tradition of Samuel Richardson and Laurence Sterne. MacKenzie's slender best-selling novel, written when the author was in his mid-twenties, relates the story of Harley, a "man of sensibility," who is placed in a chain of situations designed to arouse sharp emotional reactions in both the protagonist and the reader. The central subject of the book is Harley's emotional behavior as he falls in love, encounters old friends, stumbles into a brothel, confronts a pathetic beggar, visits Bedlam hospital, and observes the suffering of animals. In *The Man of Feeling*, and throughout the literature of sensibility, the effusive expression of emotion in appropriate circumstances, including the copious shedding of tears, is not deemed inappropriate for men.[32]

With their intertwined roots in science, philosophy, religion, psychology, and literature, eighteenth-century sensibility cults featured a new type of male, especially among the rising middle classes, in whom the fluent display of "feeling" was construed as a sign of good breeding, refined manners, and elevated morality.[33] Furthermore, mid-eighteenth-century sentimentality extended from the private to the public sphere. Sentimental fiction conspicuously participated in some of the most impassioned public controversies of the day, including the liberal-humanitarian critiques of the slave trade and of capitalist commercialism.[34] What is striking from the later perspective of Victorian Europe, with its more stringent assigning of emotional behaviors between the sexes, is that the eighteenth-century writers of sensibility constructed their emotive male characters without compromising their gender identity, that is, without fear of effeminization.

The doctrines of sensibility in the nervous culture of the Georgian age also had pronounced class connotations. Those who were better bred were widely believed to have a more refined nervous apparatus and therefore a greater sensory capacity for experiencing life's finer offerings; at the same time, unfortunately, they were more prone to nervous collapse. By restricting nervous distempers to the urban, educated, self-consciously cultured classes on the rise, eighteenth-century British physicians demarcated both themselves and their clientele from what they viewed as the crude, unschooled, lower social orders. Good blood and bad nerves went hand in hand.[35] As a consequence, a kind of medical plutocracy emerged in Georgian Britain, a nobility of the nerves endowed with natural superior sensibility and, by extension, with greater social legitimacy and political authority. By the mid-1700s, this cluster of beliefs contributed to a full-blown theory of civilization that was central to the way an elite class of Georgians conceived of themselves and their society. In the 1730s the fashionable London nerve doctor George Cheyne, with more pride than trepidation, christened the nervous distempers "the English malady." Signs of a surfeit of success and civilization, hysteria, hypochondria, the vapors, and the spleen reflected the key progressivist mentality of the age.

These attitudes and associations, moreover, directly shaped how people viewed themselves in sickness and health. Hysteria and its kindred categories operated throughout this period as an entire new way of thinking, feeling, and seeing in Georgian society. Because nervousness was thought to strike the higher social strata, which were associated with sensibility and refinement, these afflications were even cultivated in select circles. "Nervous self-fashioning" occurred in letters, diaries, memoirs, and autobiographies (and, one imagines, in countless conversations) as doctors, writers, and laypersons alike internalized the new codes of behavior.[36] Equipped with a growing medical marketplace, an increasingly print-dominated society, and a newly naturalized model for understanding their internal life, many educated eighteenth-century Britons monitored their transient psychological aches and pains as never before. It was arguably the first age of mass medicalized self-consciousness.

The treatise on the nervous disorders, a distinctively eighteenth-century British genre, is the most notable textual expression of Georgian nervous culture. The authors of these tracts were typically prominent physicians with fashionable city practices, precursors of the Victorian "nerve doctors" and twentieth-century private-practice psychiatrists. Their writings catalogue symptoms, reel off remedies, and speculate widely and wildly about the causes of the distempers.[37]

While Georgian treatises on the distempers are not centrally concerned with gender, the large majority of them discuss the nervous hygiene of both sexes. Richard Blackmore (1654–1729), who was known as much for his bad epic verse as his forward-looking medical ideas, served as physician to both William III and Queen Anne. In his *Treatise of the Spleen and Vapours, or Hypochondriacal and Hysterical Affections* (1725), Blackmore assigns the primary cause of these infirmities to "laxity of the abdominal fibers" that allows "peccant juices" to percolate through to the bloodstream and adulterate the animal spirits formed in the brain. Blackmore emphatically classifies female hysteria and male hypochondria as varieties of a single morbid affliction: "The Symptoms that disturb the Operations of the Mind and Imagination in Hysterick Women, are the same with those in Hypocondriacal Men, with some inconsiderable Variety."[38] He identifies a great range of hysterical symptoms— including "Fluctuations of Judgment . . . Absence of Mind, want of self-determining power, Inattention, Incogitancy, Diffidence, Suspicion, and an Aptness to take well-meant Things amiss"—that may supervene without discrimination in men and women.[39]

Blackmore's colleague Nicholas Robinson conjectured that the distempers arose from defective elasticity of the nerve fibers. In *A New System of the Spleen, Vapours, and Hypochondriack Melancholy,* published in 1729, Robinson endorsed the Sydenhamian notion that hypochondria is the masculine analogue to hysteria. In Robinson's experience, the male and female distempers were so jumbled together as to make distinctions impossible:

> From the best and nicest Observations I have been able to make, I cannot discover any other Difference between the Spleen and Hypochondriack Melancholy, than that the Hip. is the Spleen improv'd on the Constitution, through a longer Continuance of the Disease: the Vapours are so nearly related to the Spleen, that whatever can, with any Propriety, be alleg'd of the one, with a very little Variation, may be inferr'd of the other.

Robinson then enumerates the symptoms of mind and body that may be shared by both sexes, concluding that "what the Vapours are in Women . . . the Spleen is in Men."[40]

Another medical writer of the period, Richard Browne, dismissed as obsolete the old gendering of these diagnoses. In *Medicina Musica,* which includes an addendum on the distempers, Browne in 1729 unhesitatingly asserted his medical modernism: "It was the Opinion of the Ancients, that the Spleen was the Seat of this Disorder in Men as the Uterus in Women, and that consequently this Disease in the two Sexes was really and essentially different. But this ridiculous ungrounded Notion has long since been confuted." Only custom, Browne surmised, caused physicians to continue to use separate terms. "I think it undeniably evident, if we strictly observe the Rise and Progress of the Symptoms, that there is no Difference in the essential Properties of the Disease . . . and therefore these different Denominations are only imaginary Distinctions and really imply but one and the same Disorder."[41]

As physician and physiologist, professor at the Edinburgh Medical School, Royal Society Fellow, and medical adviser to King George III in Scotland, Robert Whytt (1714–1766) was probably the most distinguished of the Georgian nerve doctors. Like his medical colleagues, Whytt determinedly defended the parallel between female hysteria and male hypochondria.

> It is true that in women, hysteric symptoms occur more frequently, and are often much more sudden and violent, than the hypochondriac in men; but this circumstance, which is only a consequence of the more delicate frame and sedentary life . . . by no means shews the two diseases to be, strictly speaking, different.[42]

Whytt proceeds to stress the role of intense emotions, especially fear, grief, and anxiety, in male and female cases alike. He notes additionally the absence of hysteria in prepubescent girls and autopsied women with organic uterine diseases, as well as the presence of hysterical symptoms in postmenopausal women, and then links these clinical facts with both a critique of the uterine theory and a defense of masculine hysteria. Moreover, Whytt cites two cases of nervous phenomena in men—that of Francis Bacon, who was said to have fainted when he once observed an eclipse of the sun, and a young Dalmatian man who, upon witnessing an epileptic seizure, suddenly lapsed into a fit himself.[43]

The most explicit statement in early modern British treatises of the nervous distempers is found in Andrew Wilson's *Medical Researches: Being an Enquiry into the Nature and Origin of Hysterics in the Female Constitution, and into the Distinction between that Disease and Hypochrondriac or Nervous Disorders,* published in 1776. A London asylum doctor, Wilson launches his treatise with a short but remarkable chapter titled "The Identity of the General Nature of the Sexes." "There is nothing, so far as respects diseases or morbid affections, peculiar to males, or to which females are not exposed in common with them. As individuals of the same species, they have a common constitution reared and supported upon the same general animal principles and laws, and are subject to the same infirmities and affections which are accessory to the generating of diseases." This is exactly the type of observation that would vanish from European medical discourse during the first half of the nineteenth century. Wilson goes on to assert not just the similarity but the identity of the nerves, fluids, vessels, membranes, and glands in adult men and women.[44] In a later chapter of *Medical Researches,* he examines the clinical relationship among hysteria, hypochondria, and the nervous disorders: "I call these [disorders] synonymous," he decides, "because wherein they may be supposed to be distinguished, the difference is only in degree." Speculating on the physiological mechanism of symptoms in hysteria sufferers, Wilson uses the male pronoun. And turning to remedies, he cites several measures that are effective in young people, "especially males."[45]

Nervous culture spread to the northwest of England, too. John Ferriar was a prominent physician and public health reformer at the Manchester Royal Infirmary. Writing near the end of the century in his *Medical Histories and Reflections* (1795), Ferriar contends that even the most stylized hysterical symptoms can occur in males: "Fevers often terminate in hysterical disorders, especially in women; men too are sometimes hysterically inclined, upon recovering from typhus, for they experience a capricious disposition to laugh or cry and a degree of the globus hystericus."[46] In an earlier edition of the work, Ferriar related the case of "J.C.," a seventeen-year-old male who had consulted him in the spring of 1789, "affected with regular hysteric fits, in consequence of continued vexation and anxiety." "J.C." reported "great dejection of spirits, sighing, and uneasiness around the praecordia" and said that "he felt the globus hystericus at the approach of each paroxysm." In addition, Ferriar observed of the patient that "his pulse was weak . . . his tongue somewhat foul, and his countenance timid." The young man's fits subsided after downing an emetic and some opium pills.[47]

The nervous maladies, including hysteria, became prime subject matter in eighteenth-century imaginative literature as well, while the Georgian literary hypochondriac evolved into a recognized cultural personality. Novels, poetry, drama, and dialogues from the period are replete with references to the nervous ill-health of male authors and their male characters.

Alexander Pope's famous mock-epic poem *The Rape of the Lock* (1712; 1714) draws on contemporary medical theory to heighten the psychological complexity of its characters.[48] Lyric poets like William Collins and Christopher Smart described themselves, and were diagnosed by others, as mad, melancholic, or hysterical. And the fictional literature of sensibility showcased at least as many male as female characters. The satirical Scottish novelist Tobias Smollett, for example, who was a practicing surgeon as well as a novelist, depicted male and female "hysterical" characters in his *Life and Adventures of Sir Launcelot Greaves* (1762), which is partly set in a madhouse. Laurence Sterne likewise drew extensively on medical sources in his novel writing, and Henry Fielding, Samuel Richardson, and Jane Austen employed for artistic purposes the vocabulary of nerves, sympathy, sensibility, and distemper.[49] Medical and literary authors alike poetized about the nervous distempers.[50]

Eighteenth-century autobiography also registered the theme of nervous introspection. Between 1777 and 1783, the famous writer and biographer James Boswell churned out some seventy monthly essays in *The London Magazine* under the pseudonym "The HYPOCHONDRIACK." Similarly, in his celebrated multi-volume diary, Boswell endlessly and obsessively records his own ever-shifting nervous and mental states.[51] Recalling a breakfast conversation with a friend in 1787, he observes laconically that "we hypochondrized mutually," as if discussing the distempers were a mode of sociability.[52] This same idiom of suffering made its way into the letters and diaries of nonliterary authors. The journal of Joseph Farington, the landscape painter and London socialite, brims with references to doctors, health, and sickness. On August 6, 1810, Farington recorded that his friend Horace Hone had been in "a very nervous, Hysterical state, the effect of anxiety of mind."[53] In much the same vein, Edward Jenner, the surgeon and anatomist acclaimed for his discovery of inoculation for smallpox, was afflicted with a curious symptom in the final year of his life: "a morbid sensibility to sharp sounds," such as that of common kitchen utensils scraping against cups and plates, that "annoy my Nerves in this distressing way." Writing several months before his death to his friend and fellow physician Alexander Marcet, Jenner acknowledged the likely nature of his quirk. "In a Female I should call it Hysterical," he frets, "but in myself I know not what to call it, but by the old sweeping term nervous."[54]

The most interesting and instructive case involves David Hume

(1711–1776), scion of the Scottish Enlightenment. During his late teens and early twenties, Hume abandoned his studies in the law and entered upon a far more precarious career in philosophy. In the spring of 1729, following a period of intense intellectual exertion, Hume's mental and physical stamina suddenly evaporated. He felt emotionally disoriented; he found it nearly impossible to concentrate on the book he was trying to write; and he experienced heart palpitations, skin ulcers, and stomach pains. For nearly five years these troubles, at times disabling, lingered.[55] When Hume finally emerged from the turmoil, he immediately proceeded to write *A Treatise on Human Nature* (1739–1740), his first attempt to construct a full-fledged philosophical system. In retrospect, this youthful neurotic episode appears to have been a classic "creative malady" preceding a period of great artistic or intellectual creativity.[56]

Tracking his own mental and emotional health closely, Hume wrote often in letters to family and friends at this time about his "distemper." He frequented local spas, rode daily into the countryside, and visited the family doctor, who prescribed "a Course of Bitters and Anti-hysteric Pills" along with "an English Pint of Claret Wine every Day."[57] Most revealingly, in Hume's literary estate scholars located a lengthy letter, dating from the spring of 1734, that Hume wrote to a prominent London physician detailing his nervous vulnerabilities.[58] Hume probably never dispatched this letter but rather wrote it for himself as part of a personal therapeutic effort. In it, he provides "a kind of History of my Life" with attention to "the present Condition of my mind." Hume narrates his evolving symptomatology beginning in September 1729, including "lowness of spirits" and a debilitating exhaustion that cruelly kept him from his desk: "all my Ardour seem'd in a moment to be extinguisht, & I co'd no longer raise my Mind to that pitch, which formerly gave me such excessive Pleasure." He rules out various bodily diseases, and he resists the idea that he suffers from "common Vapours"; but he cites his local physician's verdict that "I had fairly got the Disease of the Learned." Hume thinks that his predicament might better be compared with the mental state of the French religious mystics: "I have often thought that their Case and mine were pretty parallel, and that their rapturous Admirations might discompose the Fabric of the Nerves and Brain, as much as profound Reflections."[59]

To counter "these Motions of the Mind," Hume resolves upon a life of greater worldly activity. Completing his long self-analysis, he ends his report to the anonymous medical recipient with a set of urgent inquries: "whether among all those Scholars you have been acquainted with you have ever known any affected in this manner? Whether I can ever hope for a Recovery? Whether I must long wait for it? Whether my Recovery will ever be perfect, and my Spirits regain their former Spring and Vigor, so as to endure the Fatigue of deep and abstruse thinking?"[60] In his *Life of David Hume,* Ernest Mossner describes the young Hume as "a scholar-philosopher afflicted with the 'vapours'" and characterizes this uniquely self-revelatory letter as "at once the most intimate and the strangest that he ever wrote, partaking of the candor of the consulting room and perhaps even of that of the confessional."[61] In contrast to Boswell, Johnson, and many others in the Georgian intelligentsia, however, Hume's nervous infirmity was episodic; by all indications, his self-ministrations worked, and he went on to a life of good health and fluent productivity.

## Enlightenment Hysteria

Several features emerge from the eighteenth-century British literature on nervous health and sickness. First, the Georgian medical community abandoned almost completely primary gynecological explanations of hysterical pathology. Given the millennium-long dominance of these theories, this was not a negligible development. Although a few exceptions remained, by and large Enlightenment physicians in Britain dissociated the nervous distempers from the womb and envisaged them instead as organic disorders with a mixed mental and physical symptomatology that arose from the nervous system and was mediated by the abdominal viscera.[62] Many medical writers openly ridiculed the uterine theory as laughably old-fashioned. By the middle decades of the century, this seems to have become in part an ideological stance—a self-consciously modern assertion on the part of the little flock of medical *philosophes*.[63]

The extensive application of the nervous distemper diagnoses is another feature of note. Georgian nervous culture was effectively restricted to the middle and upper social strata, but within these circles, contemporaries believed the disorders flourished widely. Burton rejected the dichotomy between sanity and insanity and asked plangently, "Who is free from melancholy? Who is not touched more or less in habit or disposition?"[64] Alluding to Willis, Blackmore maintained that the nervous distempers were as common as fevers and estimated that one-third of all people "are destroyed or made miserable by the Diseases."[65] Cheyne endorsed Blackmore's estimate, labeling these ailments "English maladies," as if the entire nation were prone. And in France, Joseph Raulin contended that the vapors constituted "a veritable social plague, an endemic disease in the cities" of Europe.[66] The number and popularity of medical treatises on the nervous distempers, the social prominence of nerve specialists, and the vast pharmacopoeia for ministering to them suggest just how widespread these ailments were believed to be.

Precisely because clinical nervousness was believed to be so prevalent, the nervous individual was perceived to be as much a cultural type as a medical patient. Nervous suffering was viewed not so much as a disease to be combated and overcome but as a permanent part of *la condition humaine*. Accordingly, British medical discourse of the period is comparatively free of the sort of stigmatizing, value-laden rhetoric that became so common in the following century. The hysteric and hypochondriac were at times subjected to derision or caricature; but this was the worst of it, and they were just as likely to be regarded as victims of real physical and emotional distress. In contrast to Victorian medical moralizing, which linked nervousness to a contemptible lack of will and a hereditarian scheme of degeneration, there was notably little condemnation of the nervous patient in the 1700s.

Another outstanding trait of Georgian medical culture is the interconnectedness among the scientific, literary, philosophical, and religious discourses on hysteria. Burton, an Oxford clergyman, drew on a mass of scientific and nonscientific learning to produce his treatise. Locke, the preeminent psychologist, epistemologist, and political philosopher of the late Stuart era, was trained in medicine and was a friend and associate of Sydenham. And the principal novelists of sensibility, as we have seen, were conversant with the new physiologies of the day. Smollett had attended the Edinburgh School of Medicine, and Sterne was an Anglican clergyman. Cheyne hobnobbed with Pope, Wesley, Hume, and Johnson. In addition to his clinical activities, Blackmore wrote voluminous verse and prose. A significant percentage of prominent men of letters, poets, and intellectuals of Georgian England were medical practitioners by training and practice, while a striking number of scientifically knowledgeable figures contributed to the literary, religious, political, and philosophical life of the time.[67]

One consequence of this interplay between medicine and the

cultural arts was a blurring of demarcations between genres of commentary about the nervous distempers, in men and women alike. Theology and psychological autobiography merged; autobiography was pressed into the service of science; and clinical case histories read like short stories. Before the formation of C. P. Snow's "two cultures," these domains cohabitated comfortably and were regarded as complementary, rather than conflicting, methods of inquiry and understanding. Together, they generated a single repertoire of words, ideas, images, and associations about health and illness, the mind and the emotions, sensibility and suffering, from which everyone could draw in the formation of a shared medico-literary culture.

Yet one topic is conspicuously absent from the Georgian literature on the nerves, and that is sexuality. In the century-long succession of medical texts from Mandeville to Ferriar, references to sexual excess or promiscuity as a cause of nervous breakdown occasionally appear; but in general eighteenth-century British writing on this subject, in sharp contrast to classical, renaissance, Victorian, and Freudian discourses, is notably de-sexualized. As cause, symptom, and behavior, sexuality was not theorized as a primary, determining force or factor. With the formulation of less sexualized models of the nervous disorders, and the turn away from gynecological and demonological theories, the conceptual obstacles to the equalization of the diagnosis between the sexes were negligible.

Correspondingly, masculine nervous susceptibility in the medical and nonmedical writing of Georgian Britain was only rarely associated with effeminacy and never with homosexuality. Eighteenth-century Britons conceptualized manliness largely in moral, rather than physical, terms;[68] they regarded wisdom, virtue, rectitude, sympathy, and responsiveness as key "manly" attributes. In contrast to Victorian proscriptions on public male emotionality, the cultivation of true feeling, especially when aroused by religious, ethical, or aesthetic circumstances, was construed as a masculine quality. An excess of partying, gaming, and womanizing, on the other hand, as well as overindulgence in the new material luxuries of the day, might be viewed as unmanly. Likewise, the decadent, unproductive aristocrat and the foppish, affected dandy were often considered effeminate.[69] But in Georgian society, nervous suffering was not seen to compromise virility.

## Mandeville, Cheyne, Johnson

Three works written by major British authors at different times during the 1700s illustrate Enlightenment views on hysteria. In these texts, either a physician with a serious literary avocation or a medically steeped literary intellectual probes and portrays human mental life. Each author takes the suffering of men's psyches as his central subject and highlights a different style of nervous self-representation.

Dutch by birth, Bernard de Mandeville (1670–1733) received his medical education in Leyden and then settled in England in 1691. While Mandeville is best remembered for his popular, ingeniously subversive poem *The Fable of the Bees,* published in 1705, in his consulting practice he specialized in disorders of the gut and the nerves. Mandeville's *Treatise of Hypochondriack and Hysterick Passions, vulgarly called Hypo in Men and Vapours in Women,* which appeared in 1711, was easily the most widely read of the early Georgian tracts on the nerves.[70] The treatise takes the unique form of three long, interlocking dialogues between an imaginary physician, Philopirio, and a male patient, Misomedon, with each dialogue representing a day's conversation between the figures. Mandeville states at the outset that he has assumed the doctor's persona. He intends the treatise primarily as an attack on two contemporary *bêtes noires:* rationalist medical systematizing and excessive therapeutic meddling. In the process, however, he explores the state of medical understanding of the nervous maladies, dramatizes the interaction between doctor and patient, and underscores the subjectivities of nervous anxiety.

In effect, Mandeville's treatise is a book-length case history of a fictional upper-middle-class patient. Misomedon quickly takes control of the exchange and presents his medical history at length. Morbidly self-preoccupied, he produces a breathless, 30-page catalogue of symptoms from the past decade, including headaches, vertigo, insomnia, irritability, excitability, nightmares, and endless gastrointestinal upsets.[71] This leads to the patient's self-diagnosis: "Hypochondriacus Confirmatus."[72] Philopirio then re-enters the discussion, offering his own philosophy of medical practice while sagely continuing to indulge his patient's self-absorbed loquacity. By the dialogue's end, Misomedon is palpably happier, and it becomes apparent that their conversation itself has been therapeutic. Mid-twentieth-century scholars have inevitably dubbed it a pre-psychoanalytic "talking cure."

The second dialogue, the longest of the three, moves from autobiography to medical theory.[73] This section chiefly consists of an intricately detailed discussion between gentleman-philosophers about the range of past and present theories of hysteria and hypochondria. The lion's share of praise goes to Willis, Sydenham, and the Italian physician Giorgio Baglivi—all early advocates of the idea of hysteria in men. Philopirio then takes up Misomedon's own case, which he classifies as an obstinate example of "the Disease of the Learned," the Burtonian synonym for male hysteria. He surmises that the patient's complaints are seated in the stomach, but mediated through a nervous system discombobulated by "the irregularities of youth," excessive conjugal venery, "labour of the brain," and Galenic malpractice.[74]

The third and final dialogue of Mandeville's book begins with a cornucopia of diets, procedures, and medications that compose the "physick" of their day. This leads to the introduction of Misomedon's wife, Polytheca, who in turn relates the story of their hysterical teenage daughter who has been smitten by "the fits" for years.[75] At this point, it becomes clear that Misomedon is part of an acutely dysfunctional family of neurotics. The intrusion of the wife and daughter allows Philopirio to hold forth on the similarities and differences between "the Hysterick Passion in Women" and "the Hypochondriack in Men."[76] He suggests different causes for nervous affections in women, including thinner blood and greater physical delicacy and emotional lability. Nevertheless, he judges male and female cases to be the same malady, and throughout the treatise he uses the terms "vapours," "hysteria," and "hypochondria" interchangeably. He also cites cases of other male patients from his practice who are similarly afflicted.[77]

Mandeville's dialogues, written in the generation immediately following the deaths of Willis and Sydenham, initiated the eighteenth-century British tradition of the treatise on nervous disorders. Just over two decades later, in 1733, George Cheyne's *The English Malady* made its appearance.[78] Cheyne (1671–1743) came from a family of clergymen; he was an amateur mathematician and Fellow of the Royal Society who maintained highly fashionable medical practices in London and Bath. Cheyne's book represents the gentrification of the Georgian nervous disorders at its height. His treatise was clearly conceived and written for an audience of private, well-off clients—hence the distemper's later nickname, "affluenza." Cheyne's achievement lies in formulating and popularizing the idea that the distempers were linked to the progress of civilization, thereby obtaining for them not only social legitimation but cultural cachet. Among the best-known and most influential books of the mid-Georgian age, *The English Malady* went through several quick editions and was easily the most widely read of all the eighteenth-century treatises on the nerves.[79]

Cheyne was above all a skillful synthesizer. In his system, nervous maladies result from weakness or laxity of the nerves, which in turn is brought about by bad heredity, poor diet, excessive luxury, and too much book reading. The doctor favored an unrelenting therapeutic regime of tonics, milk, vegetables, and physical exercise. Most noteworthy is the long third section of *The English Malady*, which is devoted to illustrative cases drawn from Cheyne's thriving practice in Bath, the elegant Georgian spa town in Somerset.[80] Notably absent in his case presentations is any sense whatsoever of gender specificity in the nervous disorders. Aside from the occasional citation of menstruation or pregnancy as complicating factors, Cheyne discusses the backgrounds, symptoms, and treatments of his male and female patients on equal footing. He presents eighteen case histories of "the English malady"—ten of men and eight of women. All the male cases involve gentlemen with respectable, even distinguished, professional backgrounds. The first case relates the story of "a tender young gentleman of great Worth and Ingenuity here in our Neighbourhood" who suffered from "a most violent Nervous Headach, which returning at certain Periods, overcame and sunk him to Extremity and even sometimes approached near to Epileptick Fits."[81] The third case tells of a Scottish man "eminent in the Law, and of great Honour, Probity, and fine Parts." He too was blighted by "nervous headach" as well as "Want of Sleep," "Loss of Appetite, and Inquietude," and "constant extreme lowness, oppression, and . . . the greatest Difficulty to attend his Studies or to apply to the Business of his Profession."[82] A later chapter introduces some of Cheyne's more severe cases, including "the Case of the learned and ingenious Dr. Cranstoun" in which Cheyne reproduces a letter from the doctor-patient detailing his

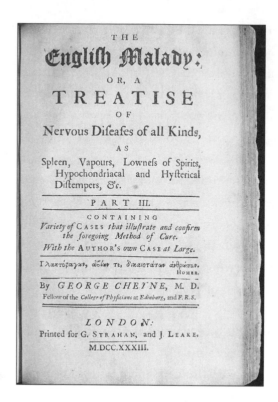

Frontispiece of the first edition of George Cheyne's *The English Malady* (1733), which includes the author's own case history.

condition. Cheyne adds that Cranstoun's case is by no means rare and that he, Cheyne, currently has under his care similar patients, including "several Gentlemen of the [medical] Faculty."[83]

Whereas Mandeville integrated autobiography into his treatise by alternately assuming the voices of the physician and the protagonist-patient, Cheyne achieves much the same result by presenting nothing less than his own extended medical autobiography. His book's remarkable final chapter is headed "The Case of the Author."[84] Like Burton a century earlier, Cheyne professed to suffer from the disease of which he wrote; he often refers to himself as a "valetudinarian," and in the dedication he asserts that his work is directed toward "my Fellow-Sufferers." In this forty-page excursus, the most popular nerve doctor of mid-eighteenth-century Britain reports minutely on his own florid and evolving neurotica from the time of his youth up to the present. In his early twenties, for example, Cheyne was stricken inexplicably with "a sudden violent Head-ach" and "extream Sickness in my Stomach." His state of mind deteriorated as "Fright, Anxiety, Dread, and Terror" flooded in. He wondered if anyone had ever endured "so atrocious a nervous Case" as his own, and he remained bedridden for months.[85] For guidance, Cheyne read Sydenham—including the passages on hysteria[86]—and consulted friends, doctors, and clergy.

> At last, my Sufferings were not to be expressed, and I can scarce describe, or reflect on them without Horror. A perpetual Anxiety and Inquietude, no Sleep nor Appetite, a constant Reaching, Gulping, and fruitless Endeavour to pump up Flegm, Wind, or Choler Day and Night: A constant Colick, and an ill Taste and Savour in my Mouth and Stomach, that overcame and poisoned every Thing I got down; a melancholy Fright and Pannick, where my Reason was of no Use to me.[87]

Like Freud during the 1890s, in correspondence with his physician-friend Wilhelm Fliess, Cheyne formulated his ideas about nervous prostration by moving regularly between his own case and those of his patients. To be sure, Cheyne's auto-observations are less penetrating than Freud's, and his suffering is less credible than Burton's or Samuel Johnson's. In an entrepreneurial attempt to attract patients, Cheyne was clearly placing himself in the same personal circumstances as his clients in order to show empathy. Nevertheless, the degree of emotional self-reportage is impressive. *The English Malady* of 1733 contains the lengthiest autobiographical case history in an eighteenth-century medical text, and it deals frontally with a male hysteric.

Samuel Johnson is a figure of yet a different order. Poet, essayist, critic, and lexicographer, Johnson (1709–1784) is judged the leading British literary intellectual of his generation. With him, it is less a single text that is pertinent than an entire life and oeuvre.

Johnson's experience with sickness throughout his adulthood has been documented copiously.[88] Compelled for financial reasons to leave Oxford before taking his degree, failing in a venture to set up a secondary school near his home in Staffordshire, and dealing with the recent death of his father, the young Johnson sank into depressed lethargy. In 1729, at the age of twenty, he found himself, as his famous biographer Boswell put it, "overwhelmed with an horrible hypochondria, with perpetual irritation, fretfulness and impatience; and with a dejection, gloom and despair, which made existence misery. From this dismal malady he never afterwards was perfectly relieved. That it was, in some degree, occasioned by a defect in his nervous system," Boswell added, "appears highly probable."[89] In subsequent years, Johnson's symptoms proliferated. He developed eccentric mannerisms, including peculiar tic-like motions, and he was riddled with phobias. He suffered physically, too, being afflicted with gout and chronic bronchitis. He doctored himself obsessively and became morosely self-absorbed. His desperate fear was that his depression might collapse at any moment into full-fledged insanity.[90]

The Johnson/Boswell correspondence, one of literary history's most famous epistolary exchanges, forms a running quasi-medical dialogue. Johnson refers to his "morbid melancholy" and "disturbances of the mind very near to madness," while Boswell speaks of "the hypochondriacal disorder that was ever lurking about him."[91] Not coincidentally, Johnson was exceptionally well versed in the medicine of his time. He knew prominent medical personalities and was "a great dabbler in physick," recognized for his extensive reading in both classical and contemporary medical texts.[92] Interestingly, he was an avid reader of Robert Burton's works—he once insisted that *The Anatomy of Melancholy* was the only book that ever got him out of bed early—and he knew Cheyne's *English Malady*.[93] Johnson even wrote a brief "Life of Dr. Sydenham," which was widely reproduced in collections of Syndenham's works during the eighteenth and nineteenth centuries.[94]

Throughout these writings, Johnson acknowledged the nervous disorders in men and women without hesitation or inhibition. In a letter dated Saturday, June 12, 1779, written to his close friend and medical confidante Hester Thrale, Johnson consolingly responded to the news that Thrale's husband had undergone some sort of attack: "Your account of Mr. Thrale's illness is very terrible, but when I remember that he seems to have it peculiar to his constitution, that whatever distemper he has, he always has his head affected, I am less frightened. The seizure was, I think, not apoplectical, but hysterical, and therefore not dangerous to life."[95]

Johnson's discussions of nervous health and illness were by no means limited to epistolary chatter about himself and his friends. Rather, they lie close to the center of his literary art. Johnson's most penetrating exploration of the operations of the mind, written during his mother's terminal illness, came in 1759 with *The History of Rasselas, The Prince of Abyssinia*.[96] At the heart of this pessimistic philosophical novel is the long cautionary tale of the mad astronomer of Cairo, expounded by the mentor-narrator Imlac to the young prince of the kingdom who aspires to study and master the natural philosophy of the day.[97] For forty years, the astronomer studied the motions and appearances of the celestial bodies, striving to calculate them precisely. However, in his solitary and obsessive quest, he developed the conviction that, God-like, he controlled the earth's weather. With Imlac's story, Johnson constructed a charming Newtonian parable of unriddling the heavens pursued to the point of pathology. Like Hume in his early manhood, Johnson's astronomer is a "man of learning" in the age of reason driven to madness by the search for knowledge.

Imlac's long presentation of this "case" and its causes in *Rasselas* is a substantial exposition on the nature of nervous and mental disease. In it, Johnson writes from the dual perspectives of the observer and the insane man,[98] presenting the obsessions and delusions of the astronomer both as observed by Imlac and as experienced by the astronomer. In a further innovation, he reconstructs the experience of going mad as a process of progressive mental deterioration. The novel also includes insights into the accompanying psychological states of guilt, anxiety, and depression. The "clinical," "pre-Freudian" qualities of Johnson's writing, in *Rasselas* and elsewhere, have long been noted.[99] Nineteenth-century British asylum doctors were even in the habit of citing his fictional descriptions of human behavior for their textbook-like fidelity.

Johnson's account of the growth of the astronomer's disorder, and of the origins of madness in excessive imagination, is highly convincing. His understanding of the mental processes was inextricably bound up with his own troubled mind, including deep fears about his own sanity.[100] It seems evident that Johnson's interest in medical matters was not limited to individual texts but rather suffused his world view. At times, his own condition—operating alternately as a personal motive, subject of analysis, and source of insight—contributed to the creation of artistic and intellectual works of high caliber. With *Rasselas,* we find ourselves once again in Georgian Britain, at the intersection of science, psychology, literature, and autobiography, and in the presence of a male author and male fictional characters.

THE SEVENTEENTH- AND eighteenth-century English and Scottish medical literature on the nervous distempers can be viewed as a sort of pre-psychiatric discourse on male hysteria. From Robert Burton's anatomizing of his melancholic debilities to Dr. Johnson's brilliant, brooding ruminations on his nervous miseries, from Bernard de Mandeville's fictional dialogue between doctor and patient to George Cheyne's nervous self-display, male authors described the psychological travails of other men. Although physicians in Britain in this period stated officially that hysteria developed more often in women, the actual textual record of Enlightenment hysteria devotes a good deal more space to the disorder in its male incarnations. Even at their most superficial—as a publicly cultivated, self-indulgent sick role or a *maladie à la mode*—the Georgian nervous disorders were shared by both sexes. Moreover, the major Enlightenment-era theorists of these infirmities were, as we have seen, among the most academically well-established physicians of their age. It is not today's psychiatric writing about post-traumatic stress disorders, nor the medical commentary on "shell shock" during the First World War, but the early modern discourse on the nervous distempers that represents the first instance of the medicalization of male emotional suffering in the European West. Although significant gender asymmetries undoubtedly remained in these writings,[101] the eighteenth-century diagnosis of hysteria and its kindred states was a far more egalitarian diagnosis than what preceded and followed it. No longer a reproductive failing or demonic curse, and not yet a form of moral profligacy or constitutional degeneracy, nervous disease in Britain during these generations was widely construed as a sign of refinement and sensibility. Because emotional self-display involved no violation of the approved way of being an adult male in society, a nonderogatory model of masculine nervous illness was possible. Doctors, philosophers, poets, novelists, and clergymen meticulously described the genteel disorders of melancholy, hypochondria, hysteria, and the spleen in their clients, their characters, and themselves. For millennia of medical history, the disease of the wandering womb had been envisioned as the female condition par excellence; but in Great Britain for a full century following the 1688 revolution, the male hysterias flourished.[102]

CHAPTER 2

# The Great Victorian Eclipse

A GREAT WAVE of amnesia regarding the nervous disorders descended upon European medicine around 1800. During the three-quarters of a century running from 1790 to 1860, medical science and practice were aggressively pressed into the service of discovering and maintaining a regime of difference between the sexes. A new drive to base the putatively pervasive differences between the sexes in nature developed, and biomedical knowledge that emphasized the contrasts and oppositions between men and women came to the fore. Conversely, anything that called into question the new gender dichotomies—theories of causation, clinical practices, diagnostic categories—was officially ignored, discredited, or despised. Not surprisingly, the concept of hysteria in the male sex during these years became submerged, rhetorically and ideologically, appearing only as the story of evasions, resistances, and silences. In dramatic contrast, discourses of female hysteria during the first half of the nineteenth century thrived as never before.

---

AFTER TWO HUNDRED years of recording the varieties of nervous experience in men and women alike, the medical profession in one European country after another abandoned this line of clinical inquiry and denied the similarity of nervous susceptibility between the sexes. The fact that a new dichotomized view of the sexes set in during the years 1790 to 1820, a period of great turmoil across the European continent, is scarcely a coincidence. The wholesale suppression of the idea of male hysteria during these decades was in fact an epiphenomenon of larger changes whose real centers lay elsewhere in social, political, and military events—events that sparked intensely negative, at times reactionary, responses.

The force of the European Enlightenment brought a powerful egalitarian message. From Locke and Montesquieu to Rousseau and Jefferson, Enlightenment thinkers cast their reformist message in the gender-neutral language of natural civic law and inalienable human rights.[1] The fact that citizenship was granted during this period to other previously disempowered groups, such as French Jews, and that some contemporaries sought to extend the new rights to European women and Caribbean slaves, illustrated the emancipatory possibilities of Enlightenment thought and practice. The subversive implications of enlightened ideology were reflected in the role of women in high society. A coterie of women from the liberal aristocracy organized many of the leading salons, where debates about social, intellectual, and scientific issues occurred within the political culture of late absolutist France.[2] Critics of the revolution cited as sources of French national instability the improper intellectual autonomy, indirect political influence, and alleged sexual promiscuity of women in Old Regime France. These apprehensions were greatly amplified by the course of French political history after 1789. The "moderate phase" of the French Revolution empowered middle-class professional men at the expense of king, nobility, and church. But the momentous possibilities for other social and political transformations unleashed by the storming of the Bastille prison, the abolition of the feudal system, and the promulgation of the First French Republic quickly became apparent.

With the publication of Marie-Olympe de Gouges' manifesto-like *Declaration of the Rights of Woman* in 1791, a small but articulate group of French urban women sought a place for the female half of the nation in the expanded liberal democratic public sphere. In Britain, Mary Wollstonecraft's famous *Vindication of the Rights of Woman* (1792) likewise drew its arguments from the Enlightenment vocabulary of universal reason, nature, and law. Beyond their well-known role in certain insurrectionary *journées,* women were bold actors in nearly every stage of those extraordinary six years of French history. By 1795, they had fought for a spectrum of rights— suffrage, divorce, inheritance laws, property and tax laws, child custody, job security, educational opportunities—which amounted to a campaign for full legal and political equality between the sexes.[3]

As so often happens, however, the challenge of liberalization was met with an effort at renormalization. This reaction—the first anti-feminist "backlash"—was vehement and very successful. The overwhelming majority of articulate adult males (and of French women, especially in the more pious provinces) were staunchly opposed to women's rights at every stage. The National Constituent Assembly passed its constitution of 1791 without serious consideration of the petition for female suffrage, and the national legislature rejected all subsequent pleas for women's rights. As events became more radical, women were legally barred from participating in the Paris Commune and the section assemblies. The Société révolutionnaire des femmes républicaines was outlawed in October 1793. A victim of the Jacobin Terror, Olympe de Gouges was sent to the scaffold for political sedition in November 1793; other politically active women were flogged, arrested, or exiled.

Nor did the reaction against rebellious women end in 1795. For all intents and purposes, women played no official role whatsoever in French politics during the eras of the Directorate, Consulate, First Empire, and Bourbon Restoration. In Britain, Wollstonecraft, who had observed part of the revolution firsthand in Paris, was vilified throughout the nineteenth century. From Louis DeBonald to Jules Michelet to Hippolyte Taine, nineteenth-century conservative male commentators depicted revolutionary *citoyennes* as crazed and murderous harridans. For his part, Edmund Burke numbered among the Revolution's greatest evils its attempts to emancipate women, which in his view served to debase marital authority and destabilize domestic order. The charge most frequently leveled against the French by Britons during the 1790s was that their women had attained undue and overweening influence.[4] When France then began to threaten directly the territorial integrity of Britain and continental Europe, anxieties about national military readiness brought further social and gender retrenchment. Not coincidentally, Britain, which was deeply involved in both the critique of the French Revolution and the military struggle to contain Napoleon, spearheaded the gender counter-revolution.

Reacting in part to the perceived excesses of the revolution, with its programmatic anti-clericalism and egalitarianism, and in part to the alleged libertinism of the Directorate, Napoleon promulgated the Concordat with Rome in 1801 and the Civil Code in 1804. While his motivations for returning France to Roman Catholicism were various, he was in part attracted to the Church's emphasis on the stability and sanctity of the family, which he regarded as an indispensable aspect of reestablishing social order. The

Concordat fostered a generation-long revival of Catholicism in French society, culture, and thought, and the Civil Code formally restored the privileges of masculinity and patriarchy.[5] For the countries occupied by Napoleon, including the German states and parts of the Hapsburg Empire, the Code also became a legal model. It is little wonder that academic physicians appointed by the governments of Napoleon and the restored Bourbon monarchy were the most culturally conservative in the entire nineteenth century.[6]

The post-1814 Restoration era was the quintessential period of political counter-revolution; in both political theory and practice, classic British and European conservatism emerged quite directly as a reaction against the perceived excesses and instabilities of the preceding generation. After twenty-five years of war and revolution, the powers that triumphantly opposed Napoleon sought a peace that above all would prevent radical events like the French Revolution from occurring again anywhere in Europe. The four major victors—Austria, Great Britain, Russia, and Prussia—that met at the Congress of Vienna in 1814–1815 restored royal and aristocratic governments across the continent. Louis XVIII, brother of the executed French king, was restored to the throne, and post-Napoleonic monarchs launched a half-century drive to prevent reform of any sort from spreading to other countries and social groups, especially to the working classes.[7] Censorship tightened across Europe. Democratic uprisings in Spain, Greece, and Russia between 1820 and 1825 were aggressively stamped out. According to the Holy Alliance, advanced by the ultra-conservative Tsar Alexander of Russia, European states should conduct their affairs according to Christian teachings. The Congress of Vienna enshrined European politics not only as an elite realm of socioeconomic privilege but also as a purely masculine domain.[8]

Reinforcing European-wide reactions against the political and intellectual upheavals of the 1790s were the waves of Protestant religious enthusiasm, both Anglican and nonconformist, that swept across England in the late eighteenth and early nineteenth centuries.[9] Godliness, self-discipline, and a moral seriousness were the human qualities that Evangelical ministers prized most dearly. In its earlier phases, exemplified by figures such as William Wilberforce, Hannah More, and Lord Shaftesbury, the Evangelical ethos encouraged tenderness, self-expression, and sympathy toward the deserving poor.[10] Beginning in the 1820s, however, a narrower and more severe version of Evangelicalism took hold that placed an unrelenting emphasis on duty, earnestness, and will power. The majority of Victorians grew up during the height of Evangelicalism's influence, in the middle decades of the nineteenth century, and were profoundly affected by the moral climate it shaped. A combination of piety, prudery, and propriety characteristic of Victorian times can be traced back to the Evangelical sensibility.[11] From Charlotte Brontë to Samuel Butler, later anti-Victorian critics alternately assaulted and satirized Evangelicalism as the root cause of the middle-class cult of respectability and conformity.

Predictably, the Evangelical ethos was highly conservative on matters of sexuality, gender identity, and the family, stressing the virtues of obedience, chaste love, and marital fidelity within a stable and unchanging patriarchal family structure.[12] The rise of evangelical Christianity in Britain and the United States also helped to transform attitudes about female sexuality, encouraging an ideology of female "passionlessness" in the pursuit of the ideal of moral purity.[13] The ideal of Christian manliness emphasized the traditional roles of adult men as husbands, fathers, and upholders of the social order. Conversely, it frowned upon what it regarded as idleness, playfulness, and sensual pleasures, and it became ever more intolerant of masculine emotional self-expression.[14] In the Evangelical view, the ideal masculine character was tough, sober, and industrious, a view that left little room for nervous or emotional vulnerability.

At the same time, the period between 1790 and 1870 brought the advent of mechanized industrialization to many European settings. With the first waves of industrialization, many adult males left their households, where they had previously worked as part of an integrated family unit, in order to work in or near cities in centralized industrial settings.[15] To be sure, women continued to work in the textile industry as well as in artisanal trades and family-run shops. But mining, metalwork, construction, railroading, and large machine factory work were exclusively man's work, and the new trade unions were dominated by males. Among the middle classes, management in the market manufacturing world was also monopolized by men. Correspondingly, the home increasingly became a feminine preserve. A key signifier of bourgeois status during the nineteenth century was that wives did not have to work outside the home.[16]

Accordingly, the class dimensions of our story shift during the Victorian decades. The nervous indisposition of Georgian-era gentlemen had partly been an aristocratic affectation. But the industrial revolution was fueled by the new "middling classes" that were concentrated in the growing cities of Britain and continental Europe. With the coming of "the bourgeois century," the commercial and professional classes emerged as by far the most politically ambitious, economically dynamic, and culturally influential sector in society, and with them came new behavioral standards. Nineteenth-century industrialization was a crucible for the formation of both working- and middle-class masculinities, as work—rather than pedigree, sex, family, or character—became the key factor in defining manhood.[17] Discipline, productivity, and self-mastery were the qualities most admired under the competitive and acquisitive capitalist regime. It is significant that physicians, including specialists in the nervous disorders, emerged predominantly from the professional middle classes during the nineteenth century, and they inevitably imbibed the values and attitudes of their class.

The new model of bourgeois masculine behavior that took shape during the first half of the nineteenth century left comparatively little room for noncomformist character types. In capitalist society, the victims of nervous invalidism were compelled to withdraw from the all-important public arenas of power and productivity, unable to contribute to the various economies of the day, whether national, familial, or sexual. "Sensitive nerves no longer implied quickness of mind or acuteness of sympathy, as in the past," Janet Oppenheim has observed, "but a virtual assurance that the man so cursed would be unable to play his allotted part on the public stage."[18] The old "culture of nerves," in short, undercut the emergent claims to middle-class manhood.

THESE COMBINED HISTORICAL forces—anti–Enlightenment sentiment, post-revolutionary reaction, Christian Evangelicalism, the bourgeois family structure, gendered nationalism, and capitalist industrialization—decisively shaped nineteenth-century middle-class perceptions of men and women. Sanctioned by Christianity, the bourgeois family was assumed to be the primary unit of social organization, and social and gender roles were neatly assigned between husband and wife, parents and children.[19] Men were seen as rational, resolute, and self-restrained, whereas women were emotional, tender, and intuitive. Men's destiny was to work in the competitive public arenas of politics, law, business, or the military as citizens, soldiers, entrepreneurs, and professional experts. Spectators rather than participants in the public arena, women inhabited the private domestic domain as wives, mothers, and caretakers. Men were seen to possess the reason and willpower to surmount the emotions and passions to which women succumbed. Within the household, husbands and fathers were naturally in charge while wives, children, and servants were expected to obey. In the sexual domain, men were presumed to be dominant and desirous whereas women were passive and modest.[20] Of course, this historical picture of the "separate spheres" needs to be sharpened and qualified, as several historians have emphasized.[21] Nevertheless, a highly demarcated world of gender extensively shaped the medical discourse of the day.

Over the course of the nineteenth century, the more expressive moments of the early Evangelicals became in turn unacceptable, incomprehensible, and contemptible. The eighteenth-century acceptance of manly emotion in the face of an appropriate moral, religious, or cultural stimulus faded. Likewise, public expressions of homosocial affection became ever more problematic, and there was an attendant increase in policing homosexuality.[22] By the end of Victoria's reign, the spectrum of emotions deemed appropriate for adult men in Britain had greatly diminished, as the familiar historical image of stoical insensibility and the stiff upper lip emerged and hardened.[23]

Throughout the 1800s, the ideological work of masculinity played out on several reinforcing levels. Ideals of middle-class manliness served to ensure the authority of husbands and fathers within the patriarchal domestic economy. Among the professional and business classes, self-consciously manly behaviors established a man's class credentials, especially in contrast to what was perceived to be the decadent and nonproductive aristocratic class and the brute and profligate manual working orders.[24] Not least important, Victorian codes of masculinity, with their emphasis on emotional self-control and sexual sublimation, fueled Britain's long and astonishing ascendancy over the Third World throughout this period. Particularly during the last third of the 1800s, British imperialism required the projection of power and control from the tiny, geographically remote British Isles outward across the globe. As a consequence, many Britons at this time came to perceive gender deficiencies not simply as individual eccentricities; rather, such shortcomings risked undermining the family, the capitalist marketplace, middle-class authority, and the nation's all-important imperial project.

## Hysteria in French Medical Thought, 1790–1860

During the revolutionary and early Napoleonic years, hardly any medical writing at all about hysteria was published in France. Perhaps with hysteria assuming overtly political forms—with it running wild in the streets, so to speak—doctors could not observe or perceive the phenomenon in the clinic. When a medical commentary on the topic re-emerged, during the early years of the new century, it had changed profoundly.

Several features marked the new post-revolutionary discourse about hysteria. Georgian physicians had regarded social class as the key variable for susceptibility to the nervous distempers. On both sides of the English Channel, however, early nineteenth-century physicians saw gender as the primary agent of pathology and relegated social class to the status of a predisposing factor. Femaleness itself became the key determinant of hysterical illness, and physicians increasingly defined women's nature as inextricably bound up with their reproductive anatomy and physiology. Any deviation from the prescribed norm of sexual moderation—virginity, masturbation, overindulgence, sterility, prostitution—was interpreted as a possible cause of nervous collapse.

European medical writing about hysteria during the first half of the nineteenth century became saturated with sexuality. In contrast, Sydenham had abandoned references to sexuality, and in early modern British medicine generally, sex rarely appeared in case histories of the hysterical distempers. Likewise, readers of the entries on "Hysteria" and "Vapors" in Diderot and D'Alembert's epic-making *Encyclopédie* found that avant-garde scientific opinion on these topics in the 1760s said little about sex.[25] From the early 1800s onward, however, sexuality, both as an etiology and a symptomatology of hysteria, takes center stage. When in the mid-1820s the Viennese phrenologist Franz Joseph Gall referenced hysteria, he situated the disorder in the human cerebellum because this part of the brain, he believed, was the seat of carnal love.[26]

A further mutation in European hysteria discourse concerns a change in genre. Around 1800, the treatise on the nervous distempers, as a type of medical literature, began to disappear.[27] For the next half-century, hysteria was addressed either through chapters in textbooks on insanity—a change that denoted a greater degree of pathologization—or in general reference works of medicine. Both sources were cast in technical, scientistic language directed largely to fellow medical practitioners. At the same time, a new type of professional figure emerged to explain hysteria and minister to its victims: the state-appointed and salaried specialist, including the public asylum doctor or alienist, who now succeeded the private practitioner of Cheyne's day with a specialty in the nerves.[28]

Anglo-French hysteria literature after 1800 also displayed a marked change in tone. Seventeenth- and eighteenth-century medical writers believed that the nervous and psychological suffering of their clients was real, and by and large they responded—partly for financial reasons—with sympathy and supplication. Their nineteenth-century successors, however, saw things differently. In the early-nineteenth-century process of "the moralization of medicine," the figure of the hysteric fared poorly.[29] With only a few exceptions, medical writings about hysteria between 1800 and 1870 display a palpable antagonism between the professional author and his hysterical subjects. Contempt and condemnation rather than consolation and collaboration marked the doctor/patient relationship during these years. In this far more moralized scientific discourse, hysteria was reconfigured as a kind of character flaw, the lamentable result of a lack of will power, a pathetic excess of emotionality, or constitutional degeneration.

Feminization, sexualization, pathologization, and moralization: in the transformed European discourse of hysteria during the late eighteenth and early nineteenth centuries, these were key processes. Together, they constitute the greatest rupture in the entire discursive history of hysteria. And what of male hysteria in this complex process? In French and British medical texts of the period, the male hysteric is nowhere and everywhere. The fate of the male hysteric during these generations was indissolubly linked with the extravagant fantasies of femininity that dominated the male medical imagination. Characterized only in oppositional terms, scientific representations of the male hysteric now appeared either as the fleeting specter of emotional and psychological effeminacy, to be sternly extirpated by doctors and patients, or as a social, clinical, and semantic impossibility.[30]

Two French physicians working immediately after the turn of the century inaugurated this new phase of medical thought. The first is Philippe Pinel (1745–1826), the legendary "founder of modern psychiatry." In his *Medical and Philosophical Treatise on Mental Illness*, which heralds the famous "moral treatment" of madness, Pinel did not address hysteria. He devoted much of his later career, however, to disease classification. In the first 1798 edition of his au-

thoritative *Philosophical Nosography,* Pinel includes a two-page discussion of hysteria, occurring exclusively in women, in which he
associates the pathology with disordered menstruation and sexual
deprivation. He classifies hysteria alongside hypochondria, under
the rubric of "the nonfeverish insanities," separated from the "aph-
rodisiacal neuroses" like nymphomania and priapism.[31] However,
beginning with his fourth edition of the work that appeared in
1810, Pinel recategorized hysteria. Writing during the Napoleonic
wars, Pinel brushed aside the entire category of "the nervous distempers"—a slap at Sydenham. Instead, he now separated hysteria
from hypochondria and reclassified it under the "Reproductive
Neuroses" and the sub-section "Genital Neuroses of Women."[32] Pinel listed hysteria's causes as "an acute physical or psychological
sensibility, abuse of the venereal pleasures, strong and frequent emotional experiences, lubricious reading and conversation . . . the
diminution or suppression of menstruation." Most surprisingly, he
voiced the old classical refrain: "The original source of hysteria, as
its name indicates, appears to be the uterus."[33] Subsequent editions
of the work up to 1818 repeated this classification, as did an influential dictionary article that Pinel coauthored in 1819.[34] Thus the
most influential clinical classification of disease in early nineteenth-
century France captured and codified the new gendered medical
conceptualizations of the age, including the re-eroticization of the
hysteria diagnosis, that marked the post-revolutionary moment.

The second influential medical statement at the opening of the
century came from Jean-Baptiste Louyer-Villermay (1776–1837),
whose voice, at least on hysteria, was louder and more resonant
than Pinel's. Half a generation younger than Pinel, Louyer-Villermay
had never known the liberal cosmopolitanism of the late Enlightenment. Born in Brittany and employed as a surgeon at the Rennes
hospital, Louyer-Villermay had briefly been imprisoned by the

Revolutionary Tribunal during the Terror for allegedly allowing hospital patients to escape during the royalist counter-revolutionary uprisings in western France. Before 1789, his father-lawyer had been a member of the conservative Breton parliament. Eventually Louyer-Villermay *fils* moved to Paris, where he completed his training and practiced medicine for many years under Napoleon, Louis XVIII, and Charles X. He published on very few subjects other than hysteria; nor did he gain a permanent hospital appointment. In light of these facts, his influence is instructive.[35]

Louyer-Villermay first enunciated his theories of hysteria in his medical dissertation (Pinel was among his professors) completed in 1802, the year after Napoleon signed the Concordat with Rome.[36] In 1816, two years after the Bourbon line had been re-established, he produced a greatly enlarged, two-volume version of the dissertation under the title *Treatise on the Nervous Maladies and Vapors, especially Hysteria and Hypochondria*. And in 1818, he wrote a 40-page summary of his views in the multi-volume *Dictionnaire des sciences médicales,* the leading French-language reference work of medicine for its generation.[37]

Published in the immediate post-Waterloo period, these last two texts became the founding statements for the neo-Hippocratic hysteria tradition, which held sway in French medical thought throughout the Restoration and the July Monarchy. Eighteenth-century British physicians had embraced Willis, Sydenham, and Boerhaave for inspiration. In contrast, Louyer-Villermay and his followers enlisted the ancient Greeks, and in particular Hippocrates, whose teachings were then the subject of a brisk revival in French medicine.[38] For Louyer-Villermay, hysteria's synonyms include "suffocation of the uterus," "ascension of the womb," and "uterine strangulation."[39] According to his modernized womb theory, the uterus is a dark, mysterious, all-powerful presence. He observes that whereas the male genitalia are small and external, the female reproductive apparatus occupies a much larger portion of a woman's body, embedded in deep proximity to vital internal organs. In Louyer-Villermay's imagination, the uterus not only exercises tremendous power over women's bodies and minds but also invites political analogy: "the empire of the reproductive organs" has its "imperious laws," and female puberty is a "local revolution in the uterus."[40] Prone to pathological malfunction at the least provocation, and surrounded by a vast plexus of supersensitive nerves that radiate outward, the uterus in this conception telegraphically transmits the slightest stimulus from the pelvic region across the entire field of the female body.[41]

Louyer-Villermay also summarizes the etiology of hysteria: "Absolute and involuntary chastity is the most common cause of this malady," he states confidently. Hysterical breakdown, he adds, is common "in women who once enjoyed the pleasures of the hymen" but who are suddenly deprived of sexual gratification.[42] Among other causes, sexual and romantic factors predominate, including "onanism," "the abuse of venereal pleasures," "an ardent and lascivious uterine system," "an unruly periodic flow," and "an overly tender or excitable heart."[43] He then describes the specific provocations that may evoke hysterical symptoms, including "bed sheets pressing against the genitals," "tight clothing," "lukewarm baths," and "excessive or habitual consumption of foods that . . . have an especially exciting effect on the genital area."[44] The hysterical fit is a sort of "spasm of the uterus."[45]

Nothing if not consistent, Louyer-Villermay's theories of etiology, symptomatology, and therapeutics mesh neatly. Hysteria "almost always gives way to sexual union," he asserts in 1818, repeating the tried and true Platonic topos.[46] He describes the case of one of his patients by saying straightforwardly that "she chose a young and very loving husband, soon became pregnant, and recovered perfectly."[47] Wed, bedded, impregnated, and domesticated, the women under his care found symptomatological relief, if not existential happiness. It was not without reason that Pierre Briquet, writing forty years later about Louyer-Villermay's treatise, quipped that the book "ought to be dated 1500 rather than 1815 [sic]."[48] Nevertheless, the French academic community embraced Louyer-Villermay: in 1832 his two weighty volumes on hysteria were republished verbatim, and in 1836, the year before his death, he was elected President of the Academy of Medicine.

In the preceding 150 years, leading European physicians had adduced the reality of male hysteria specifically to counter ancient uterine theories. Louyer-Villermay therefore devoted a great deal of energy to refuting the idea of hysterical sickness in the male sex. It was no longer a question, as in the previous century, of determining the comparative ratio of male to female cases of hysteria. "If we demonstrate that a malady exists whose seat is the uterus, and that is quite distinct from any disorders of the male genital organs, will it not be obvious that this is an exclusively female ailment?" Louyer-Villermay asked rhetorically.[49] Men, simply put, can't be hysterical; they don't have uteruses.

The first physician in France to write at length about hysteria in the new century, Louyer-Villermay was determined to refeminize hysteria,[50] but to succeed in the task he had to refute the arguments of his British predecessors of the preceding century. Enlightenment medicine had been marked by continual cross-Channel interplay.[51] Following the French Revolution, however, this tradition of exchange came to an end as the two countries were locked in national rivalry. Louyer-Villermay feigns surprise that the medical early moderns were ever allowed to prevail over the august Hippocrates and Galen. He reviews several past cases of adult males diagnosed with hysteria and acknowledges that their clinical profiles offer "an almost perfect analogy" to hysteria in female cases, but he ultimately judges their affliction to be something other than hysteria. "No corresponding malady exists among men," he concludes reassuringly.[52] Louyer-Villermay remained the major authority on hysterical disease in France during the Napoleonic and Restoration periods, when his ideas dovetailed neatly with the general social and political conservatism of the age.[53] However, early in the 1820s a counter-current appeared, fleetingly, before again being submerged under the dominant uterinist discourse.

Étienne-Jean Georget, born in 1795 near Tours in the heart of château country, was a generation younger than Louyer-Villermay. In 1816 Georget came to the French capital for his clinical internship at the Salpêtrière, where the elderly Pinel still practiced and where he became J. E. D. Esquirol's assistant. By all accounts, Georget was a brilliant clinician with a gift for lucid exposition and diagnostic discrimination. He was also a notably independent thinker. In 1821, Georget produced a two-volume study of the physiology of the brain and nervous system, which included a substantial chapter on hysteria. He was twenty-six years old. A few years later, he contributed all the entries on mental and nervous illnesses for the *Dictionnaire de médecine*, a shorter competitor of the *Dictionnaire des sciences médicales*.[54] He is best known today as the author of *De la folie* (*On Madness*, 1820) and as a pioneer of legal psychiatry.

Temperamentally, Georget was a young Turk who minced few words: "The notion of locating the seat of so-called hysterical symptoms in the uterus seems to me so absurd and ridiculous that I would scarcely bother to combat it were it not regarded by modern authors as a truth," he states forthrightly at the outset of his book.[55] Time and again, Georget brushes off the uterine hypothesis as "a capital error" and mocks "received opinions" that trace a riotous array of symptoms to the uterus. He brands Louyer-Villermay, whose treatise had appeared five years earlier and whom Georget seems especially to dislike, a "dogmatist" and "absolute partisan" of the neo-Hippocratic school.[56] Firmly rejecting his predecessor's overwrought vision of the primordial, pathogenic uterus, he observes that in an unimpregnated condition the uterus is in fact quite small and that the organ serves the modest functions of containing and expelling the fetus and channeling menstrual flow.[57]

In place of Hippocrates, Galen, and Areteus, Georget returned to Willis and Whytt (and the Italian Lepois) as the authorities. Like them, he contended categorically that the brain and spinal cord are the primary seats of hysterical dysfunction.[58] Accumulating clinical evidence, Georget maintained that unbiased clinical observation failed utterly to support the dominant neo-Hippocratic interpretation: many hysterical patients reveal no postmortem uterine pathology; most women with organic uterine problems aren't hysterical; and some women who have had hysterectomies remain hysterical. Hysteria, he concludes curtly, is "an affliction of the brain that does not have the least connection to the uterus."[59]

In transforming hysteria from a uterine to a cerebral—or, more precisely, psycho-cerebral—ailment, Georget was arguing inferentially that it was not sex-dependent. Several neo-Hippocratic ideas crop up in his writings, illustrating how difficult it was for even the most original thinkers to break free of the Greco-Roman heritage. Nevertheless, the young Georget voiced a set of ideas that were notably forward-looking. Nymphomania, he declares, has nothing whatsoever to do with hysteria.[60] Although hysteria is commoner in women than in men, the reason for this is a scientific mystery. And because of its misleading etymology, Georget advocates abandoning altogether the word "hysteria" and replacing it with the gender-neutral term "convulsive cerebropathy" or, simply, "attack of the nerves."[61] He scoffingly rejects the idea of marital coitus as a cure-all.[62] While his medical contemporaries repeatedly sought to mask their scientific uncertainty, Georget acknowledged on numerous occasions the state of ignorance about the nature and causes of hysteria.[63]

In keeping with these innovations, Georget was the one French physician writing during the first half of the 1800s to endorse the idea of male hysteria enthusiastically and without qualifications. "The malady under study is scarcely exclusive to the female sex," he observes. "Every day in society, we hear speak of men as well as women who have nervous attacks." Georget goes on to praise the eighteenth-century French authors who wrote about the vapors for their recognition of the nervous disorders in men, and he reports that he personally has observed cases in many adult males.[64] To develop the point, he revives the Sydenhamian tradition by pairing his dictionary article on hysteria with an entry on hypochondria.[65] Georget's 1824 encyclopedia article is the earliest text in Western medical history to use plural masculine or neutral pronouns in discussing hysterical patients—for instance, "les malades," "ils," and "eux"—rather than exclusively feminine pronouns.[66]

Despite their power and precocity, Georget's writings failed to establish a full-fledged counter-discourse of hysteria. Various forces militated against him. In 1822–23 the French Department of the Interior had conducted a purge of the Paris Medical Faculty, dismissing nearly a dozen professors (including the elderly Pinel) for propounding ideas that the royalist government deemed radical, materialist, or anti-clerical.[67] Also at play were cultural and professional pressures to embrace a specifically French theory of the disorder. Most decisive was the fact that the gifted Georget died of pulmonary tuberculosis in 1828, at the age of only thirty-three, and thus was unable to defend or extend his ideas.[68] During the two decades following Georget's premature demise, Louyer-Villermay's neo-Hippocratic nonsense flourished without challenges.

Several years after Georget's death, Achille Louis Foville (1799–1878) provided a frontal assault on the new psycho-cerebral paradigm. Another Esquirol protégé, Foville served as professor of physiology in Rouen. His close connections with the royal Orléanist family later earned him choice positions as Esquirol's successor at the Charenton asylum and as personal physician to Louis-Philippe's son. In 1833, Foville continued the battle of the encyclopedia articles: his entry on hysteria in the *Dictionary of Medicine and Pratical Surgery* is a spirited, polemical performance written to disprove the gifted but (in his view) misguided Georget.[69] Foville here rejects out-of-hand Georget's impertinent proposal to replace "hysteria" with a new term. He maintains that Georget "forgets how remarkable the changes are in women at puberty . . . and the role the sensual passions exert in the life of so many women."[70] He proposes further that if some hysterical symptoms trace to the brain, as Georget asserted, the brain itself, in a hypothetical looping action, is adversely affected by the reproductive organs:"I don't hesitate to call the uterus the true *point de départ* of the phenomena that together constitute hysteria."[71] It would be difficult to find a clearer exercise in resistance to intellectual innovation than Foville's article.

The same year Foville published his piece, Frédéric Dubois D'Amiens (1799–1873) weighed in with a 550-page restatement of the Galeno-Hippocratic model. In *Histoire philosophique de l'hypochondrie et l'hystérie* (1833), Dubois D'Amiens returns to the subject of Louyer-Villermay's 1802 dissertation and seeks definitively to discredit the diagnostic cluster of hysteria/hypochondria, which since Sydenham had bedeviled proponents of the uterine model.[72] After a pompous, positivistic introduction linking the progress of the human species with the march of science, the author declares flatly that hysteria is exclusive to women. Contrary to Georget, "the brain has nothing to do with hysteria."[73] The disease develops solely between puberty and menopause, he claims.[74] It is caused by an emotional shock to or organic disturbances of the genital system; preeminent among the former are *chagrins d'amour* of various sorts and among the latter, "uterine irritation acting through the cerebro-spinal axis."[75] In an inspired passage near the close of his bloated book, Dubois D'Amiens observes quaintly that whereas nervous sensibility is spread equally throughout the male body, in women it is concentratred explosively in the pelvis.[76] "So-called hysterical symptoms indicated in men" are dismissed by the author as misdiagnoses.[77] As if to confirm this hypothesis as universal truth, the Royal Medical Society of Bordeaux awarded Dubois D'Amiens's treatise their Civrieux Prize. Later, as "perpetual secretary" of the Paris Academy of Medicine from the late 1840s to the early 1870s, Dubois D'Amiens became a prominent figure in the Parisian medical elite.

During the second quarter of the nineteenth century, two medical authors in France sought to conjoin the neo-Hippocratic tradition with cultural Romanticism, which was just then peaking in France. Julien Joseph Virey (1775–1846) was born near Langres, overlooking the Marne River in eastern France. He became first a senior pharmacist at the military hospital of Val-de-Grâce in Paris and then professor of Natural History at the École militaire. Virey was highly prolific, publishing one volume after another during the 1820s and 1830s on a wide range of health-related topics. As the author of entries on "Homme," "Femme," "Virginité," and "Pudeur" in the *Dictionnaire des sciences médicales,* he was a significant voice on issues of gender in his time.

In Virey's *On the Physiological, Moral, and Literary Aspects of Woman*

(1823; reprinted in 1825 and 1834), the discourse of nineteenth-century hysteria merges with the courtship and marriage manual, the French Romantic treatise on women in the manner of Jules Michelet, and the mildly pornographic novel in the late Enlightenment tradition.[78] The book is full of quotatable, symptomatic assertions. Virey composes a picture of absolute anatomical and physiological opposition between men and women: "Differences between the sexes are not limited only to the organs of generation in man and woman," he instructs. "Rather, every part of their bodies, even those parts that seem unrelated to the sexes, experience some influence."[79] Virey proceeds to describe how men's and women's voices, posture, complexion, bone structure, hair texture, heart rate, blood viscosity, and even cellular organ tissues differ. Cumulatively, "males live by the head, the heart, the extremities, and the upper portions of the body; women live by the uterus, abdomen, and tissue of their breasts, as well as by their lower, internal organs."[80] Virey, needless to say, is not enthusiastic about gender-bending: "A man with an effeminate constitution is not a picture of beauty; a masculine woman revolts the senses."[81]

Virey sprinkles comments about hysteria throughout his fanciful treatise. He is uninterested in the current debate about the anatomical localization of hysteria. His book, rather, is littered with references to the authors and events of ancient Egypt, Greece, Babylonia, and Assyria. Unfulfilled, the uterus "becomes a furious and insatiable animal."[82] Hysteria is most likely to afflict "young women who are completely celibate, or young, childless widows, or even sterile women who lost their virginity for nothing."[83] Among other therapies, Virey endorses the application of malodorous substances on the pelvis and "foul-smelling fumigations applied to the vulva."[84] He expresses the view that hysteria is basically an intensification of femininity itself. Women are endowed with a capacity for passion

and feeling, which if channeled in moderation is ideal for their domestic and maternal duties but which constantly spills over into
excess: "While the symptoms of hysteria disturb the health of so
many women, how many other *mental hysterias,* which remain secret, unknown, ferment in their tender souls, provoke those violent
whims, those temporary enthusiasms, those passing exaltations that
others just as fugitive have replaced, caught in this never-ending
fickleness."[85]

Jean-Louis Brachet (1789–1858), the second French Romantic
theorist of hysteria, was professor of physiology at the Lyon Medical School, where he distinguished himself with work on the action of the heart muscle and the function of the ganglionary nervous system. Unlike Pinel, Georget, Voisin, and Foville, he was not
an alienist.[86] In his *Traité de l'hystérie* of 1847, Brachet promisingly
echoes Georget in contending that hysteria is "a spasmodic disease
of the cerebral nervous system." Also à la Georget, he proposes a
new name, "cerebral neurospasmia," for the disorder.[87] Nevertheless, Brachet grafts onto Georget's model the Romantic gender
ideology of Virey, Michelet, and Senancour. Under Brachet's pen,
the hysteria treatise becomes a paean to total difference—anatomical, physiological, moral, temperamental, even metaphysical—between the sexes.[88] Women, Brachet maintains, have "a special mod-
ification of the nervous system" that causes a predisposition to
hysteria. "In man, the intelligence comes first, and the impression
next," he explains, whereas "sensibility constitutes the whole of the
woman."[89] Echoing Rousseau in *Émile,* Brachet is not content simply to gender the nerves and senses: "It is not only through the
uterus that woman is what she is. . . . She is such in her whole constitution. From head to foot, outside and inside, whatever part of
the body you examine, you will find that everywhere she is the
same."[90] He then proceeds to discuss how each organ and opera-

tion of the woman's body is different than in the man's body, including circulation, digestion, perspiration, urination, and excretion.[91]

In his 1847 treatise, Brachet then incorporates hysteria into this all-encompassing vision of femaleness. "Hysteria," he announces in his Preface, "is the exclusive appanage of their [women's] sex"; it is "her special malady."[92] Earlier authors in the French textual tradition sited hysteria variously in the uterus, the viscera, the nerves, the brain, and the senses. For Brachet, the very state of being female is the determining factor. Here the treatise on hysteria becomes less a clinical monograph on a disease than a philosophical study of femininity, female nature, and female sexuality.[93] In one of those memorable epigrammatic formulations at which the Gallic mind excels—"Je pense, donc je suis," "Après moi, le déluge"—Brachet encapsulates the gendered world of nineteenth-century French hysteria by asserting that "L'hystérie, c'est la femme—Hysteria *is* woman."[94]

Interestingly, Brachet rejects Louyer-Villermay's and Dubois D'Amiens's idea of hysteria's female exclusivity.[95] The last of the eighteen clinical cases he presents involves a male—a thirty-five-year-old tailor named "M. T."[96] But the author's caveats about the case undercut his own concession. Hysterical breakdown in men, Brachet rushes to inform readers, occurs only "very rarely." He estimates that less than one male hysteric exists for every 100 female hysterics.[97] In fact, he finds the idea so counterintuitive that he in effect suggests a hysterical male is not a man at all:

> If a man experiences the circumstances that subject his nervous system to the same physiological state similar or analogous to that of a woman, the man will also become subject to hysteria. This is why the man who is feminized by his constitutional

predisposition, whether innate or acquired, by his education, by some prolonged or special illness, by a soft and overly sentimental life, by too many sensual pleasures, and so forth, that is why, I say, this man, who seems to have eyes, feet, and hands only *ad honores,* will be prone to experience hysteria.[98]

The final major statement in the French neo-Hippocratic tradition is Hector Landouzy's *Complete Treatise on Hysteria,* which, like Brachet's book, appeared near the end of Louis-Philippe's constitutional monarchy.[99] The most professionally accomplished author in the tradition, Landouzy (1812–1864) was also one of the few French hysteria doctors to pass his entire career in the provinces. Born and educated in the historic cathedral city of Reims, Landouzy did his internship in Paris before returning to his native city in the Marne. He held professorships at the Reims Medical School in anatomy and physiology and in general clinical medicine before being appointed Rector of the Reims Medical School.

Why Landouzy, whose work previously focused on typhus and pneumonia, took up the topic of hysteria is unclear—perhaps because the Paris Academy of Medicine, whose attention the provincial Landouzy no doubt wished to catch, sponsored a competition in 1845 for the best monograph on the subject. Whatever the reason, Landouzy's treatise, more than any other publication on hysteria during the first half of the nineteenth century, includes a number of features that physicians today might admire. Landouzy provides the fullest discussion before Charcot of hysterical paralyses of the extremities, and he discriminates diagnostically between hysterical attacks and epileptic seizures better than anyone had before.[100]

But Landouzy's clinical acumen was compromised by his general theory of hysteria, which was based on an inflexible, sectarian devotion to the uterine model. An orthodox neo-Hippocratic, Landouzy often cites the ancient authorities with uncritical awe. He restricts hysteria's onset to the period between puberty and menopause. Menstrual symptoms are common in his cases, and hysteria and nymphomania are allied disorders. Like Louyer-Villermay, he records a list of synonyms for hysteria—women's asthma, widow's melancholy, uterine epilepsy, utero-cephalgia—that underscore the malady's true origins in his view.[101] "Care for the uterus and hysteria will disappear" was his message.[102]

Landouzy embraced the aims, methods, and language of the dissecting room more than previous theorists had. For him, it was not strong emotions, or bad living habits, or reading novels, or too little or too much sex that caused hysteria; it was "organic lesions" of the female reproductive system. Willis in the 1670s and Georget in the 1820s had dissected patients diagnosed as hysterical, and found nothing. But Landouzy was trained in the 1830s, when French pathological anatomy was being bolstered by improved microscopic techniques. Moreover, Landouzy may have sensed that in the current scientific environment, with its emphasis on localizable tissue pathologies, the absence of a structural correlate for hysteria was beginning to call into question the uterine hypothesis. Whatever the reasons, out of 67 patients diagnosed as hysterics in his book, Landouzy reports that no fewer than 55 revealed postmortem evidence of "material alterations of the reproductive apparatus," including tumors, lesions, inflammations, ulcerations, deformities, occlusions, and swellings of the uterus or ovaries.[103] In three other hysterical patients, he claims to have found brain lesions. For those patients in whom he was unable to locate any appreciable organic defect, he expressed confidence that a tissue lesion would be found if the appropriate investigative tools were available to science.[104]

It will come as no surprise that a medical thinker who regarded *strangulatio vulvae* as a synonym for hysteria did not embrace the notion of male hysteria. Landouzy describes the question of hysteria in men as "one of the most delicate points of science."[105] In a single declarative sentence, he admits the theoretical possibility of masculine hysterical disorders;[106] but he is even more dismissive than Brachet. When "hysteriform incidents" do occur in men, he traces them to "the ganglionary genital apparatus of man analogous to that affecting woman."[107] Gathering case-historical data had familiarized Landouzy with the record of medical history, which from the seventeenth and eighteenth centuries rather awkwardly included over 30 cases diagnosed as male hysterics. In an extraordinary retrospective exercise, Landouzy proceeded with all 30 male cases either to rediagnose them as other ailments (epilepsy, tuberculosis, meningitis, "convulsive asthma," among others) or to reject them as inconclusive.[108] So intent was Landouzy on securing the sex-specific uterine hypothesis—and, by inference, denying male hysterical illness—that he sought systematically to purge medical history itself of all contradicting clinical evidence.

Hector Landouzy's treatise was without doubt the most widely read and cited work on hysteria between Louyer-Villermay's encyclopedia article of 1818 and Pierre Briquet's study at the end of the 1850s. In November 1845 the Paris Academy of Medicine, the most prestigious medical body in France, crowned Landouzy's *Traité complet de l'hystérie* with its Civrieux Prize. Later in his career, the author was honored as a "Chevalier de la Légion d'Honneur" in recognition of a lifetime of achievements. The provincial Landouzy had indeed captured the attention of the Parisian academic medical establishment. It is not hard to guess why the conservative, all-male Academy of Medicine embraced Landouzy. More than any previous publication on the subject, Landouzy's treatise not only confirmed traditional prejudices and preconceptions about female sickness and male health; it also aptly cast this reconfirmation in the up-to-date scientific language of pathological anatomy, differential diagnostics, and quantitative methodology. Landouzy succeeded in modernizing the neo-Hippocratic tradition so that, in the profession's eyes, it was at once accurate, authoritative, and au courant.

Only by reconstructing the rich and extravagant traditions of seeing and conceiving hysterical sickness in women can we appreciate the glaring absence of such a tradition in men. The conditions for the impossibility of a discourse of male hysteria during the first three-quarters of the nineteenth century are now apparent. Because hysteria was characterized definitionally as a female disorder, there was no conceptual or theoretical space for male hysteria in French medical culture throughout this long period. For seventy years, academic medical communities in both Paris and the provinces stood united in rejecting early modern teachings about hysteria, returning to the theories of Plato and Hippocrates, and passionately regendering hysteria as a female malady grounded in reproductive anatomy and physiology. Doing so meant containing Georget's upstart critique of the mid-1820s and disregarding a few obscure medical writings on the topic that appeared during this period.[109] But these tasks proved relatively easy to accomplish.

## British Hysteria Theory, 1790-1870

The transfer of the seat of all hysterical manifestations from the uterus to the brain by Jorden, Willis, and Sydenham had constituted a major turning point in the history of hysteria. Similarly, the culture of nerves and sensibility in eighteenth-century Britain encompassed extensively, if not quite equivalently, men and women. Thus it is reasonable to expect that nineteenth-century physicians would build on these impressive precedents and practices. But this was far from the case. By the end of the 1700s, the English and Scottish tradition of the treatise on the nervous distempers, with its literate synthesis of medicine, literature, and autobiography, was vanishing. The lively and unified Georgian discourse of the nerves splintered into separate models of hysteria—gynecological, neurological, characterological—the last two of which bore a closer resemblance to contemporaneous French medical thought than to the ideas of scientific savants in early modern Britain. Most conspicuously, in contrast to their continental coevals, doctors in Britain from the late Enlightenment through the long Victorian era shied away from hysteria altogether as a topic of inquiry. Throughout the nineteenth century there were fewer British than French theorists of hysteria, although they speak with voices that are more distinctive.

We see the beginnings of the shift as early as the 1760s in the celebrated Edinburgh clinician William Cullen (1710–1790). Working against the backdrop of the Scottish Enlightenment and the high point of literature on the nervous distempers, Cullen's vision of these maladies departed significantly from that of his countrymen. Known for coining the term "neurosis," Cullen established it as a significant pathological category and placed the nervous system at the center of the somatic process that determined health and disease. Unlike Mandeville, Cheyne, and Whytt, he did not produce a general treatise on nervous disorders; however, in his influential *Synopsis Nosologiae Methodicae* (1769) Cullen classifies hysteria under the "spasmodic neuroses," and his *First Lines of the Practice of Physic* (1776–1784) includes a chapter entitled "On the Hysteria, or the Hysteric Disease."[110] "These affections have been supposed peculiar to the female sex; and indeed they sometimes, though rarely, attack also the male sex; never, however, that I have observed in the same exquisite degree," Cullen observes in the latter source. But after this promising beginning, he turns solely to hysteria in women, which he links to reproductive physiology. "In the female sex," he continues, "the disease occurs especially from the age of puberty to that of thirty-five years. . . . At all ages, the time at which it most readily occurs is that of the menstrual period. . . . It affects the barren more than the breeding women, and therefore frequently young widows."[111]

Cullen's ideas about pathology are transitional: hysteria first breaks out in the gut, he contends, reflecting the Georgian preoccupation with digestive turmoil, but then it quickly shifts its locus: "Although the disease appears to begin in the alimentary canal, yet the connection which the paroxysms so often have with the menstrual flux, and with the diseases that depend on the state of the genitals, show that the physicians have at all times judged rightly in considering the disease as an affliction of the uterus and other parts of the genital system."[112] Cullen, in short, segues from a nongendered to a gendered etiology.

Cullen further divorces hysteria from hypochondria and in its place links the disorder to a diagnostic neologism then emerging from France. "It [the hysteric passion] occurs especially in those females who are liable to the Nymphomania; and the Nosologists have properly enough marked one of the varieties of the disease by the title *Hysteria Libindinosa*."[113] Writing in the later 1770s, Cullen in effect overturned Willis and Sydenham, his illustrious medical countrymen of the preceding century, and resexualized the concept of hysteria in the French manner. According to the *Oxford English Dictionary*, the first printed indigenous instance of the word "Nymphomania" in the English language appears in Cullen's *Nosology*.[114]

After the silent interlude of the revolutionary decade, just as Pinel's writings first appeared in Paris, the Scottish naval doctor

Thomas Trotter (1760–1832) took up his pen. Born and raised near the Scottish-English border, Trotter received his medical education at Edinburgh, where the elderly Cullen was one of his teachers. Trotter is best known today for his 1804 *Essay on Drunkenness,* now regarded as the first text to interpret excessive drinking as a medical condition rather than a character flaw.[115] In the late 1770s, Trotter went to sea and seems to have had something of a swashbuckling career, serving as ship's surgeon on a private slave ship in the West Indies and on government frigates in naval battles against the French. Beginning in 1794, he worked as "Physician to the Channel Fleet," where he was responsible for the health conditions of thousands of sailors aboard some forty warships.[116]

Trotter regarded *Medicina Nautica* (1797–1803) as his most important publication. A wide-ranging, three-volume collection with chapters on typhus, dysentery, and syphilis, this text reveals a strong awareness of what we would today call psychosomatic causation. It narrates numerous cases involving symptoms that seem to be caused, amplified, or prolonged by psychological distress, cases that Trotter again and again likens to hysteria. In the second volume of *Medicina Nautica* (1799), he includes excerpts from his journal on the health of the British fleet. The following entry is dated August 25, 1797:

> There appeared an unusual despondency and dejection of spirits among the patients in the different sick berths. . . . When some of these cases were moved to the hospital ship, we found not a few of them subject to very frequent fits of hysteria; and where this singular affection recurred with as much violence of convulsion as we have ever marked it in female habits, attended with globus, dysphagia, immoderate risibility, weeping, and delirium. The same sympathy seemed to extend from one to an-

other, as is often met with in the fair sex. Three or four [of them] were sometimes in a fit at once.[117]

In the third volume of *Medicina Nautica,* published in 1803, Trotter not only returns to this topic but devotes a full and remarkably candid chapter to it. Under the heading "spasmodic affections," he notes a direct, undeniable comparison between nervous symptoms in hard-bitten career sailors and in fragile high-society women:

> That a body of men, by education and habit accustomed to adventure, braving danger in every hideous form, and surpassing hardship, famine, and fatigue in every shape . . . should be subject to complaints more nearly allied to the tender female than the robust masculine constitution, would appear a paradox, did not daily experience confirm the fact. . . . The hero and the infant here unite: the athletic male and the hysteric woman; for we have often seen their complaints so much alike that no distinction could be drawn between them.[118]

Trotter goes on to observe that these nervous episodes may afflict officers and seamen alike. He pinpoints heredity, hard drinking, and physical illness as predisposing causes. He speculates on the circumstances peculiar to ship life that are conducive to nervous debility, and he notes that emotional distress—including nostalgia for home, death of a family member, "disappointments in the tender passion," fear of death, or thwarted ambition—often underlies these breakdowns. There is no sense in Trotter's remarks that these morbid outbreaks compromise the masculine identity of his sailor-patients. To the contrary, Trotter draws on the classical military past to find an honorable lineage for this suffering: after citing Xerxes and Alexander, who broke down under the emotional stress of bat-

tle, he concludes grandiosely that "the British naval hero, not inferior to Greek or Persian name, may there be allowed to exemplify
the same extremes of the great and the little, in his composition, in
his pleasures, in passions, and diseases."[119]

These remarkable passages in *Medicina Nautica* from the period
1799–1803, however, do not represent Thomas Trotter's final thinking on the subject. In 1807, Trotter published *A View of the Nervous
Temperament*.[120] This later book of Trotter's powerfully illustrates the
historical link between war, nationalism, and gender conservatism.
Like Louyer-Villermay's medical dissertation published in Paris
several years earlier, Trotter's *View of the Nervous Temperament* marks
the end of the eighteenth-century discourse of the nervous distempers and the advent of a cluster of ideas and characteristics that
would eventually constitute Victorian gender ideology. In this text
Trotter's medical scope is much narrower than in his earlier work,
his tone quirkier and more opinionated. Good student of Cullen
that he was, Trotter opens *View of the Nervous Temperament* by en-
dorsing the neurocentric model of the human body rather than the
old physiology of fluid balance. He then introduces with great fan-
fare the phenomenon of "nervousness," a hodgepodge of symptoms from hiccups to hemorrhoids, and including *globus hystericus*
and *clavus,* which he endows with the status of a coherent clinical
syndrome. To Trotter's great concern, these nervous cases, he believed, were now proliferating wildly: "In the present day, this class
of diseases forms by far the largest proportion of the whole which
come under the treatment of the physician. . . . At the beginning of
the nineteenth century," he exaggerates further, "we do not hesitate
to affirm that nervous disorders . . . may now be justly reckoned
two thirds of the whole with which civilized society is afflicted."[121]

Trotter proceeds to flesh out his construction of "nervousness"
in several ways that are new in the British medical discourse of hys-

teria. Nervous maladies are not simply a source of individual un-
happiness, he states; rather, they have become "an epidemic" that
afflicts "the national character." What's more, the increasing prevalence of the nervous disorders threatens the well-being of the
country as a whole. According to Trotter, rampant nervous debility
poses a threat to British commercial prowess, political independence, and military preparedness. Continually blurring clinical reportage and cultural diagnosis, Trotter's alarmist rhetoric in places
becomes apocalyptic: "If not restrained soon," he admonishes, "[the
epidemic] must inevitably sap our physical strength of constitution,
make us an easy conquest to our invaders, and ultimately convert
us into a nation of slaves and idiots."[122] During an era of relative
security and stability, eighteenth-century doctors and patients had
styled themselves as nervous as a sign of sensibility and civilization.
But by 1807, when a French land and naval invasion of the British
Isles seemed imminent, Trotter was interpreting the same traits as a
grave issue of homeland security.

For Burton, Mandeville, Cheyne, and Whytt, the distempers
were largely limited to the rich, the clergy, and literary and seden-
tary individuals. Trotter, in contrast, insists that the current wave of
nervousness affects the community at large. Hysteria in the lower
classes, which Trotter recognizes but attributes stereotypically to
drunkenness, holds little interest for him. The contagion he fears,
and the subject of his most hyperbolic condemnation, is the spread
of nervousness to the ascendant middle classes. A member himself
of a bourgeois profession on the rise, Trotter sees the new middle
orders as the architects of Britain's growing urban centers, capitalist
economy, and imperial infrastructure.[123] The agents of Britain's future greatness must be kept happy, healthy, and productive.

Most pertinent to our story is Trotter's gendering of nervousness. In *Medicina Nautica,* hysteria is seen as a male as well as a fe-

male malady. Not so in *A View of the Nervous Temperament*. In the 1807 text, Trotter has no truck whatsoever with the notion, recently resurrected by Louyer-Villermay, of the uterine origins of hysteria. Trotter's hysteria manifests a more general "femininity," which he construes not anatomically but as a diffuse pejorative category that is at once behavioral and cultural. In this light, the current contagion of nervousness, an "inheritance of the fair sex," is inflicting a loss of masculine virility on both individual men and the British nation as a whole.[124]

The specter of the nervous middle-class British male haunts this war doctor's text. Regarding nervous men, Trotter charges that "these persons are commonly pale and sallow, soft-fibred, and of a slender make. Not a few of them behind the counter approach in external form toward the female constitution; and they seem to borrow from their fair customers an effeminacy of manners, and a smallness of voice, that sometimes make their sex doubtful."[125] As this passage hints, it is especially the worlds of commerce and politics that have the most to fear, in Trotter's mind: "Could an army of man-milliners defend the British islands against the ruffians of Bonaparte?" Trotter wonders. From Thomas Carlyle's cultural diatribes of the 1860s up through Wyndham Lewis's misogynistic rants between the two world wars, conservative male British commentators have fretted about "the softening of European manners," which they envisioned as a general feminization of the West. Trotter voiced this same anxiety at the very beginning of the nineteenth century, using the distinctive medicalized language of hysteria.

It is difficult to ascertain at this remove why Thomas Trotter was so agitated in this later book. (The second half of Trotter's career seems to have been troubled. A physical injury in addition to the death of his patron, Admiral Howe, forced him out of the navy at mid-career without a pension.)[126] Whatever its origins, this book brings sharply into focus the differences between discourses of hysteria before and after the great revolutionary divide. In 1733, Cheyne had proudly portrayed excessive nervous sensitivity as a national malady, and as late as 1790, Burke uninhibitedly recorded his gush of tears upon the sight of Marie Antoinette at Versailles. But by the time of Trotter, just a decade and a half later, the status of the nervous maladies has changed profoundly: under the combined effect of personal misogyny and national warfare, an abundant capacity for feeling in men is reconstrued as weak, feminine, and threatening.[127] The same behaviors that Georgian gentlemen cultivated through "nervous self-fashioning" are now seen, in Trotter's transvaluation, as signs of serious pathology and a fearful demasculinization. Moreover, hysteria in Trotter's presentation has expanded beyond the specialized communities of clergy, artists, and scholars and now infects the middle classes at large, with the most dire political and military implications. "Effeminacy" and "unmanliness" also make their historical entrance into considerations of hysteria, with both categories entailing distillations of stereotyped female characteristics, irrationally projected onto men and then interpreted, contemptuously, as compromising some alleged ontological essence of male identity.

During the 1820s and early 1830s, a number of prominent British "psychiatrists" published influential but wholly traditional statements about hysteria.[128] In 1837, under very different historical circumstances than those of Trotter's time, Benjamin Brodie's *Lectures Illustrative of Certain Local Nervous Affections* appeared.[129] Professor of comparative anatomy and physiology at the Royal College of Surgeons and private physician to the royal family, Brodie (1783–1862) was one of the most eminent medical men of his time. He was the only nineteenth-century British hysteria doctor to be knighted. In his short book, he reports on a class of perplexing cases from his practice in which patients suffered long-term articular pain and swelling but in whom postmortem examination revealed no deterioration of the bone or cartilage. Brodie observes further that many of these conditions were preceded in the life of the patient by a minor physical injury or an upsetting emotional experience. He interprets these cases as "local nervous affections" patterned, often in exquisite detail, on neurological diseases. His initial observations involved deformities of the joints—"hysterical knee," "hysterical hip," and so forth—but he goes on to present hysterogenic cases of paralysis, back pain, chorea, edema, torticollis, loss of voice, and urinary retention.

In contrast to the French neo-Hippocratics of the day, Brodie confidently asserts that "hysteria belongs not to the uterus but to the nervous system."[130] Nevertheless, throughout his presentation, he exclusively uses the female pronoun when discussing hysterical patients—a group, he contends, that is very numerous: "I do not hesitate to declare that among the higher classes of society at least four fifths of female patients who are commonly supposed to labour under diseases of the joints labor under hysteria, and nothing else."[131] Brodie had a keen appreciation of the mind's influence over the body, a phenomenon, he knew full well, by no means limited to one sex. But where are Brodie's male hysterics?[132]

Thomas Laycock (1812 1876) wrote more voluminously about hysteria than any nineteenth-century British physician. In 1855, he secured the Chair of the Practice of Physic at Edinburgh University—this was Whytt's and Cullen's post from the previous century—and he is recognized today as a founder of "physiological psychology" and an early advocate of evolutionary psychology.[133]

Laycock launched his publishing career in 1838–1839 with a detailed study of hysteria in the *Edinburgh Medical and Surgical Journal,* followed by the publication of *An Essay on Hysteria* (1840) and

*A Treatise on the Nervous Diseases of Women* (1840), the work on which his early reputation primarily rested.[134] Laycock presents his work as a comprehensive clarification of hysteria's forms, causes, and course. He sets out four axioms: hysterical disorders are anchored in the nervous system; the sexual organs act deleteriously upon the nervous system; females are principally prone to these ailments; and the danger years are between puberty and menopause.[135] Laycock introduces these points as the common sense of his day, quite beyond the need for clinical evidence or logical argument; thus his book is full of phrases like "it is universally known that" and "as everyone acknowledges."

Unlike Trotter, Laycock was little concerned with the nervous ill-health of the nation. (Great Britain faced no major external threat when he wrote in the later 1830s.) Nor was he preoccupied, as were his French pathoanatomical contemporaries, with locating the "lesion of hysteria." Rather, Laycock's view of hysteria is the older one, that of an individual affliction caused by female reproductive structure or function gone awry. "The most exclusive and universal liability of the female sex to these affections and their evident connection with the generative organs, have induced all the ancient, and a large majority of the modern, writers on these diseases to attribute their origin to some morbid state of the uterus," he asserts, in the process selectively misreading his own nation's medical history.[136] Drawing on recent research of the British anatomists Charles Bell and Marshall Hall, Laycock then argues that the matrix of nerves surrounding the uterus enervates the entire female body, and since the nerves go everywhere, the hysteric might suffer in any organ of her body.[137] The result is that female physiology is forever prone to malfunction, particularly during the biological rites of passage—menstruation, parturition, lactation, and menopause.[138]

Reflecting new research from the Continent, Laycock declares the ovaries to be the key hysteria-producing organs. He calls menstruation a "type of hysterical hemorrhage."[139] Reminiscent of Landouzy, he includes in his two books some 67 case histories. A tally of symptom profiles reveals that globus hystericus, pseudoparalyses, anesthesias and hyperesthesias, swelling of joints, heart palpitations, and nausea in fact appear most often. In his interpretations, however, Laycock emphasizes symptoms related to ovarian hormones, like menstrual pain, tender breasts, and hoarse voice.[140] He notes that boys and girls are equally susceptible to bouts of hysteria. Characteristically, however, he claims that the hysterical impressionability of children of the two sexes diverges at puberty: "We may infer ... that the affectability of childhood is diminished in the male on the approach and by the accession of puberty, while in the female it is only altered in proportion as more vigorous vital powers influence the system."[141] Laycock includes a progressive polemic against the practice of bleeding to treat hysterics, but he mouths other superstitions, including the belief that "the best cure of hysteria is for the patient to marry and bear children."[142]

Like Landouzy during this same period across the Channel, Laycock's ideas are premised on a belief in the absolute difference of male and female, a view he buttresses with extensive pseudozoological data.[143] Laycock is not entirely silent on hysteria's male incarnations. "Hysteria most unquestionably occurs in the male," he states promisingly. But his actual clinical observations of hysteria in men are highly qualified:

I think I have seen three cases in the hospital, the symptoms of which, if they had been observed in females, would certainly have entitled their history to a place in my collection. The first was that of a small delicate youth, aged 14. He had paroxysms of violent palpitations and dyspnea, occurring regularly every night for two or three weeks together. To these were occasionally added spectral illusions, delirium amounting sometimes to furious mania, cephalaea, diminished secretion of urine, pain in the loins, constipation, and . . . an unconquerable dislike of animal food. He recovered as he approached puberty. The other two cases were those of fat, pale-faced, effeminate-looking men. In the one, the affection was attributed to malaria, and he had flabby wasted testicles, with very scanty secretion of urine, globus, borborygmi, colic, and paralytic affection of the arm.[144]

One of Laycock's three male patients, in other words, isn't a real case of hysteria at all but one of malaria, and in the other two cases hysteria equates with a degree of demasculinization that borders on a complete loss of gender identity. In the first of the three cases, the symptoms vanish with the advent of phallic manhood.

Thus from Cullen in the late 1760s to Laycock in the early 1840s and beyond, British medical authors envisioned the hysterical disorders as fundamentally female afflictions. A few physicians summarily rejected the very possibility of hysteria in males, reasoning that men were anatomically immune. Most British medical statements during this long period consist of one or two sentences that abstractly cite the idea of masculine hysteria without either theoretical elaboration or case-historical illustration. In general, British physicians from the 1790s to the 1870s hastened to dismiss rather than to detail and dramatize the incidence of hysteria among members of their own sex. Time and again, they did so either by stressing hysteria's exceptional rarity in men, which allowed them to reject individual cases as statistically and therefore interpretively negligible, or by linking it dismissively with femininity and effeminacy, an exercise in circular reasoning that allowed them to argue away the very clinical data that might have compelled them to revise medical orthodoxy.

## Two Mid-Century Exceptions

There were two less conformist voices within the Anglo-French medical world between the 1790s and 1860s. Both authors wrote in the 1850s, and the story of their ideas, as well as the professional reception of those ideas, is instructive.

After a decade of silence, two works on hysteria appeared on the British medical scene in the early 1850s: William James Anderson's *The Causes, Symptoms, and Treatment of Eccentric Nervous Affections* (1850), and Robert Brudenell Carter's *On the Pathology and Treatment of Hysteria* (1853).[145] A Laycockian restatement of the utero-ovarian doctrine, Anderson's book is unoriginal. Carter's volume, however, may well be the single most intriguing text on hysteria in British medical history. The book's interest lies in its remarkable compression into a short space of so many forward-looking and backward-looking attitudes by an author who was still very youthful.

The son of a major in the Royal Marines, Robert Brudenell Carter (1828–1918) received his medical training in London. Carter's 161-page *On the Pathology and Treatment of Hysteria* was his first book, which he wrote when he was only twenty-five. In the mid-1850s, Carter worked as an army surgeon during the Crimean War and later, back in England, as a country practitioner. At the age of forty, he returned to the capital where he spent the remainder of his career first at the Royal South London Hospital and then at St. George's Hospital, where he specialized in ophthalmology. He founded the Nottingham Eye Infirmary in 1859. During the 1870s and 1880s, he was a leading figure in British ophthalmology as well as a staff writer for the *Times* and the *Lancet*.[146]

In light of his age when he wrote *On the Pathology and Treatment of Hysteria,* we have to wonder where Carter gained his clinical experience; already in his mid-twenties he possessed detailed and pungent ideas about the nervous disorders that he was motivated to set down in print. In this book Carter largely rejects the physicalist bases of hysteria theorized by his predecessors Cullen, Laycock, and John Conolly. In their place, he formulates what Ilza Veith regards as the first psychological interpretation of hysteria.[147] It is not irritable ovaries or overactive uteri that produce hysterical symptoms, but intense emotions. In particular, "the sexual emotions," as Carter calls them, are decisive: it is "the universal consent of the medical profession that the sexual passion is more concerned than any other single emotion, and, perhaps, as much as all others put together, in the production of the hysteric paroxysm."[148] Men and women differ, however, in how they experience these passions, according to Carter. "If the relative power of emotion against the sexes be compared in the present day, even without including the erotic passion, it is seen to be considerably greater in the woman than in the man, partly from that natural conformation which causes the former to feel, under circumstances where the latter thinks."[149]

Carter proceeds to elaborate a line of argument first hinted at by Conolly. It is not just emotions but emotions that have for one reason or another been restrained, unnaturally withheld from expression, that are injurious. Furthermore, in present-day society, Carter reasons, this cause weighs especially heavily on the middle-class woman, who is "more often under the necessity of endeavouring to conceal her feelings." Carter's implied critique of society encompasses the contemporary roles prescribed for men as well as women:

When sexual desire is taken into account, it will add immensely to the forces bearing upon the female, who is often much under its dominion; and who, if unmarried and chaste, is compelled to restrain every manifestation of its sway. Man, on the contrary, has such facilities for its gratification, that as a source of disease it is almost inert against him, and when powerfully excited, it is pretty sure to be speedily exhausted through the proper channel.[150]

Presumably a reference to pre- and extra-marital sex, including prostitution and mistresses, Carter's "facilities for gratifying" the sex drive keep men, unlike women, healthy and unhysterical.

The final chapter of Carter's book, titled "Hysteria in the Working Classes," breaks more new ground. Carter here argues at length that "all the varieties of hysteria are of frequent occurrence among the poorer classes."[151] Unlike the pre-industrial Cullen, or Trotter at sea, or Laycock in provincial York, Carter worked in metropolitan London during the 1850s when a large-scale, mechanized, industrial economy was rapidly taking shape, and when working-class political and social movements were emerging. As a consequence, he in effect proletarianizes the nervous disorders. In Carter's short 1853 tract, hysteria is a universal malady that can affect anyone up and down the socioeconomic scale.

Carter's critique of the socio-sexual system of his time looks forward to such anti-Victorian critics as George Bernard Shaw and Lytton Strachey, and his rudimentary notion of emotional and sexual repression brings to mind Breuer and Freud's *Studies on Hysteria* of 1895. Likewise, his closing chapter on working-class hysteria anticipates Charcot's research on "traumatic hysteria" among French artisans and factory workers, as well as World War I shell shock among working-class infantrymen. Taken together, these features tempt us to see Carter as a man ahead of his time who was free of the prejudices of his day.[152]

He may well have been. But other parts of Carter's book are not only a good deal less innovative but are outright reactionary. Carter contends commendably that "the existence of many well-authenticated instances of masculine hysteria" renders the uterine and ovarian models "utterly untenable"—a direct challenge to his distinguished senior contemporary Laycock. He further suggests that in earlier times, when the conditions of life were hardier, men never succumbed to hysteria, but that with the advent of modern civilization "the circle of masculine emotions" had widened, thereby creating more and more cases in males.[153] Despite these pronouncements, Carter goes on to discuss "the greater proclivity of the female sex to hysteria and . . . the absolute rarity of its occurrence in man." He bases these assertions on men's and women's fundamentally different emotional identities: "On the whole, it appears reasonable to ascribe the comparative immunity of man, not so much to the failure of emotion, when excited, in producing its legitimate effects; as to the fact that in him strong emotion is a matter of comparatively rare occurrence, scarcely called forth except to demand immediate and energetic action of some kind."[154] Unlike women, in other words, men are fundamentally unfeeling, and thus insulated from nervous susceptibility.

In Carter's chapter on therapeutics, running to 60 pages, we find the most detailed and impassioned discussion of the doctor-patient relationship in the history of hysteria before Freud's papers on therapy of the early 1900s. But instead of the attentive, empathic listening of psychoanalysis, Carter advocates a skeptical, authoritarian mastering of patients, whom he sees as petulant, deceitful children requiring stern discipline. In these pages, it is clear that he regards his female hysterical patients as medically blameworthy and morally reprehensible. He contemptuously charges that many hysterical women have learned to fake their illnesses in order to get emotional sympathy and sexual attention from physicians. In one passage, he warns his colleagues against performing vaginal examinations on hysterical women.[155] Carter portrays the doctor's encounter with his female patients as a titanic power struggle between two combatants equally matched in skill, resourcefulness, and determination to fight. Treatment requires that the physician reveal to the patient her "vicious propensity" and "deadened moral sense."[156] Throughout his discussion, Carter refers to the hysterical patient as "she," thereby giving the entire doctor-patient encounter the aura of a grand battle of the sexes. Utterly absent from the second half of his book are the nascent sensibility and perceptive appreciation of women's social constraints that characterize the early parts of the work. Likewise missing—despite "the many well-authenticated instances" acknowledged earlier—is any reference to male patients.

Another partial exception to the dominant nineteenth-century European discourse of hysteria is found in the work of the Parisian internist Pierre Briquet (1796–1881), who wrote about hysteria several years after Carter. Briquet was born in the immediate aftermath of the French Revolution and died during the early years of the Third Republic. He worked throughout his long career at the Hôpital de la Charité in Paris. Like Carter with his prominent later career in ophthalmology, Briquet was mainly recognized for his work on infectious diseases; he was heavily involved in public health campaigns to contain the cholera epidemics that periodically plagued the French capital throughout the 1800s. Unlike his predecessors Louyer-Villermay, Georget, Brachet, Dubois D'Amiens, and Landouzy, Briquet was not an alienist. Nonetheless, in 1859—midway through his career and at the end of the first,

repressive decade of the Second Empire—he published his enormously ambitious *Traité clinique et thérapeutique de l'hystérie*.[157]

Briquet is in fact a figure of premier importance in the intellectual history of hysteria. He begins his 720-page treatise by firmly
centering hysteria in the brain, conjecturing that a part of the human brain is reserved for emotional or "affective sensations," as opposed to motor control and intellectual operations. He then specifies that "hysteria is an illness consisting of a neurosis of the part
of the brain destined to receive affective impressions and feelings."[158] He goes on to maintain that the disorder is caused by the
complex and highly individual interaction of many disparate factors, including age, gender, emotional disposition, family history,
mode of education, previous physical illness, and psychological
stress. The malady develops temperamentally, he claims, in individuals with an "affective predominance." Among the emotional
causes, Briquet highlights traumatic domestic events such as the
death of a spouse, anxiety over the health of children, or physical
spousal abuse. He distances himself from what he regards as past
prejudices about the disease by repeatedly downplaying any association with sexuality.[159]

Hysterical sickness, Briquet hypothesizes, has the capacity to affect every part of the physical body. He proposes a connection between individual symptoms of the disease, whether physical or psychological, and specific emotional experiences: "If one takes any
hysterical symptom, one will find always its model in an act that
constitutes a manifestation of emotion. . . . Hysterical phenomena represent the more or less troubled . . . manifestation of painful
sentiments, and emotions and passions that are sad or violent."[160]
These are insightful observations, formulated thirty-five years before the psychoanalytic notion of psychological conversion and

seventy years before William B. Cannon's work on the actions of the autonomic nervous system.

Previous authors had floated theories of the disorder derived from dominant medical philosophies or from a small number of representative cases. Briquet, in contrast, conducted what can only be called epidemiological research. He claimed that he personally gathered information over a ten-year period on 430 new clinical histories of hysteria, and he analyzed this material for medical and sociological correlations involving age, gender, occupation, family background, social class, educational level, sexual life style, and prior physical and mental health. With many of his patients, he even collected a kind of follow-up data on their condition from six months to four years after their date of discharge.

After his introductory remarks, Briquet chooses to begin the main body of his book with a 40-page discussion of hysteria in the adult male—the very first discussion of its kind in a nineteenth-century medical text.[161] Briquet's motives for including this discussion are manifestly polemical. He explains that upon undertaking his clinical study,

> To my great astonishment, it didn't take me long to see that the clinical facts I was discovering were entirely different from those found in the most traditional authors. I soon realized that hysteria had never been studied like other diseases, by observing first and concluding thereafter. In all that had been written on the subject, I found far more imagination than verifiable fact.[162]

Over and over, Briquet briskly dismisses previous medical commentaries on hysteria as errant nonsense. He argues strenuously against the view that "the uterus is everything in the woman," and he reacts with angry incredulity to the revival of ancient doctrine by his colleagues, from Louyer-Villermay to Landouzy. Of masculine hysteria, he observes pointedly that "it is likely that up to the present people did not see hysteria in men because they did not want to see it."[163] Briquet never loses an opportunity to declare that the overwhelming majority of cases of hysteria involve no disturbance of the structure or function of the male or female genitalia, adding that "an error maintained for so long about a matter so easy to illuminate demonstrates in what spirit past scientific observation was practiced."[164] In an extraordinary passage, he compares at length the sexual anatomy of males and females, emphasizing analogous structures and functions as well as similarities in sensory innervation; he concludes that these are so alike that they cannot possibly explain gender differences in the prevalence of hysteria.[165] Briquet even comes to the defense of the hysteric's integrity and character: "By blaming everything on the ovary and uterus . . . doctors have made hysteria into a disease of promiscuity and a shameful sickness, which has tended to turn hysterical patients into objects of disgust and pity."

Briquet estimates that male and female cases occur in a ratio of 1 to 20.[166] In his opening chapter, he then introduces the seven adult men among his patients diagnosed as hysterical. In these pages we meet the following individuals: Ernest Langlois, a 29-year-old baker who, following a violent argument with an ex-girlfriend, suffered "une attaque de nerfs avec perte de connaissance et convulsions assez fortes [a nervous attack with loss of consciousness and rather powerful convulsions]"; Émile Laroche, a 29-year-old cook who, upon the death of a close friend during a cholera epidemic, began vomiting his food and experiencing headaches, stomach pain, and a loss of sensation on the left side of his body; Derue, an 18-year-old mechanic who spontaneously collapsed into a hysterical attack following coitus; Jean-Baptiste Tissier, a 39-year-old house painter who, after barely escaping execution by the Mobile National Guard during the 1848 revolution, experienced convulsions and outbursts of anger; Leon Bongor, an 18-year-old printer's apprentice who endured "a strong constriction of the throat" and the sensation of a ball moving upward through his body; Rendanne, a 29-year-old house painter who, after being caught in a thunderstorm, gradually lost much of his muscular strength as well as his senses of hearing and speech; and Grasson, a 25-year-old typesetter who, following a bad turn of financial events, suffered "attacks of nerves" and "loss of sensation on the lower part of the face."[167] In all seven cases, the hysterical symptoms were set in motion by purely emotional experiences.

Yet, for all his modernity, Briquet represents only a partial exception to the dominant discourse of hysteria in nineteenth-century Europe. Although Briquet mounted a full-throated assault on the French neo-Hippocratic tradition of his time, he simultaneously articulated the views and attitudes of French cultural Romanticism. For instance, he genders as female and then sexualizes his own notion of "the emotional brain." Throughout his book, he uncritically assumes that women are more highly developed morally and emotionally—he prefers the term *impressionnable*—and that males have an innate intellectual superiority. "Woman is made to feel, and to feel is the essence of hysteria; in contrast, Man is made to act."[168] Abandoning his early emphasis on sameness between the sexes, Briquet increasingly affirms that "the differences between men and women depend on the respective roles assigned to them in society."[169] Moreover, he proposes that, in light of their much greater affectability, a quarter of all women in the world at one time or another in their lives fall prey to hysterical neurosis. Hysteria is always transmitted matrilineally, he claims, and the disease "is in a sense then the appanage of the female sex."[170]

Despite his brave opening inclusion of the seven extended cases in men, Briquet subsequently comments that the male may become "epileptic, insane, hypochondriacal, but he only rarely becomes hysterical."[171] Oddly, throughout the remaining hundreds of pages of his treatise, he never again references masculine hysteria. Furthermore, at a later point in his exposition he ponders directly the serious societal implications of male hysteria:

> Let us imagine a man endowed with the faculty of being affected in the same way as a woman. He would become hysterical and consequently unfit for his predestined role, namely, that of protection and of strength. *Hysteria in a man means the overthrow of the laws constitutive of our society.*[172]

Here Briquet lays bare the high stakes involved in the exploration of male emotional and nervous vulnerability: in the end, striving to defend traditional gender identities in the manner of earlier French hysteria doctors, Briquet appeals not to Nature or to God, but to "the laws of society." Furthermore, he chooses to use a term associated with social and political subversion—the hysterical male would bring the "overthrow" *(renversement)* of society. By the end of Briquet's long and authoritative exposition, an adult man capable of "affective impressions" is seen not only as sick and abnormal, but also as a deviation from, and a menace to, the bourgeois family order.

When Briquet's volume appeared in 1859, he was an established figure in the Parisian medical community with a prominent hospital appointment. His weighty tome could not be ignored. The *Traité clinique et thérapeutique de l'hystérie* was reviewed favorably in the medical press, and the next year Briquet was inducted into the Academy of Medicine. But by the late 1860s, leading French alienists were dissenting from Briquet by name and insisting, again, that hysteria and hypersexuality were inextricably linked. Most tellingly, the 1860s, the decade when Briquet's ideas should have been spreading widely, were the very years when a new characterological view of hysteria, marked by overt misogyny and a categorical denial of male hysteria, flourished.[173] The exception was Charcot, who beginning in the early 1870s cited Briquet's arguments in his own efforts to establish the reality of male hysteria. With the rise of psychoanalysis after the turn of the century, however, Briquet's book was eclipsed and remained so until the late twentieth century. Neither his nor Carter's original and enlightened analyses of the nervous disorders were particularly influential in their own time, and both failed to discredit the durable tradition of gynecological determinism.

## Hysteria's Two Cultures

At the Enlightenment's end, a major bifurcation of the scientific and artistic commentaries on mind and body began to develop within European culture. This split was part of a larger, metacultural fracture that occurred in many domains of Western life and thought and that over time give rise to what C. P. Snow in the late 1950s famously labeled "the two cultures" of art and science.[174] Hysteria, too, has its two cultures. Whereas European physicians between 1790 and 1870 were resolutely unwilling to take up the male psyche as a subject of systematic investigation, cultural savants of the age, especially men and women of letters, engaged in the most probing exploration of male psychological subjectivity in the European West up to that time.

During the same decades, the congeries of processes lumped together under the term "professionalization" rapidly expanded in western and central Europe. In medicine, the age-old practices of self-medication, household doctoring, and neighbor consultations declined as ever larger numbers of people sought treatment by trained and certified caretakers. Physicians strove increasingly to separate themselves from "quacks," "empirics," herbalists, and "officiers de santé." The first clinical specialties—dermatology, dentistry, ophthalmology, and psychiatry among them—emerged, and from the 1830s and 1840s onward, specialty journals proliferated. In France during the revolutionary 1790s, mandatory state-sponsored systems of training, examination, and licensing were instituted. By the mid-nineteenth century, the interrelated concepts of the academic physician and the teaching hospital had appeared. Needless to say, these developments from the later eighteenth century onward were accompanied by a rapid rise in the status and prestige of medical practitioners.

Conspicuously, women were excluded from these professionalizing trends. It is now widely acknowledged by scholars that women played a significantly larger and more varied role in medical practice during the seventeenth and eighteenth centuries—as nurses, hospital administrators, druggists, midwives, bone-setters, and lay healers as well as doctors' wives and widows—than they did during the nineteenth century. The legal requirement of a degree from a university medical school in order to practice medicine, at a time when women were barred from admission to universities across Europe, had the effect of marginalizing or outlawing women from medical practice.[175] With the rise of "male midwifery" (that is, obstetrics), female midwives were increasingly squeezed out of even the traditional practice of childbirth.[176] For all intents and purposes, modern European medicine as a professional collectivity was founded to a substantial degree on the exclusion of the female.

Even more fundamentally, science itself, as both an intellectual system and a professional activity, emerged during this era as a strictly masculine domain. Expert knowledge came to be seen as a male possession. Both factually and symbolically, medicine's leading venues—the study, the clinic, the laboratory, the university lecture hall—became masculine enclaves. Likewise, the new sartorial self-fashioning of academic physicians—a brotherhood of bearded men in black—was intended to connote the masculine virtues of sober, rational authority. The male medical profession that took shape in the early decades of the 1800s self-consciously sought to pursue a "modern," "scientific" methodology; that methodology rested on mutually reinforcing qualities, such as objectivity, rationality, detachment, empirical research, and intellectual mastery. More and more for nineteenth-century "men of science," to be objective meant to distance oneself as far as humanly possible from the distorting perspective of one's own personal presuppositions, to keep apart the prejudices of the self from the investigation of the external world. To put it differently, the very grounds for achieving knowledge of the natural world in the emerging positivist world view involved a radical and unrelenting separation of the object and subject of investigation.[177]

We can glimpse this process of the masculinization of knowledge in several new aspects and attitudes of nineteenth-century European medicine. From the 1820s onward, the anatomico-pathological method, seeking to correlate symptoms and lesions posthumously, became the hallmark of avant-garde clinical medicine as the modern concept of "scientific medicine" took hold. Patients were increasingly envisioned not so much as individual sufferers but as exemplifications of universal disease types. Populations of sick people at large city hospitals became commodified as "clinical material" for scientific investigation. The autopsy, the most impersonal relation to the body and death, and animal vivisection, requiring an insensitivity to pain in sentient creatures, were repeatedly cited as indispensable methods of medical science. Even styles of medical writing reflected the new ethos: by the early 1800s, the narrative content of medical case histories had become notably more technical and scientistic, addressed solely to a limited readership of male medical elites. In one field after another, the rhetoric and ideology of detached impersonality infiltrated European medical discourse and praxis.

Conversely, any semblance of subjectivity in medical science and practice was deemed inappropriate. Medicine came more and more to be defined as a science rather than an art. In case-historical writing, references to the physician's own life—along the lines of Mandeville's fictional dialogue of patient and physician or George Cheyne's long exercise in self-observation—now vanished from clinical discourse. More generally, nonempirical modes of experience and apprehension—philosophical speculation, psychological intuition, personal introspection—came to be seen not as complementary but as contradictory to rational objective analysis and were therefore shunned as insufficiently *wissenschaftlich*. Reason itself came to be gendered as masculine, whereas emotion was evermore associated with the feminine.[178] To the positivist physicians of this "heroic" era, emotion, passion, and sensibility were construed as inferior human faculties—the negative repudiation of reason—that contaminated the pursuit of real knowledge. As a cognitive style, objective analysis itself became a key component of masculine intellectual culture.[179]

These overlapping cultural developments provide an important context for understanding why nervous vulnerability in men was studied so rarely by European medical men during the first seventy-five years of the nineteenth century yet at the same time became an utterly absorbing subject for literary and artistic intellectuals. It is not surprising that the members of an emergent masculinist professional culture, whose intellectual methods, professional identity, and cultural authority relied on the personal cultivation and public display of strict, dispassionate objectivity, would fail to take the subjective, psychological aspects of their own gender as an object of study. On the contrary, the medical community during these years exerted itself systematically and with great resourcefulness to suppress these very aspects of masculine nature from public view. At this historical juncture, medical discourses broke from their early modern moorings, abandoning their former alliance with literary styles and sensibilities in order to develop an independent, strictly scientific identity.

AMONG THE COMPLEX of ideas and attitudes that constituted Romanticism was a celebration of the creative powers of imagination and intuition, faculties that had allegedly been neglected by Enlightenment thinkers. Romantic artists envisioned imagination as the royal road to knowledge and experience. The belief was especially fervent in the Wordsworthian strand of British literary Romanticism, with its worship of nature. What interested the Romantics above all was the generative capacity of the artist/poet/seer for whom imagination was a protean creative force, in contrast to the sensibility of the Georgian gentleman, who was now deemed silly and effete. Romantic aesthetic ideology sought a much greater awareness of the subjectivities of perception and consciousness, which they experienced as forms of Romantic self-consciousness.

Romanticism also brought bold experimentation with artistic form. In creative literature, the Age of Reason had been an age of prose, so Romanticism meant poetry in Britain and new forms of poetic prose in France. Changes in genre and gender went hand in hand: the "manly" genre of the epic, with its grand narratives of history and heroism, went into eclipse during the early 1800s, while the "feminine" pastime of poetry became the archetypically Romantic instrument of imaginative labor. The dominant image of the Romantic artist/genius was invariably male. Yet the male Romantics, who tended to view women as inferior intellectually, nonetheless admired the qualities of sympathy, perception, and feeling that women were historically believed to possess more than men. In their quest for a "poetry of feeling," Romantic male writers believed they should embrace the elements of mental and emotional femininity that they innately lacked.[180]

In *Lyrical Ballads* (1798), a key text of early British Romanticism, Wordsworth experiences strong elemental states of emotion—joy, love, passion, tenderness, grief—and then communicates these sentiments either by assuming the role of a female narrator or by presenting "feminized" states of feeling in his own voice.[181] The goal in this poetry is always to heighten the expressive capabilities of the male poet. Wordsworth was dependent on his sister Dorothy's journals for inspiration in writing his long autobiographical work *The Prelude, or, Growth of a Poet's Mind* (1850).[182] Furthermore, throughout Wordsworth's poetry, men express strong emotion in the face of nature, beauty, and art without the stigma of unmanliness—that is, they speak in voices that contrast starkly with the stern self-control and inexpressive rationality that defined ideals of masculine selfhood in other contemporaneous domains of British society, such as law, politics, business, and medicine. In his *Defence of Poetry* (1821; 1840), Percy Bysshe Shelley similarly speaks of incorporating female empathy into the poet's masculine sphere, and Samuel Taylor Coleridge is quoted as contending that "a great mind must be androgynous."[183] Although John Keats wrote no "Ode to Hysteria," a great deal of early nineteenth-century British Romantic poetry explores and exposes masculine psychological subjectivity, and it does so by pursuing a new ideal of feminized or androgynous manhood.[184] But during these very same years when Wordsworth and his literary peers were forming a rich cultural avant-garde centered on an ethic and aesthetic of masculine psychological self-exploration, British physicians were either silent on the matter or, like the reactionary war doctor Thomas Trotter, were engaged in stigmatizing male emotionality as a sign of personal weakness and national decline.

A somewhat similar situation obtained in France. Rousseau's major autobiographical works, the *Confessions* and the *Reveries of the Solitary Walker*, appeared in print between the early 1780s and early 1790s. As a consequence, "l'esprit Jean-Jacques" pervaded French Romanticism during the first third of the nineteenth century. The cult of Goethe's young, lovesick protagonist in *The Sorrows of Young Werther* (1774) likewise spread through continental Europe during the late eighteenth and early nineteenth centuries. The late Enlightenment autobiographical tradition was then refracted through the events of the revolution and the empire to create the blend of intimate subjectivism, brooding self-consciousness, and psychological disenchantment that distinguished French Romanticism.

François-René de Chateaubriand's short, semi-autobiographical novella *René* is a key French text here.[185] Completed in 1802 (a year before Louyer-Villermay's medical dissertation) and set in the lush wilderness of colonial Louisiana, *René* is part travelogue, part youthful idyll, and part nature reverie. Chateaubriand's literary tone poem relates the story of a wistful, world-weary youth who has abandoned his patriarchal heritage in France in order to live among the Natchez Indians of French North America. But the content of the story, Chateaubriand explains at the outset, will be "not the

adventures of his [René's] life, for he had never had any, but the in-
nermost feelings of his soul"—his spiritual and existential ponder-
ings, his reveries amidst the beauties of nature, his emotional yearn-
ings and frustrations.[186] It is little wonder that doctors during the
age of Charcot considered Chateaubriand diagnosable.[187]

Chateaubriand's troubled, introspective protagonist became the
archetype for a whole gallery of melancholy male protagonists who
populated the creative literature of the French Romantic era.
Senancour's *Obermann* (1804), Benjamin Constant's *Adolphe* (1816),
Alfred de Vigny's *Poèmes antiques et modernes* (1826), Félicité Robert
de Lamennais's *Paroles d'un croyant* (1834), and Alfred de Musset's
*Confession d'un enfant du siècle* (1836) all embroider on Chateaubri-
and's version of the modern masculine hero, a figure who refuses
or fails to adopt the orthodoxies of the virile, militarist masculinity
that was glorified by Napoleon and reinforced by the conservative governments of the Restoration and July Monarchy.[188] Again,
the contrast with contemporaneous medico-scientific discourse
couldn't be sharper. The imaginative productions of Chateaubri-
and, Senancour, Vigny, Lamennais, Lamartine, and Musset, like the
literature of British Romantic poetry, offer another instance of a
new masculine subjectivity that is altered or expanded for creative,
expressive purposes. Their fiction emerged precisely during the decades when French neo-Hippocratic physicians were methodically
suppressing the idea of male hysteria, and with it the vulnerable,
"feminine" aspects of masculine psychological identity.

Back in Britain, the novels of the mid-Victorian era dramatized
this contrast still further. The figure of the male nervous invalid
populated British novels of the 1830s, 1840s, and 1850s, which
were written notably by both male and female authors. Mid-
century "narratives of nervousness" by Charlotte Brontë, George
Eliot, Wilkie Collins, Mary Braddon, and William Gilbert reflect

critically on the new ideal of middle-class manliness that was be-
coming prevalent in England during the first decades of Victoria's
reign.[189] *The Professor, The Lifted Veil,* and *The Woman in White* are
studies in male consciousness in which the novelist represents self-
consciousness simultaneously as a virtue, a necessity, and a curse.
On the one hand, the self-induced and undefined nervous symptoms of these male characters are depicted as mysterious, pitiful,
even contemptible. On the other, the vagueness of the characters'
suffering underscores the failure of medical science to master this
category of disease. In contrast to the growing masculinist rhetoric
of health, extroversion, and self-mastery that animated science, politics, industry, and empire, these novels feature male protagonists
who do not conform to prescriptive norms of social productivity
and biological reproductivity.[190] In the process, Brontë, Eliot, and
Collins challenge the gendering of nervous illness itself as formulated by biomedical science and institutionalized in society.

Meanwhile, the scandal-provoking *Madame Bovary,* Gustave
Flaubert's first and best-known novel, appeared in book form in
the spring of 1857 in Paris, two years before Briquet's *Clinical and
Therapeutic Treatise on Hysteria.*[191] In a well-known review of Flaubert's novel, the poet Charles Baudelaire labeled Emma Bovary
as "hysterical." Baudelaire also explored the intense and intimate
identification of Flaubert with his female fictional creation, in the
process probing what today would be called the gender identities
of both male artist and female protagonist. Baudelaire perceived a
subtle but deep psychological and emotional symbiosis between
Flaubert and Emma Bovary, and he implied that the immense artistic success of Flaubert's novel was the result of this fleeting union
between the male and the female.[192]

It is a commonplace that all fiction writing is in some measure
autobiographical, especially an author's first novel. Baudelaire's re-

view, with its emphasis on the androgynous and autobiographical elements in *Madame Bovary*, was the one commentary on the book that Flaubert is said to have approved of.[193] In correspondence with friends written during his composition of the novel, Flaubert at times used the pronoun "I" when speaking of Emma Bovary. Also interesting in this light is the author's much-quoted account of the gestation of the novel. Later in his career, Flaubert was repeatedly asked on whom in real life he had patterned Emma's character. At least once he is reported to have said, "Madame Bovary, c'est moi; d'après moi."[194] Analogously, in his private epistolary self-representations, Flaubert chose to discuss his mental and emotional vicissitudes in the language of contemporary medical diagnosis, in several instances openly labeling himself "hysterical."[195]

Romantic and Victorian autobiography is another literary source of significance. The first citation of the word "autobiography" in the *Oxford English Dictionary* dates from 1797, and the German *Selbstbiographie* predated the English term by a decade.[196] Reflecting the general growth of Western individualism, autobiographical writings of all varieties—memoirs, confessions, lives and letters, novelistic autobiographies, epistolary and first-person novels—glutted the literary marketplace during the 1800s. Although it is difficult to generalize about such a diverse corpus of writing, the psychological content of nineteenth-century European autobiography is conspicuous.[197] These self-narratives are nearly always more than recitals of biographical fact. Unlike many examples of the genre preceding Goethe and Rousseau, Romantic and Victorian life histories are conceived as formats for presenting, probing, and even creating individual psychological identity, usually in their male authors.[198]

British middle-class autobiographies in particular often struggle openly with a range of intimate experiences, including emotional relations with parents, internal conflicts about career, the loss of religious faith, and sexual and gender identity. Several of the best-known texts in the nineteenth-century autobiographical canon report on episodes of nervous and mental collapse and recovery in the author's life. Among the Romantic autobiographers, Wordsworth, De Quincey, and Coleridge chronicle their vulnerable emotional states. And during the Victorian decades, Mill, Ruskin, Faraday, Spencer, Darwin, and Galton, among others, discuss personal depressive experiences in their published letters, memoirs, and autobiographies—all part of a project of masculine self-representation.[199]

Inevitably, John Stuart Mill (1806–1873) occupies a special place in this story. The case is well known. James Mill, the Utilitarian thinker and doctrinaire Benthamite, took control of his eldest son's education from early childhood. Young Mill was schooled in Greek at the age of three, Latin language and literature at six, and British political economy at fourteen. His precocity was astounding, and by his late teens, he had not only mastered these materials but was steadily publishing his own work. Readings and activities that the severe and overweening father deemed frivolous were prohibited. The fact that Mill was schooled at home, that his mother was apparently silent, and that Jeremy Bentham himself lived for a period in the household must have made the adolescent Mill feel trapped.[200]

Intellectually overworked, emotionally starved, and psychologically browbeaten, Mill in the fall of 1826, at the age of twenty, broke down. He relates the story in his autobiography's famous fifth chapter, titled "A Crisis in My Mental History."[201] Likening the experience to a religious conversion, Mill came to realize that his father's Utilitarian philosophy and Benthamite program of reform were not the all-sufficient system of thought he was raised to believe and could not provide a comprehensive blueprint for either social improvement or personal happiness.[202] A kind of robotic reasoning machine, Mill in young adulthood lacked the capacity to feel. Throughout "the melancholy winter of 1826–1827," he was in a continual state of "depression," "dejection," and "a dull state of nerves," he tells us. His earlier activities, both social and intellectual, were drained of meaning. He struggled to free himself from his "irrepressible self-consciousness," but could barely get through his daily activities.[203]

The source of Mill's eventual solace was unexpected. After a year and a half of misery, he reports, "a small ray of light broke in upon my gloom."[204] Mill had an epiphany when reading the memoirs of the French historian and writer Jean-François Marmontel, and he came to see a way out of his paralyzing despair: through the careful and systematic cultivation of the emotional and aesthetic side of his nature, he would gradually enrich his prior training in "the analysing spirit." "The maintenance of a due balance among the faculties now seemed to me of primary importance. The cultivation of the feelings became one of the cardinal points in my ethical and philosophical creed."[205] To this end, Mill turned to the culture of European Romanticism that was flourishing around him—specifically, Wordsworth's and Coleridge's poetry, the writings of Goethe, and German Romantic music—as a complement to his earlier hyperrationalistic faith and a tonic for his psychological suffering. Henceforth, he wrote to a friend in 1832, he would not neglect to cultivate "his inner life," which he now christened "the chief part of his life."[206]

In his short and highly selective autobiography, written some twenty-five years after the fact and long after the death of his father, Mill was not obliged to include a chapter on this experience at all, or he might have just noted the incident in passing. Instead, Mill includes the story as a lengthy and dramatic chapter that is central to the book. Even at the peak of his professional fame and intellectual maturity, the recollection of his youthful nervous malady remained crucial to Mill's own sense of his life. Furthermore, despite the stereotype of Mill's prose as controlled and colorless, the chapter brims with emotional energy and psychological observations.[207]

As is well known, Mill maintained a remarkable emotional and intellectual partnership with Harriet Taylor (1808–1858), who was his steady (if platonic) companion for two decades after they met in the early 1830s and then his wife from 1851 until her early death in 1858. Not least in the *Autobiography* itself, Mill claimed time and again that his wife decisively influenced what he thought, wrote, and published, particularly on issues of social justice, personal liberty, and the oppression of women. Some scholars, like Mill's enemies in his own day, charged either that Mill's assessment of his wife's role was ludicrously idealized or that her influence was decisive but deleterious. But recent scholarship demonstrates persuasively that Taylor's own writings, and her role in Mill's intellectual life, were indeed much more substantive than previously appreciated.[208] Mill's wife in fact oversaw the writing of the bulk of the first draft of the *Autobiography*, composed during the early years of their marriage, and Mill accepted the majority of her editorial interventions.[209] Not coincidentally, Mill's brave and celebrated broadside *The Subjection of Women*, which remains the most impressive philosophical defense of women's rights to come out of Victorian Britain, was written in 1861 and published in 1869, the same year he finished the autobiography. Mill's candid and in-depth account of his father as the cause of his nervous collapse doubles as a critique of the paternal authority and rationalist ideal of masculinity that underpinned middle-class Victorian patriarchy. In its place, the new model of human nature and education that Mill promotes entails a union of reason and emotion that was sharply at odds with dominant gender practices and beliefs.

The prominence of the cultural arts in Mill's account is also per-

tinent. Mill first encountered Marmontel's memoir, with its revela-
tory effect, and then, in an attempt to diagnose his condition, he
turned to Coleridge, "in whom alone of all writers I have found a
true description of what I felt."[210] A few sentences later, Mill in his
search for self-treatment brings in another English poet: "Advice,
if I had known where to seek it, would have been most precious.
The words of Macbeth to the physician often occurred to my
thoughts. But there was no one on whom I could build the faintest
hope of such assistance."[211] After Marmontel, Coleridge, and Shakespeare, Mill introduces Wordsworth's ode "Intimations of Immor-
tality," which "proved to be the precise thing for my mental wants
at that particular juncture." Mill furthermore pronounces himself
"a Wordsworthian"; he defended Wordsworth's poetry in a public
debating society, and in the 1830s he made personal pilgrimages to
meet the Lake Poet.[212] By the chapter's end, Mill has seen fit to mention no fewer than ten figures from the cultural arts whose work
was relevant to the self-presentation of his youthful mental crisis.

It is common to observe that as a despondent twenty-year-old,
Mill was unable to turn either to his family or to religion for assistance during the crisis months of 1826–27. But another omission is
equally glaring: at no point in his 30-page account does Mill mention the medical psychology or the medical profession of his day.
Neither when he actually underwent the crisis, nor in 1853–54
when he and his wife drafted the autobiography, nor in 1869 when
he reworked the text for posthumous publication did Mill cite a
single medical text, author, or theory. To be sure, Mill employs
medicalized language throughout his narrative. (He refers to "my
case" and diagnoses himself with "depression" and a "mental malady." Wordsworth's poems are "a medicine for my state of mind,"
and after reading them he "was in process of recovery.")[213] We know
that several prominent British physicians—Trotter, Reid, Conolly,

Brodie, Laycock, Carter—wrote about nervous disorders during Mill's lifetime, and that the French medical literature on hysteria published during the 1820s, 1830s, and 1840s would have been readily available to the Francophonic Mill. Nevertheless, at no time does Mill appear to have read a work of medicine or consulted a physician for solace or insight.

Mill's actions in this regard contrast strikingly with those of his British philosophical predecessor David Hume. At the age of eighteen, Hume had undergone his own crisis of the mind. Like Mill, Hume overcame his youthful neurotic episode and went on to lead a life of exemplary productivity and creativity. Just as Hume's subsequent philosophy of human nature was enriched by his acknowledgment of the role of the passions in human reasoning, so Mill eventually produced a far more flexible and humane Utilitarian philosophy than his predecessors had. Hume, Mill, and Freud are in fact the historical prototypes of young intellectual males who were radically altered by hysteria. But Hume's and Freud's quests for cures differed markedly from Mill's. Hume repeatedly sought medical counsel, and his efforts to regain his equilibrium included writing the lengthy and self analytical "Epistle to Dr. Arbuthnot."[214] For his part, Freud confronted his profuse neurotic symptoms during the later 1890s in conversation with his Berlin medical colleague Wilhelm Fliess. Mill, however—the leading philosopher of Victorian Britain, whose life work was predicated on the lucid and methodical application of rational analysis to one human problem after another—did not turn to the psychological medicine of his day during his hour of greatest need.

IN GEORGIAN LONDON and Edinburgh, as we have seen, a broad, unspecialized nervous culture contained within it an extensive discourse on male hysteria. With the end of the eighteenth-century

Enlightenment and the seismic upheavals of the 1790s, however, this synthesis fragmented; the scientific and the artistic explorations of the human psyche went their separate ways. It was medical science itself that forced this cultural divorce when it embraced an exclusionary objectivist ideology, banned women from its professional ranks, and cultivated a new professional persona that was rigorously masculinist.

As a consequence, the idea of exploring male psychological subjectivity fared very differently in the "two cultures" during the period 1790–1870. Building cumulatively on eighteenth-century precedents, Anglo-French literary texts of these generations—including Romantic poetics, confessional literature, novels of sensation, and Victorian autobiography—eagerly took up the challenge of investigating the inner life of male characters, including the psychology of the author himself. In the process, these works often questioned the inherited models of gender, including the gendered divisions of reason and passion, science and art, and masculine and feminine. At times, this literature also entailed a challenge to the accuracy and sufficiency of medical models of human nature. European cultural discourses of hysteria during these years are open, creative, and exploratory. Their authors are both male and female. Moreover, some of the most powerful male-authored explorations of male psychological subjectivity during these eighty years were accomplished by literary intellectuals in conversation with women—William and Dorothy Wordsworth; Gustave Flaubert, Louise Colet, and George Sand; and John Stuart Mill and Harriet Taylor.

These features are absent from the medical literature about hysteria produced during the same years. Reflecting the continuing power of ancient medical theories as well as the enduring misogyny of Western science, physicians from Cullen and Boissier de

Sauvages in the 1770s to Carter and Briquet in the 1850s re-embraced various heritages of gynecological determinism. Although a handful of medical statements about masculine hysteria did emerge from this eighty-year period, they form only a fraction of what was written about the male maladies during the early modern and fin-de-siècle periods or about female hysteria during the nineteenth century. No European physician during this protracted period conceived of the field of male hysteria as a way of explaining or exploring interior experience. None saw it as a venue for self-reflective theoretical analysis, or as an opportunity to query cultural or clinical concepts of masculinity and femininity. Not least, where we encounter an open, varied, and vibrant discourse of hysteria in Romantic and early Victorian literary culture, in the medical-scientific realm we find silence. Medical writing on the subject is much less diversified than literary reflections are, and needless to say, every piece of medical writing about hysteria appearing between 1790 and 1870 was produced by a male author. In a real sense, masculine hysteria became a "forgotten knowledge" that had to be "rediscovered" at a later time under cultural and psychological circumstances that were more propitious. In his youth, John Stuart Mill was unable to seek psychiatric counsel because the mental medicine of his day had nothing whatsoever to offer him: it did not recognize, much less treat sympathetically and theorize insightfully, male nervous suffering.

The new doctrine of separate spheres of hysteria that prevailed during these years was not the result of new factual knowledge. Rather, nineteenth-century scientific constructions of nervous disease were the consequence of extrascientific circumstances, demonstrating clearly how social prejudice and cultural assumptions can structure theory choice, research programs, and clinical observation. Throughout this period, hysteria theory rationalized and reinforced a hierarchical relation between men and women that everywhere in Europe accompanied the ascension of the bourgeoisie. The much-vaunted masculine strength enshrined in this new social order could not be reconciled with the idea, much less the reality, of extensive nervous vulnerability in males. Promoters and upholders of the dominant masculinist culture, European physicians buttressed this world view through a model of gender-specific mental and nervous pathologies. The results were inevitable: the male authorial self found in nineteenth-century medical texts remains concealed beneath the opaque and impenetrable surface of medicine's official rhetoric of science. Throughout the period, male hysteria is a subject in search of an author.

# CHAPTER 3

# Charcot and
# *La Grande Hystérie Masculine*

EUROPE DURING THE LAST QUARTER of the nineteenth century produced three gifted and enormously productive scientific intellectuals who devoted a substantial part of their lifework to an in-depth and systematic study of hysteria: Jean-Martin Charcot, Pierre Janet, and Sigmund Freud. Charcot led the way, and in the process he ushered in the golden age of what he liked to call "the great neurosis."[1]

A native Parisian, Charcot (1825–1893) rose from a humble family of artisans to the apex of the French medical elite.[2] His teachers recognized his abilities and industry early on, and as a result his career advanced rapidly. He received his M.D. from the University of Paris in 1853 with a dissertation on arthritis. In 1860, he was named associate professor in medicine. Two years later he was appointed head of a hospital service at the Salpêtrière, the historic hospital complex near the Seine River in the thirteenth arrondissement, where he would spend the remaining thirty years of his career. Against the backdrop of Napoleon III's Second Empire, Charcot in the 1860s published books on infectious illnesses, geriatrics, and diseases of the lungs, heart, liver, and kidneys. In 1872 he was elected to the Paris Medical Faculty, the most prestigious body in French academic medicine, as professor of pathological anatomy.

With the advent of the Third Republic in 1870, Charcot turned increasingly to the emerging discipline of neurology, which he helped carve out of the larger field of general internal medicine. He produced an outpouring of publications in this new field, including classic descriptions of multiple sclerosis, Parkinson's disease, aphasia, locomotor ataxia, tabetic arthropathies ("Charcot joints"), Tourette's syndrome, and amyotrophic lateral sclerosis (Lou Gehrig's disease).[3] Because he practiced at the same institution as Pinel and because Freud was briefly one of his students, Charcot is sometimes misclassified today as a psychiatrist or alienist, but in fact he never treated or wrote about the insane.

Charcot achieved the peak of his fame in the 1880s, a decade of political and social liberalization in France. Politically engaged at a time in French history when many physicians served in the government,[4] Charcot had powerful allies in the republican government, including Léon Gambetta, president of the Chamber of Deputies, and Jules Ferry, the Minister of Public Instruction and two-time Prime Minister of France. Along with Claude Bernard and Paul Broca, Charcot was part of a self-fashioned coterie of young progressive physician-scientists who admired the rising German sciences and sought to modernize French medicine. For his medical accomplishments and reformist zeal, he was rewarded in 1882 with the creation of the Chair in the Diseases of the Nervous System, the first such professorial post in the world.[5] The Ministry of the Interior also granted him extensive financial resources to establish a neuropathological institute at the Salpêtrière, equipped with the latest medical technologies as well as a special ward for the

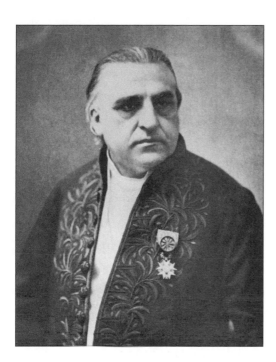

The great French
physician Jean-Martin
Charcot, looking rather
ghoulish, in his formal
garb of the Institut de
France.

treatment of nervous and neurological infirmities. The overwhelming majority of Charcot's patients, and thus the clinical repository
from which his theories derived, came in the last two decades of
his career from this Clinique des Maladies du Système Nerveux.
His voluminous writings were gathered into a nine-volume set
of collected works,[6] and he was elected an honorary member of
learned medical and scientific societies across the Western world.
The wealthy, including European aristocracy and royalty, sought his
therapeutic counsel.

Charcot was extremely successful at recruiting loyal and talented
students, both within and outside France. Working closely with his
pupils, he founded several influential medical journals and exer-
cised control over a sizable publishing empire, through which he
was able to disseminate his ideas quickly and widely. Reinforcing

his reputation as a founding figure of the new discipline was the *Archives de neurologie,* one of the first international journals in its field, which he founded in 1880.[7] The patron system in the European professions was then at its height; because of Charcot's use of nepotism to secure his protégés appointments in hospitals and medical faculties, both in Paris and the provinces, he tended to receive their uncritical devotion. The epic painter André Brouillet captured the "School of the Salpêtrière" in his life-size collective portrait, which hung in the Paris Salon of 1887.[8] Contemporaries cleverly dubbed the group "la charcoterie."[9] In the long run, Charcot's best-known students were Joseph Babinski and Pierre Marie in neurology, and of course Janet and Freud, who explored the under-theorized psychological aspects of the nervous disorders. Not surprisingly, ego, power, and politics combined to make Charcot by many accounts quite authoritarian. "The Napoleon of the neuroses" was one of his less flattering nicknames.

Charcot was also a presence in the cultural and political history of belle époque Paris. He and his wealthy wife, whose origins were in the fashion industry, maintained a lavish home in the Boulevard Saint-Germain neighborhood where they regularly invited prominent writers, thinkers, poets, scientists, artists, and politicians to their high-society *soirées.* For better or worse, many nonmedical individuals sought to attend Charcot's clinical demonstrations at the spacious hospital amphitheater, where he was renowned for his dramatic imitations of pathological syndromes. His medical work also provided sensationalistic subject matter for several prominent contemporary novelists.[10] A voracious reader in several languages, Charcot amassed one of the largest private medical libraries in Europe, the remnants of which are still on display in the Bibliothèque Charcot at the Salpêtrière. Politically, he was an aggressive advocate of the secularizing agenda of French republicanism; the journal *Le progrès médical,* founded by his combative pupil D. M. Bourneville, led the successful campaign to laicize French hospitals, with the result that medically trained nurses replaced Catholic personnel.[11] By the early 1890s, some colleagues began to rebel against Charcot's overt politicizing, blatant favoritism toward his students, and rather dictatorial personality. In the years following his sudden death from a heart attack in the summer of 1893, aspects of Charcot's medical work, including his fabled teachings about hysteria, were subjected to rigorous critique.[12]

BEFORE CHARCOT'S TIME, the Salpêtrière admitted only female patients, as it had done since its inception during the age of Louis XIV. The hospital was known alternatively as L'Hospice de la Vieillesse-Femmes. Therefore, when Charcot was formulating his early ideas about hysteria during the six-year period 1870–1876, he worked exclusively with female patients.[13] But he began to gather materials about masculine hysteria as early as 1878. The first instance of a male patient diagnosed as hysterical at the Clinique des Maladies du Système Nerveux appears in an informal hospital registry dating from February 1879.[14] Charcot's first printed case history of the disorder, a two-part article on hysteria among adolescent boys, appeared in December 1882 in *Le progrès médical,* the in-house polemical periodical mentioned earlier.[15] He published his final statement on the subject, a case history of a man who suffered from "hysterical sleepwalking," in January 1893.[16] Charcot's engagement with the topic, then, spanned the fifteen-year period from 1878 to 1893, the very years when he was at the height of his international reputation.

Unlike his French nineteenth-century predecessors, from Louyer-Villermay to Briquet, Charcot never produced a general theoretical treatise on hysteria, in either its masculine or feminine

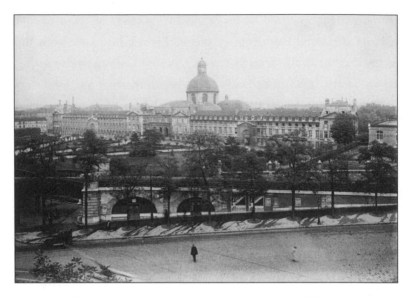

The Salpêtrière hospital in Paris, the institutional center of French hysteria studies.

versions. He had a long-standing mistrust of what he regarded as medical philosophizing. Instead, his writings take the distinctive form of book-length compilations of case histories that are intended to communicate through lucid clinical illustration and to convince through the sheer accumulation of empirical data. Reading Charcot today, one has to reconstruct a general model of disease from scores of rich clinical narratives, distinguished by eloquent and crystalline clarity.

Charcot published 61 case histories of male patients to which he assigned the primary diagnoses of "hystérie," "hystérie simple," "grande hystérie," "hystéro-épilepsie," or "hystéro-neurasthénie." His first publication in book form, which includes 21 cases that he treated between 1882 and 1885, appeared in the third volume of his *Leçons sur les maladies du système nerveux*.[17] These clinical reports initially served as formal lectures, meticulously prepared, which

Charcot delivered weekly in the teaching amphitheater of the Salpêtrière. Between 1887 and 1889, he published another 28 cases of male hysteria in his two-volume collection known as the *Leçons du mardi à la Salpêtrière*.[18] In contrast to the formal lectures, these lessons consist of informal clinical dialogues and demonstrations, conducted either at a patient's bedside in the hospital ward or in Charcot's private examining office, which were then recorded in students' notebooks and later reconstructed and printed. These spontaneous performances were a particularly French pedagogical exercise, dating back to at least the 1830s, which Charcot had apparently mastered. During the early 1890s, Charcot included several more cases in the two volumes of his *Clinique des maladies du système nerveux;*[19] and he or his students published at least four other cases involving hysterical male patients that were not included in the *Oeuvres complètes* but that appeared in medical periodicals.[20] In addition to these printed sources, the Bibliothèque Charcot contains scattered manuscript materials on a number of cases, and medical libraries outside France hold several relevant documents.[21] Finally, the Archives de l'Assistance Publique in Paris houses a fragmentary diagnostic registry for the Salpêtrière polyclinic that records biographical and clinical data on 11 hysterical patients—four women and seven men—who were treated between 1879 and 1883.[22] All in all, then, we have information on nearly 90 male patients whom Charcot regarded as hysterics. This sizable literature establishes at once that for Charcot, "hystérie mâle" was not merely a theoretical possibility, a clinical rarity, or a textbook abstraction; it was a workaday diagnosis.

Charcot's work on hysteria is more closely associated with a single hospital than that of any other physician. Within the Salpêtrière, his male patients came from a variety of locations, including the General Infirmary and a recently established outpatient clinic or *consultation externe.* Physicians who oversaw patients in other sectors of the hospital occasionally transferred a patient to Charcot's service. His newly established neuropathological institute at the hospital included such state-of-the-art facilities as a pathological anatomy museum, an electro-diagnostic laboratory, a casting workshop, a photographic atelier, and an ophthalmology consulting room. Most important among the facilities, founded in 1882, was a special wing of the hospital Infirmary for male patients. This new Service des Hommes, located along the Rue de l'Infirmerie in the Deuxième Section of the hospital, was devoted to the study and treatment of adult male patients diagnosed with transient nervous and neurological disorders. The ward initially contained twenty beds; two years later, it was expanded to fifty beds.[23] In 1885 the Clinique des Maladies du Système Nerveux itself began to accept male patients, particularly those suffering from chronic infirmities. By the first half of the 1880s, the requisite patient pool for a close and methodical study of hysterical disorders in males was at Charcot's daily disposal.

Viewed historically, these institutional changes were significant developments. Since the seventeenth century, the Salpêtrière had served as an enormous welfare institution for poor, sick, and dispossessed women, while their male counterparts were transported farther afield to the Bicêtre hospital on the southeastern outskirts of the city. The admission of the first men at this historic Hospice de la Vieillesse-Femmes neatly parallels Charcot's attempt to masculinize the traditionally "feminine" diagnosis of hysteria.

After a decade and a half of work in traditional medical fields, why did France's leading neurologist take up a subject as controversial as masculine hysteria? From long years of clinical observation, Charcot had genuinely come to believe that men and children were susceptible to the same nervous disorders as women. His personal observations in the clinic were reinforced by a reading of two important medical texts. Since his days as a intern rotating through the hospitals of Paris, he had been much impressed by the common sense and clinical acumen of Briquet's *Traité clinique et thérapeutique de l'hystérie* (1859), with its powerful opening endorsement of male hysteria. (Continuing his work at the Charité hospital, Briquet during the 1860s was an elder colleague of Charcot's in the Parisian medical community.) Charcot was also impressed with a more obscure but recent source—a short and strikingly original Paris medical dissertation entitled *De hystérie chez l'homme,* written by one Auguste Klein.[24] Published in 1880, Klein's thesis was a collation, in both written and tabular forms, of 78 cases of nervous maladies, drawn from the European medical literature of the preceding two centuries, which Klein maintained were misdiagnosed instances of hysteria in men. The young Klein, in other words, had boldly reversed the same diagnostic gesture that Hector Landouzy had undertaken in his tract during the mid-1840s. Complimentary mentions of both Briquet's treatise and Klein's thesis appear in Charcot's writings.

Charcot's attraction to the male hysteria concept was also a logical extension of his earlier general work on the disorder. His initial set of writings on female hysteria was complete by the late 1870s. During the remaining fifteen years of his career, Charcot modified the content of this construction in only minor ways. On numerous occasions, however, he broadened the scope of the theory's application to encompass other patient populations. In particular, his work on hysteria in the 1880s is characterized by a kind of nosographical inflation in which the range of clinical phenomena ascribed to the disorder expands continually. In the long run this process proved to be problematic: his working account of the neurosis became clinically over-inclusive, and thus after his death it was open to piecemeal dismantlement.[25] Be that as it may, Charcot's completion of the proto-theory of female hysteria and his first interest in hysteria in men (and children) both occurred in the late 1870s, suggesting that these patient groups offered new fields of application for his favorite diagnostic creation in its expansive phase.

To these considerations should be added the role of the cultural ideology of the Salpêtrière School. Within the medical world of late nineteenth-century France, Charcot and his entourage formed a self-conscious scientific avant-garde. They saw themselves as a cadre of latter-day medical *philosophes* determined to rout out vestiges of past error and superstition wherever they persisted.[26] Ostentatiously replacing the beliefs of earlier, "pre-scientific" times with the methods and findings of modern empirical science was a critical Enlightenment exercise that Charcot found irresistibly gratifying. Entangled for centuries with scientific ignorance, popular prejudices, and religious persecution, hysteria was a prime subject for rationalist reinterpretation. The many monographs on male hysteria coming out of France in the Charcot era typically begin with a "Historical Overview" that functions as mild ideological propaganda, chronicling the advance of the contemporary scientific understanding of hysterical illness over the crude beliefs and inhumane practices of the past.[27] The fact that French neo-Hippocratism and Romantic gender ideology, both of which Charcot rejected programmatically, had in some sense been underwritten by the governments of Napoleon I, the Bourbon Restoration, and the July Monarchy no doubt strengthened the revisionist determination of the republican Charcot.

Finally, Charcot's campaign on behalf of the existence of male hysteria had a clear intraprofessional agenda. Throughout the nineteenth century internists, alienists, gynecologists, neurologists, and surgeons all wrote about and ministered to hysteria, with each group of specialists putting forth a view of the disease and its treatment that enhanced its own explanatory authority over the subject.[28] In these rivalries Charcot was an eager and aggressive player. He organized a school of students, founded professional journals, established new hospital facilities, and lobbied for government funding of a new academic chair—all toward the goal of advancing a specifically neurological study of the *maladies nerveuses.* Integral to Charcot's efforts in this direction was his model of hysteria, with a neuropathic theory of etiology, a symptomatology that emphasized paralyses, anesthesias, and contractures, and a purely physicalistic regimen of therapy. In the drive to neurologize hysteria, the male hysteria idea was highly serviceable. From Willis and Sydenham onward, models of the disorder anchored in the nervous system (rather than in reproductive physiology or in character types) tended to be much less gendered. In his first published writings, Charcot routinely cites the existence of cases of hysteria in adult men (and, incidentally, in prepubertal children and postmenopausal women) as conclusive refutation of past and present uterine theories. In the decades following his death, Charcot's efforts to appropriate hysteria for neurology lost out to private-practice psychiatry, especially psychoanalysis; but during the 1870s and 1880s, his powerful neurological reading was embraced in the mainstream European medical world, and he challenged decisively the gynecological understanding of these cases that was resurgent in German, British, and American medicine during the penultimate decades of the century.[29]

A corollary to this last point concerns a rather specialized humanitarian issue. In Germany, Britain, and the United States, the final third of the nineteenth century witnessed the widespread practice of amputative gynecological surgery in the treatment of women with so-called functional nervous disorders. These radical interventions, which included hysterectomies, clitoridectomies, and unilateral and bilateral ovariotomies, reached their peak between 1875 and 1885.[30] Although these procedures were never as common in France as in other countries, a number of Parisian surgeons nonetheless wrote in favor of their use. Charcot and his followers argued vociferously against these surgeries, which they regarded essentially as misguided castrations, and a number of times they chose to do so in writings on male hysteria.[31] By propounding a theory of hysteria in the male, then, Charcot was also attempting to undermine a theoretical model of the disorder that had led to some of the most deplorable therapeutic practices of his day.

Thus we can see that for the male hysteria research project, Charcot had varied, multiple motivations, which reinforced one another; a self-conscious desire to challenge the gender regime of the day, it should be noted, was not among these motives.

NOT UNEXPECTEDLY, Charcot's work on hysteria in adult men was highly controversial when it first appeared. Charcot cultivated this controversy, although exactly what he was arguing for and against changed over time. At the outset, he was chiefly concerned to establish the reality and frequency of hysterical illnesses in the male sex. "In truth," he wrote, "words, and particularly words in medical nosography, mean nothing except as symbols. They cannot claim to possess the merit of a descriptive definition. Get yourself into the habit of thinking . . . that in itself the word 'hysteria' signifies nothing, and little by little, you will get used to speaking of hysteria in men without thinking in the least of 'the uterus.'"[32] What is required, he explained further, is a break with the history and etymology of the disease, a modernization in understanding that would "make you recognize and, so to speak, see for yourself the identity of the great neurosis in the two sexes."[33]

In an attempt to "modernize" the diagnosis, Charcot anticipated, and tried to refute, a number of dismissive stereotypes. He rejected from the outset, for instance, the notions that the disorder in males was limited to boys at puberty, that it existed solely in the leisured (that is, decadent) upper classes of society, and that it occurred exclusively in effeminate or homosexual men. On the question of age, he maintained that hysterical pathology could develop at any period of life from infancy to old age. Among his published cases of hysterical males, the youngest patient was 11 years of age, the oldest 56.[34] Charcot found the greatest concentration of cases in patients between the ages of 20 and 40. On the much-debated issue of the ratio of hysteria between men and women, he endorsed Briquet's mid-century figure of a 1 to 20 ratio, estimating that in reality the ratio was slightly closer than this.[35]

Concerning the social epidemiology of male hysteria, Charcot again rejected the received wisdom. European authors from Robert Burton onward believed the greatest susceptibility to nervous illnesses occurred in members of the affluent classes and blamed the pattern on either an idle, self-indulgent style of living or the excesses of urban, commercial civilization. In fin-de-siècle France, a version of these same images circulated in the writings of literary figures like Huysmans, Wilde, and, later, Proust, in which the character of the effete aristocrat, morbidly preoccupied with the cultivation of his nervous eccentricities, recurs prominently. Charcot knew the picture well, in both its medical and literary formulations, and reacted sharply against it:

> When we speak today of neurasthenia or male hysteria, it still seems that we almost exclusively have in mind the man of the privileged classes, sated by culture, exhausted by pleasures' abuses, by business preoccupations, or an excess of intellectual

exertion. This is an error that I have many times had to argue against, and against which it will no doubt be necessary to argue for a long time to come, because it appears far from being eradicated. However, it has been perfectly well-established that these same disorders, at least in the cities, may be observed on a grand scale among the workers and artisans, by those the least favored by fate and who scarcely know anything other than hard manual labor.[36]

Accordingly, the most striking feature of Charcot's male hysterical patients is their socioeconomic identity. Of the 61 men and boys described in his writings, all but five had urban or rural working-class backgrounds. Two of these five, both of whom were teenagers, came from wealthy families, while the other three were beggars or vagabonds.[37] The majority of his hysterical men were masons, bakers, carpenters, gardeners, plumbers, locksmiths, railway workers, factory workers, and the like. To be more precise, they were either laborers in new, large-scale, mechanized industries, such as the oil, rubber, or railroad industries; or members of the traditional artisanal crafts or *petits métiers* of Paris; or peasants from the countryside.[38] Furthermore, nearly all the male patients sent by other physicians from outside the Salpêtrière for consultation with Charcot came from hospitals in working-class districts of Paris, such as the Hôpital Saint-Louis near Belleville. It was specifically the inability of these men to work as a result of their nervous disabilities—that is, to perform their prescribed masculine duties in capitalist society—that appeared to define their sickness in the eyes of middle-class diagnosticians.[39]

Several circumstances help to explain the unique social constitution of Charcot's chosen patient population. The Salpêtrière was a free municipal hospital that drew much of its population from surrounding neighborhoods composed of the lower social echelons. When local people in the area fell seriously ill, they sought assistance at the nearest public medical facility. Interestingly, Charcot himself contended on more than one occasion that manual workers were more vulnerable to nervous breakdown because their work entailed greater physical exertion, emotional strains, and noxious environmental influences in the workplace. Another possible consideration—and it can only be speculative—is Charcot's personal family background. Charcot was a prime example of the "self-made medical mandarin" of the early Third Republic,[40] and his father had worked proudly as a wheelwright, designing and constructing wooden carriage wheels in central Paris. Perhaps Charcot retained an enduring interest in and filial respect for the French tradition of artisanal labor.

On three occasions, all from the late 1880s, Charcot published case descriptions of male hysteria in members of the most impoverished social classes.[41] "Where does hysteria hide?" he asked during a clinical lesson in 1889. "In the last few years, I have often shown [that it hides] in the working class and among manual artisans. We must also search for it in the gutter, among the beggars, the vagabonds, and the dispossessed, in the poor houses and even perhaps the jails and penitentiaries."[42] The grinding effects of poverty and severe social instability, Charcot implies, can act pathogenically. For two of the three cases in this social category, however, Charcot added the diagnosis of degeneration to the primary label of hysteria. This rare hybrid diagnosis in his writings does not seem to be merited by the symptomatology of the cases, suggesting that for sociological reasons he employed a more stigmatizing classification for patients who were poor, indigent, and unemployed.

Skilled artisans, industrial factory workers, peasants recently arrived in the capital city, and the down-and-out—this was Charcot's variegated clinical clientele in his publications on male hysteria. However, his patient pool was socially heterogeneous within the lower orders only. One group was conspicuously excluded: in significant contrast to the well-to-do population that eighteenth-century British nerve doctors discussed (or the urban bourgeois neurotics that Freud would shortly theorize), the social category that Charcot himself occupied at the time was not represented among his case histories. It might well have been otherwise: throughout the 1880s Charcot spent his mornings at the Salpêtrière, but he typically devoted the afternoon hours to an elite private practice in his home. Here he encountered very different, more diversified, and often far wealthier clients, none of whom appear in his printed writings. Was it social discretion in this age of respectability that excluded the sensitive stories of middle- and upper-class patients from the published medical record? Did Charcot in fact find it possible to apply the hysteria diagnosis to members of his own sex in part because the individuals he so classified issued from a social background different from his own?[43] Whatever the reasons may have been, the white male bourgeois body and psyche are emphatically not implicated in Charcot's official model of male hysteria.

Charcot's choice of patient population in the construction of his disease picture may have at least one additional explanation. Discoursing on "hystérie virile," Charcot seized every opportunity to underscore the authentically "masculine" nature of the disorder. We have already seen the lingering suspicion that he was addressing in this regard. To cite only two influential examples, the Viennese alienist Ernst von Feuchtersleben had commented in his pioneering 1845 textbook of psychiatry that "when men are attacked by genuine hysterical fits (*globus hystericus*, etc.) . . . they are, for the most part, effeminate men." Twenty years later, the English surgeon

John Russell Reynolds noted in his *System of Medicine* that hysterical disorders were extremely rare in members of his own sex. "When hysteria is found in either a man or a boy, it is to be observed that such person is, either mentally or morally, of feminine constitution."[44]

On this point, too, Charcot was arguing against the grain. "These adult men who are prey to the hysterical neurosis," he declared adamantly, "do not always present characteristics of femininity. Far from it. They are, at least in a majority of cases, robust men presenting all the attributes of the male sex, soldiers or artisans, married and the fathers of families, men, in other words, in whom one would be surprised, unless forewarned, to meet with an illness considered by most people as exclusive to women."[45] At the beginning of a set of lectures in 1885 presenting six cases of male hysteria, he elaborated even more pointedly:

> We concede that an effeminate young man, after certain excesses, disappointments, deep emotions, may present various phenomena of a hysterical nature; but that a vigorous and well-built artisan, not enervated by high culture, a train engineer, for example, not previously overly-emotional, or at least not in appearance, may ... become hysterical, just like a woman ... now there, it seems, is something that has never entered the imagination of some people. Nothing, however, is better proven, and it is a notion that we must get used to.[46]

Charcot was determined to establish the solidly heterosexual credentials of the male patients he wrote about, and his case histories are filled with amusing remarks about the "masculine" bodily and behavioral traits of the patient. Concerning a hysterical contracture in an unnamed 34-year-old blacksmith, he describes the man as "the father of four children, quite robust, and without any sign of effeminacy."[47] He introduces Antoine Charnu, a 41-year-old baker who came to the hospital in March of 1892, as "a rigorously built patient, musculature very developed" with "a very calm character."[48] And in the fragmentary notes at the Bibliothèque Charcot on the case of one Jean-Pierre Mattivet, Charcot carefully characterizes Mattivet, who was plagued by a number of severe hysterical symptoms, as "a hearty laborer" and points out that the patient had manfully undergone amputation of an arm during the Franco-Prussian War.[49]

Not surprisingly, Charcot virtually never broaches the subject of homosexuality in his writings on male hysteria. Here, too, he probably did not want the concept reduced by critics to a clinical caricature. In the *Archives de neurologie* of 1882, he did publish a lengthy (and highly moralizing) paper on the case of "Monsieur X.," a homosexual university professor from the provinces.[50] Although this case of "genital inversion" includes a number of unmistakably hysterical features, Charcot wrote the case report with Valentin Magnan, the prominent exponent of degeneration theory, and again he chose to subsume the clinical material in question under the darker and more encompassing category of "degeneration" rather than hysteria. In other words, Charcot was willing, even eager, to apply the hysteria diagnosis to members of the male sex, but not without ascribing a conventional gender identity to them. Indeed, he may well have been drawn to clinical specimens from the working classes because, in his view and the view of his age, their masculine credentials were more secure.

CHARCOT'S IDEAS ABOUT what caused hysterical breakdown in men are no less interesting and revealing. For men and women alike, his etiological theory consists of a rather uncomplicated combination of underlying hereditary constitution and short-term triggering mechanisms. Throughout the second half of the nineteenth century, French (and Italian) psychological medicine was dominated by a severe doctrine of hereditarian determinism. "Heredity will tell you almost everything," Charcot wrote summarily in 1879—including, he believed, about the origins of nervous and neurological disease.[51] Degenerationist theory in European medicine originated in the mid-1800s with a trio of French-authored texts by Lucas, Morel, and Moreau de Tours.[52] In the 1880s and 1890s, French alienists like Magnan and the Italian criminologist Cesare Lombroso extended the paradigm further until it encompassed an enormous range of human behaviors and pathologies. Degenerationism also spread outside of French biomedicine, extending for instance to creative literature; it animated Émile Zola's twenty-volume Rougon-Macquart novel cycle, which appeared between 1871 and 1893 and attracted an international readership.[53]

In this tradition, Charcot held that his hysterical patients possessed from birth a latent flaw or defect of the nervous system—a *tare nerveuse*—that at all times was waiting to be activated by an appropriate event. Grounded in the French tradition of pathological anatomy, Charcot was certain that this constitutional susceptibility to nervous disease had an organic reality in the form of a spinal lesion, chemical imbalance, or intracranial tumor. To their endless frustration, however, Charcot and his generation were unable upon postmortem examination either to locate the actual anatomical site of the abnormality or to determine the nature of the pathophysiological process. Charcot's solution to "the problem of the missing lesion" was to postulate the existence of a "functional" or "dynamic" lesion. By this term, he meant a kind of diffuse physiological abnormality of the nervous system that cannot be detected directly but that nonetheless has a physical, most likely cortical, substratum.[54] With refinements in diagnostic technique, Charcot felt certain that the organic basis of the functional neuroses would someday be discovered.

For French physicians in the period immediately preceding the rediscovery of Mendelian genetics, the exact mechanism of transmission of hereditary traits from generation to generation remained unknown; but it seemed empirically self-evident to Charcot that hysteria was carried through the family. The disease, he postulated, can pass unilinearly, without changes in form, from generation to generation; or by skipping generations (similar to our concept of recessive inheritance); or through "transformational heredity," whereby nervous defects appear in successive generations but in altered pathological forms. The notion of heredity by transformation, a nineteenth-century French innovation, allowed hysteria to occur in tandem with a remarkably wide range of other medical and social "pathologies."

French degenerationist thought reached its most inclusive form in the 1880s, just as the medical investigation of male hysteria was at its height. In 1884, the psychologist and former Charcot pupil Charles Féré detailed the myriad hereditary interrelations of hysteria with chorea, epilepsy, Parkinson's disease, multiple sclerosis, asthma, gout, rheumatism, locomotor ataxia, and general paralysis of the insane.[55] Many of Charcot's narratives of male hysterics begin with genealogical trees laden with interconnecting cases of these other illnesses as well as cases of alcoholism, suicide, criminality, and insanity. His adherence to the degenerationist outlook was unshakable, and by the end of his lifetime it became limiting and dogmatic. If Charcot cannot locate an obvious precedent in a patient's immediate parental line, he searches wider and deeper on the family tree. A suicidal sister or a grandfather with gout provides ample indication of a proclivity to pathology. When he is unable to establish a hereditary pathogenesis, Charcot attributes this to lack of information about the patient's background or suppression by the patient of embarrassing facts about family history. His male hysterics, he is certain, are part of Féré's "great neuropathic family" of society.

Charcot maintains, moreover, that within the hereditary domain of hysterical illness the neuropathic charge is especially intense in the masculine form of the disease. He argues that in the parental transmission of male hysteria, the maternal contribution is direct and the paternal indirect. An alcoholic, epileptic, or syphilitic father, through transformational heredity, can spawn hysteria in a male child; the disorder can be conveyed directly, however, only from the mother. "Thus," he pronounced in 1885, "hysteria in the mother frequently begets hysteria in the son."[56] Asserted without statistical evidence, his matrilineal model of hysteria in men joins a long line of theories, before and after his time, that trace human psychopathology in males back to pathogenic mothers.

In hereditarily predisposed individuals, the "nervous disposition" *(diathèse nerveuse)* exists from birth in a kind of indefinite dormancy. In roughly a quarter of Charcot's cases of male hysteria, the disorder occurs spontaneously. However, most of his cases involve constitutionally susceptible but previously asymptomatic individuals whose illnesses develop as the result of a precipitating event or aggravating circumstance. Thus while the primary cause of hysteria— heredity—was uniform, the secondary causes were innumerable. In 1889, Charcot's former intern Georges Guinon catalogued the disease's many *agents provocateurs.*[57] According to Guinon's 400-page inventory, physical illnesses of all sorts could present "a morbid opportunity" for the onset of hysteria.[58] Charcot and Guinon also maintained that alcoholism provides one of the most powerful provoking agents. In over a third of Charcot's male cases, excessive drink figures prominently.[59]

The greatest number of Charcot's male hysteria cases, however, are set in motion through the destructive effect of a physical injury. In his work on so-called "traumatic hysteria," Charcot combines the medical research of the British physicians Benjamin Brodie and James Paget with a French clinical sensibility and brings the two to bear on the study of hysteria in men. The nature of the precipitating physical traumas in Charcot's cases varies greatly. The patient "Mar.," for instance, a young baker's apprentice, experienced his first hysterical attack two weeks after he had been assaulted and stabbed on the street one night. "Greff.," age 31, developed an eye twitch and severe motor dysfunctions subsequent to an accident on a fishing trip in which he almost drowned. And two middle-aged males, "D...cy" and "Augustin H.," responded with psychogenic paralyses when they were caught in thunderstorms and nearly struck by lightning.[60]

In the majority of Charcot's cases, the traumatic event takes the form of a work-related accident. The single most frequent secondary cause is train crashes. Five cases involve men engaged as train engineers, freight handlers, or construction workers on the rail lines who are victims of train collisions.[61] Other men undergo traumatic experiences in comparable work settings: a blacksmith burns his hand and forearm with a hot iron; a clerk in an oil factory is nearly crushed to death by falling metal storage barrels; a bricklayer falls two floors from his scaffolding; a ditch digger is struck in the face with a shovel while unloading a wagon; a chimney cleaner breaks his wrist when he falls from a ladder. Charcot also demonstrates that certain manifestations of hysteria can result from excessive exposure to chemicals in the environment—what he terms "toxic hysteria."[62]

The cases cited above involve physical accidents; but, in each instance, Charcot ultimately judges the post-traumatic symptoms to be hysterical. Key to his diagnosis is the observation that the severity and tenacity of the symptoms bear little relation to the nature and intensity of the injury. The "traumas" in these cases range from life-threatening train accidents to a trifling cut on the finger. Symptoms sometimes disappear as spontaneously as they have arisen, in a matter of hours, while at other times they persist for months or even years without indication of organic impairment.[63] Because of their ability to incapacitate an individual for long periods of time, Charcot knew that these hysterical infirmities were as real, psychologically and subjectively, as those that entailed evident structural damage. In the period 1885–1888, Charcot's work on masculine hysteria became almost synonymous with the investigation of traumatic hysteria. A generation later, when confronted with an epidemic of psychogenic paralysis, blindness, and amnesia among soldiers on the Western front lines, military physicians during the First World War would return to Charcot's work on traumatic hysteria.[64]

Charcot's ideas about the secondary causation of male hysteria clearly mirrored the social and cultural concerns of his day. The particular pathogenic potency he ascribed to liquor, for instance, in all likelihood reflected the increase in French middle-class distress over the perceived evils of chronic drunkenness among the working classes.[65] Charcot's emphasis on railroads as a setting for hysterical collapse likewise registered contemporary cultural anxieties about the rapid spread of high-speed mechanized transportation and the uncontrollable technological change that it symbolized.[66]

Indeed, Charcot's observations about "traumatic hysteria" and industry have their own social history. As a physician in an urban hospital situated in a working-class district adjacent to the Gare d'Austerlitz, Charcot was exposed to the industrial accidents that were multiplying as the city entered a period of accelerated industrialization. Moreover, with the rise of an urbanized, industrial-capitalist society came an assertive workers' movement, which in France was achieving its first legal and political advances in the 1880s and 1890s. One plank of early socialist programs throughout Europe was legislation to protect workers.[67] During the last two decades of the century this subject was hotly debated in the French legislature, and in 1897 the *Loi sur les accidents du travail* was passed, providing many workers with a statutory right to financial compensation from their employers in the event of serious bodily injury at work.[68] By recounting sympathetically cases that demonstrated a direct link between working conditions and debilitating illness, Charcot may well have been providing reformist commentary that his medical and lay contemporaries would have understood.

In one respect, Charcot complicated his etiological theory considerably. On first reading it appears, as it did to Charcot initially, that the medical damage in these cases is the direct result of a physical accident. But in many instances, Charcot notes a number of peculiar clinical features. He is struck by the variations in the intervals between the time of the trauma and the onset of hysterical symptoms, and by the curious incommensurability of the intensity of the trauma with the subsequent symptoms. He observes further that the loss of sensation or exaggeration of sensations that many of his patients report corresponds in location and extent not to the actual distribution of nerves and muscles in the body, but to the popular segmental understanding of anatomy. These observations caused Charcot to move tentatively beyond a strictly somaticist interpretation of the disorder. In many of Charcot's cases of masculine hysteria, it is not the physical injury per se that produces the disease; rather, the mental experiencing of the traumatic episode, the emotional and ideational accompaniment to the event, carries a pathogenic charge and leads to the development of the disorder.[69] Charcot was too skillful a neurologist to ignore the possibility of real structural damage. Indeed, he enjoyed demonstrating to audiences those complex cases in which both a physical injury and its emotional concomitants contribute to produce mixed "hystero-organic" forms of the disorder.[70] But in many instances, it is the "great psychical shaking up" *(le grand ébranlement psychique)* that provides the decisive causal element:[71]

> The nervous shock or commotion, the emotion almost un-avoidably inseparable from an often life-threatening accident, is sufficient to produce the neurosis in question. The surgical effect of the traumatism, or, in other words, the causing of a wound or contusion . . . is not a necessary element for the development of the disease, although it can contribute to it taking on a grave form.[72]

Charcot pioneered this line of thinking specifically in regard to his work on masculine hysteria.

In several instances, Charcot broadened his notion of hysterogenesis still further by dispensing altogether with the threat of a physical injury. In April 1888, for instance, "Pasq.," a 51-year-old Spaniard living in Paris, was brought by his family in an agitated state to the walk-in clinic of the Salpêtrière. The patient was unable to talk—he mimed his responses to Charcot during the clinical interview—and revealed upon examination a number of bizarre sensory malfunctions. "Pasq."'s family reported that over the previous eight years the patient had also lapsed periodically into bouts of stuttering, whispering, and mutism. Charcot interviewed the man and discovered that each of these episodes had followed an emotionally unsettling experience: once when the patient quarreled violently with his wife, a second time when his wife hid their rent money for a month, and a third when she absconded with their life savings.[73] In the second volume of the *Leçons du mardi,* precipitating hysterical symptoms in male patients include the threat of a fistfight with a friend, the death of a wife and daughter, rejection of a marriage offer, viewing a cadaver in a hospital, receiving a letter of strong parental reproach, and watching a thunderstorm. In each of these cases, it is ultimately the power of an idea or emotion—fear, rage, grief, anxiety—that "causes" hysteria.

Exactly how an idea or emotion is transformed into a bodily symptom—how, in Freud's later phrase, we get "from a mental process to a somatic innervation"—was an old and very thorny question.[74] For Charcot, we sense that such a line of investigation was intellectually uncongenial. On one occasion, however, he attempted to explore the subject. In March 1886, he delivered a lecture at the Salpêtrière entitled "Two New Cases of Hystero-Traumatic Paralysis in Men."[75] One of the cases concerned "Le Log.," a 29-year-old Breton who had recently come to Paris to work as a florist deliveryman. While crossing the Pont des Invalides with a wheelbarrow one afternoon, "Le Log." was sideswiped by a passing horse-drawn carriage. He sustained only minor physical injuries but lost consciousness momentarily. When he appeared at the hospital several days after the accident, "Le Log." presented an incoherent collection of symptoms, including headaches, trembling hands, episodes of amnesia, hypersensitivity of the scalp, and complete insensitivity to heat and cold in the lower half of his body except for his toes.

After reviewing the clinical facts of the case, Charcot inquires into "the mechanism of pathology" of the paralysis. The emotional shock from the accident, he hypothesizes, created in the patient "an intense cerebral commotion," which caused a "clouding of consciousness" and a "dissociation" of "the ego." Charcot attempts to envision this mental process by drawing analogies between traumatic hysteria and the states of drunkenness, drug intoxication, and the somnambulic stage of the hypnotic trance. Precisely what transpires intrapsychically in this last, quasi-hypnotic state remains vague, and we see Charcot at this point searching for a new, non-neurological vocabulary with which to account for the process. He theorizes that, in this state of increased psychological suggestibility, the strong physical sensation associated with the trauma is somehow reproduced as a mental representation, which then becomes fixed in the mind of the individual. He refers to this physical and mental *idée fixe* as the result of "an involuntary and most often unconscious auto-suggestion," and he describes the fertile period of delay between physical trauma and hysterical symptom as "a sort of incubation stage of unconscious mental elaboration."[76]

Charcot's central scientific project, it should be remembered, is a comprehensive descriptive clinical neurology, not a theoretical dynamic psychiatry, and his consideration of "Le Log."'s symptoms is limited to a six-page passage in a single case history.[77] Nevertheless, his reflections on the case of "Le Log." do point the way toward a psychological explanation of physical symptoms, that is, a kind of theory of conversion. Viewed in historical context, these ideas provide a preliminary step in the general movement of the age from somatogenic to psychogenic models of the mind.

CHARCOT'S HANDLING OF the issue of sexuality in the production of male neurosis is nothing if not ambivalent. In his printed writings about hysteria—in contrast to the famous visual images produced by his students or by outsiders[78]—Charcot firmly rejects a primary sexual pathogenesis for hysteria. In most of his clinical reports on male patients, he never mentions sex at all. When sexual factors do come into play, it is most often in the form of physical disorders or dysfunctions of the urogenital system. Charcot routinely inspected the genitalia of his male patients and noted his findings matter-of-factly. If he detected an abnormality, such as a scrotal tumor, undescended testicle, bladder infection, inguinal hernia, or prostatic swelling, he tended to interpret it as a possible nervous provocation. He believed that syphilitic infections, which were rampant in late-nineteenth-century European cities, could serve as secondary causes of hysterical symptoms.[79] He also occasionally reported impotence, "spermatorrhoea," and anaphrodisia in his male patients. And several times he linked hysterical neuroses in males to personal habits, namely masturbation and venereal excess.[80]

What is most noteworthy in light of the history of hysteria, however, is how rare and moderate his remarks are on this subject. Throughout his writings, Charcot demotes *la vita sexualis* to the auxiliary status of an inciting factor, and in only 3 of his 61 cases does he cite masturbation as a factor—a highly surprising fact given the contemporary obsession with the practice. Furthermore, in a number of places he raises the question only to assure readers that it does not play a determining role.[81] As viewers of the glossy and sensationalistic *Iconographie photographique* well know, Charcot and his students literally *saw* a sexual component in hysteria very clearly. These volumes, produced in the new photographic studio at the Salpêtrière by two of Charcot's followers between 1876 and 1880, record in loving and lurid detail the erotic antics of several female hysterical patients.[82] Yet in the formal construction of his causal theory, Charcot demonstrated an almost willful refusal to recognize the possible sexual dimensions of his cases. Likewise, in Georges

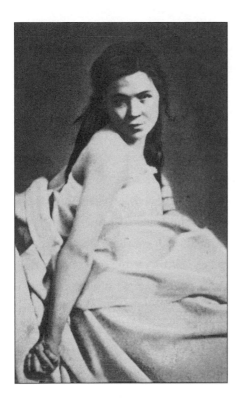

The hysterical patient
"Augustine," in an erotic pose,
as recorded in the *Iconographie
photographique de la
Salpêtrière* (1877).

Guinon's book length study of the provoking agents of hysteria, sexual factors occupy only four pages.[83] Gilles de la Tourette's thousand-page compendium, the official codification of Salpêtrière teachings, fails to mention the topic at all.

An often-repeated anecdote from early psychoanalytic history offers another perspective on this perplexing piece of theoretical behavior on Charcot's part. In the early pages of *On the History of the Psychoanalytic Movement* (1914), Freud relates the story of a dinner party he attended at the Charcot residence during his study with the French master in 1886. According to his account, Freud overheard Charcot and the renowned medical legalist Paul Brouardel discussing the case of a young married Asian couple, both of whom were beset with nervous symptoms. Charcot mentioned

that the wife was a confirmed invalid while the husband was "either impotent or exceedingly awkward," and he linked these facts
about their sexual lives to the couple's nervous travails, to which
Brouardel expressed surprise. Freud then relates Charcot's signature
comment: "Mais, dans des cas pareils, c'est toujours la chose géni-
tale, toujours, toujours, toujours" (In such cases, it is always the
genital thing—always, always, always).[84] In other words, as a young
foreign student Freud allegedly heard Charcot, during the very
years when he was investigating masculine hysteria so intensively,
utter a clear, if offhand, statement to the effect that sexuality is centrally important in the production of neurotic symptoms.

In a perceptive essay appearing in *The Alienist and Neurologist*
several years after Charcot's death, the British sexologist Havelock
Ellis hailed the recent innovative theorizing about hysteria coming
out of France, Germany, and Austria.[85] Ellis observes in the article
that Charcot in particular had sought to elevate hysteria to a subject of serious and legitimate study within the medical sciences. To
this end, Ellis continues, Charcot strove to divorce once and for all
the diagnosis of hysteria from Galeno-Hippocratic ideology, with
its age-old emphasis on excessive or apathetic sexual appetite. In
Victorian medicine and popular culture, a related stereotype had
crystallized of the lying, manipulative, hypererotic hysteric—an image, not coincidentally, that fueled the claims of gynecologists, ob-
stetricians, and psychiatrists to their authority over the subject.[86]

Ellis's observation is perceptive. The programmatic asexualism of
Charcot's published writings was not the result of medical over-
sight, or a sign of sexual hypocrisy, or a strategy for social control.
More likely, it was a calculated counter-response to ancient but
still influential etiologies of the disease and to the more recent tendency to dismiss hysterical patients because of their allegedly licen-
tious character. For Charcot, a product of the age of nineteenth-

century medical positivism, to modernize hysteria was to de-
sensationalize the diagnosis, and to scientize the diagnosis was to
de-sexualize it. There were, of course, limitations to this strategy, as
Ellis observed: "Formerly the sexual element in hysteria was somewhat exaggerated; there is now a tendency to unduly minimize
it."[87] Or we might recall here another familiar *bon mot* of Charcot's
to Freud: "La théorie, c'est bon, mais ça n'empêche pas d'exister"
(Theory is well and good, but it doesn't prevent things from existing).[88] And exist they did. Although Charcot succeeded in expelling sexuality from the causal analysis of his published cases of male
hysteria, "the genital thing" was too powerful a presence to be permanently repressed, and it inevitably burst out in other areas of his
medical commentary, in the writings of other contemporary physicians, and in unpublished medical texts from the Salpêtrière.

OF ALL THE ELEMENTS in their account of masculine hysteria,
members of the Salpêtrière school lavished the most attention
on its symptomatology. To a considerable extent, late-nineteenth-
century French doctors writing on the topic used the exhaustive
documentation of symptoms as a substitute for etiological knowledge and therapeutic efficacy. "What, then, is hysteria?" Charcot
asks in his last paper on the subject in 1892. "We do not know anything about its nature, nor about any lesions producing it. We know
it only through its manifestations and are therefore only able to
characterize it by its symptoms, for the more hysteria is subjective,
the more it is necessary to make it objective in order to recognize
it."[89] Charcot was able to get away with such a characterization because, as he envisioned it, the disease's symptoms were so diverse
and spectacular. In its French fin-de-siècle incarnation, the hysteria
diagnosis encompassed nearly the entire field of what twentieth-
century psychiatry would call the neuroses, spilling over into other

collateral clinical areas now claimed by the psychoses and various nonpsychiatric maladies.

Charcot believed that hysteria was a *névrose* (nervous disorder) in the nineteenth-century neurological sense of the term. Not surprisingly, then, signs of central nervous dysfunction figure most prominently in his symptomatological portrayal.[90] At the center of his *tableau clinique* are aberrations of sensibility, which are exhibited by 48 out of Charcot's 61 male patients (79 percent of the total). The most basic of these sensory "stigmata," as he calls them, are anesthesias and hyperesthesias, or exaggerations of sensitivity to touch, temperature, and electricity. These derangements could be cutaneous, muscular, or visceral and could affect a single organ or area—as in a facial neuralgia—or extend over the entire surface of the body. Hemianesthesias, or losses of sensation following the precise medial line of the body, were also frequent.[91] Charcot devised extensive tests to detect these sensory pathologies, and for each patient he recorded the results on printed, page-size "body maps," literally charting the external signs of hysteria on the field of the male body. To these -algias and -esthesias he added abnormalities of the five senses, especially vision, including blindness, color-blindness, reduction in light perception, double vision, and concentric narrowing of the visual field.[92] He believed that loss of the sense of taste was also common with hysteria in men.

A second major category of hysterical symptoms involves motor impairments, including paralyses, contractures, and spasms of all sorts. Twenty-nine of Charcot's male patients (47 percent) suffered from this type of infirmity. These disorders could affect a single muscle or group of muscles, or could develop as paraplegias or hemiplegias. Flaccid paralyses, in which a patient's arm or leg hangs motionless, also occurred from time to time. Contractures of the extremities, Charcot found, were for some reason particularly in-

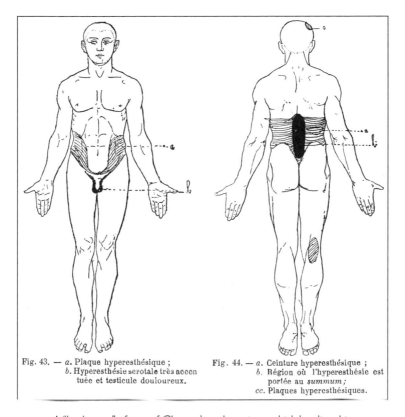

Fig. 43. — *a*. Plaque hyperesthésique ;
*b*. Hyperesthésie scrotale très accen
tuée et testicule douloureux.

Fig. 44. — *a*. Ceinture hyperesthésique ;
*b*. Région où l'hyperesthésie est
portée au *summum ;*
*cc*. Plaques hyperesthésiques.

A "body map" of one of Charcot's male patients which localizes his
hysterical symptoms.

tractable with male patients, in whom a limb could maintain a position of complete rigidity for months or even years. Furthermore,
unilateral deviations of the tongue muscles, or glosso-labial spasms,
were not uncommon.[93]

These classic neurological somatizations form the core of the
hysterias in Charcot's male patients. Beyond this, Charcot, like
Sydenham earlier, believed that hysteria was a "medical chameleon"
that could deceptively assume the form of a multitude of ailments.
In Charcot's cases, the primary symptoms listed above were at various times accompanied by a veritable kaleidoscope of complaints,

including dizziness, headaches, fevers, back pain, nosebleeds, eye twitches, diarrhea, urinary problems, rapid pulse, chest palpitations ("hysterical heart"), chest pain ("hysterical angina"), trembling of the hands and legs, pain in the joints, redness or paleness of the skin, numbness and tingling in the extremities, and increased secretion of sweat and saliva. In nearly half his male clients, Charcot discovered anesthesia of the epiglottis, a bizarre symptom that causes suppression of the gagging reflex. His writings include as well several examples of dyspnea, uncontrollable coughing, thoracic pain, and "spasms of the esophagus."[94] Charcot often isolated language disorders in these cases, such as slurring of speech, stuttering, aphonia, and mutism, all of a hysterical nature.[95] In three cases, he described in detail the phenomenon of coprolalia, characterized by an involuntary and compulsive urge to utter obscenities in public, accompanied by convulsive tics and obsessive daily thoughts and practices.[96] Conceived initially as a subcategory of male hysteria, these cases were later reclassified as Tourette's syndrome.

Needless to say, the highly neurological nature of Charcot-style hysteria presented fundamental diagnostic difficulties. Given the "neuromimetic" abilities of his patients, a responsible diagnosis required at the outset a close consideration of all possible alternative pathologies.[97] Several of Charcot's later cases of hysteria in males are in fact minor masterpieces of differential diagnosis.

The twenty-first lecture of the *Leçons du mardi,* a case in point, is a study of the hysterical simulation of syringomyelia or spinal cord cyst with a complicated combination of shifting symptoms. Charcot presents the case of "P...eyn," a 46-year-old night watchman at the construction site of the new Eiffel Tower. Following the unexpected death of his wife and young daughter, "P...eyn" developed a paralyzed right hand and wrist accompanied by swelling, skin discoloration, and loss of sensitivity to pain and temperature in the extremities. The paresis, skin problems, and dissociation of sensibility indicate a true syringomyelia. But upon further investigation, Charcot discovered that the rapid onset of the symptoms and the pattern of remissions, together with the presence of a small sensory stigmata (loss of taste on the right side of the tongue), established the case as one of hysteria rather than a degenerative neurological disorder.[98] In another case, Charcot distinguished between hysterical trembling of the legs and shaking of the extremities in cases of alcoholism, Parkinson's disease, and multiple sclerosis.[99] And in a two-part lecture delivered in March 1889, he probed the combination of epileptic seizures and epileptiform hysterical attacks in the same patient.[100]

If sensorimotor symptoms occupy pride of place in Charcot's model of hysteria, the most familiar and flamboyant expression of the disorder is of course the hysterical attack. Charcot did not believe the presence of a seizure was necessary for the diagnosis of a case as hysterical. In fact, more than a third of his male patients exhibited no convulsive behavior at all. However, when an attack did occur in male patients it tended to be intense—"a sort of storm in the hysterical atmosphere," as one doctor described it[101]—and Charcot was convinced that it followed an identical pattern in both sexes. The Salpêtrians were well known for their schematized model of the hysterical fit. The *grande attaque* commences with an *aura hysterica,* a series of premonitory symptoms including light-headedness, throbbing in the temples, a feeling of constriction of the head, and the *globus hystericus* or sensation of a lump in the throat.[102] The paroxysm proper then begins. As Charcot conceives it, the *grande crise hystérique* consists of four stages: an epileptiform period marked by tonic and clonic muscular spasms; a stage of *grands mouvements,* in which the patient assumes stylized postures such as the arched pelvis position; a phase of *attitudes passionnelles,* characterized by the hallucinatory reenactment of emotional scenes from the patient's past; and finally a lengthy and delirious period of withdrawal.[103]

Charcot's writings offer many graphic descriptions of hysterical attacks suffered by male patients, including the arched back position. In the following passage he narrates the first two stages of a seizure experienced by "Gui":

> The patient then loses consciousness completely, and the epileptoid period begins. First, the trembling of the right hand increases and is thrown forward, the eyes are convulsed upwards, the limbs are extended, the fists clenched and then twisted in exaggerated pronation. Soon the arms come together in front of the abdomen in convulsive contractions of the pectoral muscles. After this follows the period of contortions, characterized chiefly by extremely violent movements of salutation that are intermingled with incoherent gesticulations. The patient breaks or tears everything he can get his hands on. He assumes very bizarre postures and attitudes. . . . From time to time, the contortions described above stop for a moment and give way to the distinct position of the *arc de cercle*. This sometimes involves a true opisthotonos, in which the loins are separated from the plane of the bed by a distance of more than fifty centimeters, with the body resting on the head and heels. At other times, the arching is made in front, the arms crossed over the chest, legs in the air, and the trunk and head lifted upwards, with the back and buttocks alone resting on the bed.[104]

The duration of the attacks in Charcot's male patients runs from 30 seconds to 30 minutes. In some cases the fit is mild, whereas in

others, such as that of "Gui" above, the patient is violent and acro-
batic, requiring physical restraint.

The final component of Charcot's symptomatological construction is also the most exotic: the concept of the "hysterogenic zone."
This term originated with Charcot, and the idea quickly became a
distinguishing feature of the "French" theory of hysteria.[105] "These
zones," Charcot explains, "are more or less circumscribed regions
of the body on which pressure or simple rubbing produces quite
rapidly the phenomenon of the aura, and which, if you persist, may
be followed by the hysterical attack. These points or patches may in
addition be the site of permanent hypersensibility and, before an
attack, of spontaneous painful irritation."[106] Charcot believed that
these hysterogenic points were usually small, about the diameter of
a common coin, and they could be set off by touch or by electrical
or magnetic stimulation. With a number of his male patients, sensitivity was so acute that merely touching, stroking, or breathing on
these areas could evoke an attack.[107] Again, with each patient Charcot and his assistants conducted a thorough examination and then
meticulously plotted the distribution of these *points excitateurs* on
a personalized body chart of the patient. Forty-eight percent of
Charcot's male patients displayed hysterogenic zones.

Charcot believed that these hysterogenic zones could develop
anywhere on the male body. The most common places, however,
were on the top of the head, below the clavicle, in the submam-
mary region, at the bottom of the rib cage, across the anterior surface of the body trunk, between the shoulder blades, and in the
lower back. About a quarter of his male patients also presented hysterogenic zones in the pelvic region. Although Charcot rejected a
causal role for the reproductive organs in cases of hysteria, he did
acknowledge and record the extensive *symptomatological* involve-

ment of the genital area in the disorder. Accordingly, with several male patients he found that hysterical fits could be induced with the application of pressure to the groin. Seven of his hysterical males, or 11 percent, also displayed these supersensitive points along the spermatic cord, on the skin of the scrotum, or in the testes.[108]

We can see from these accounts that what Charcot banished from his reflections about causation reappeared with a vengeance in the clinical descriptions of his male hysterics. For some reason, he was particularly concerned with examining the patients in his *Service des hommes* for responses to "testicular compression." Of one patient, a 38-year-old railroad employee, he noted: "The testicle on the left side is more sensitive than the one on the right side. This is a case of testicular as opposed to ovarian hysteria."[109] In addition, he believed that in some instances pressure applied to the testes could arrest or provoke a hysterical attack. "R…eau," for instance, a traveling street-singer (and one of Charcot's three "degenerate" patients) suffered from scattered hyperesthesias in the iliac and genital regions. "The skin of the scrotum on the left side," Charcot confides, "is very sensitive to the least pressure. The testicle on the same side is still more painful and, if you press either the testicle itself or the tissues surrounding it a little harder, the patient experiences the sensation of something moving from the stomach toward the neck or he feels a sensation of suffocation" (that is, the *globus hystericus*).[110] This is hardly a surprising response. In late nineteenth-century French medical literature on male hysteria, the practice of stopping natural hysterical attacks or eliciting artificial fits through genital manipulation was quite common.[111] Men were not exempt from the "laying on of hands" that Michel Foucault highlighted in regard to female hysterics in Charcot's medical practice.[112]

Furthermore, two of Charcot's male patients engaged in a fascinating act of clinical cross-dressing. "C...cy," a middle-aged worker originally from the French Caribbean, became terrified one day when he was nearly struck by lightning during a thunderstorm. A second, unnamed figure, "a peasant of great rusticity," had recently come to Paris to work in a railway station, where he was once nearly killed in a freight car accident. In addition to several other sensory stigmata, both men developed unmistakable hysterogenic zones in the area of the lower abdominal wall corresponding exactly to the position of the ovaries in the female body.[113] Other doctors at the Salpêtrière found similar symptom-formations in their male patients. In fact, Gilles de la Tourette was so impressed by this phenomenon that he labeled these areas "les zones pseudo-ovariennes" of the male body. He believed that these points occur frequently, that they form unilaterally or bilaterally, and that they appear most often on the left side of the body.[114] Although Charcot vehemently rejected ovarian theories of hysteria, he was willing, in the descriptive realm of symptomatology, to integrate into his picture of the disease what for all intents and purposes was an element of a gynecological model of hysteria. With remarkable anatomical literalness, he then transposed the notion of ovarian hysterogenic points directly onto his male hysterical patients of the 1880s.

Whether the *points pseudo-ovariens* that Charcot located in his male patients reflected the theoretical imagination of the doctor, which was then replicated iatrogenically in the patients' behavior, or whether these were creative sympathetic reactions on the part of male patients to their female counterparts, is open to speculation.[115] Whatever their origin, for Charcot and his circle these symptoms were not metaphors for general stomach distress but rather exact anatomical analogues to the female condition. Doctors realized, of course, that these sensations "correspond to no particular organ" in men.[116] Yet the source of sensation, they insisted, is internal, not cutaneous. Pseudo-ovarian hyperesthesias are precisely located in these men and, upon compression, can produce all the symptoms of the hysterical aura and attack. As one physician at the Bicêtre hospital wrote of a man with a persistent spot of pain on the left side of his lower abdomen, it is "exactly as if there had been an ovary hidden behind the abdominal wall."[117]

GENERALLY SPEAKING, the account of hysteria that emerges from Charcot's collected writings is similar for male and female patients. In both sexes, the malady is a hereditarian-degenerative disorder of the nervous system with an extensive quasi-neurological symptomatology, a volatile pattern of development, and a largely unfavorable prognosis. Many times, Charcot insists on the essential congruence of hysterical disorders in the two sexes.[118] If we analyze the individual elements of his two diagnostic paradigms, however, we find several divergences. Although he posits a primary constitutional origin for hysteria in both sexes, statistically women remain far more prone to the disorder than men (the 1 to 20 ratio). Similarly, Charcot believes that women serve as the sole parental agents of direct transmission of hysteria to male offspring. Both of these discrepancies suggest that in Charcot's time, hysteria in the male medical imagination remained essentially a female affliction.

In most of Charcot's cases involving women, a hereditarily tainted individual becomes sick as the result of an overpowering emotional experience. Most common among these experiences, in order of frequency, are marital turmoil, unrequited love, religious ecstasy, superstitious fear, and death of a family member. As Charcot relates the histories of these female patients, we can see that these cases usually occur in domestic settings. By contrast, Charcot's adult male patients generally develop hysteria following a physically traumatic event, usually one occurring in the public workplace. The outbreak is often compounded by prior venereal infection or alcoholic excess. Charcot's writings on hysteria following a physical trauma only occasionally deal with female patients. When hysteria in males is precipitated by a purely emotional force, it is often elicited by such "manly" emotions as rage, jealousy, or agitation. In other words, knowingly or unknowingly, Charcot formulates an essentially separate set of secondary causal factors that are consonant with prevailing notions of masculine and feminine natures: women in his writings fall ill as a result of their vulnerable emotional natures and inability to control their feelings, whereas men get sick from working, drinking, or excessive fornication. Hysterical women suffer from an excess of "feminine" behaviors, hysterical men from an excess of "masculine" behaviors.

We can detect a related pattern in Charcot's projected symptom profiles. Charcot provides remarkably little information about the *mental* state of his male patients. By and large, his case histories involving men are precise, technical, descriptive narratives of the somatic symptomatology of the disorder, with little reference to psychological matters. With his female patients, neurological description also predominates, but it is typically accompanied by the mention of symptoms such as extravagant mood shifts, attacks of anxiety, fits of crying, and threats of suicide. Such emotional self-displays only occasionally complicate Charcot's male cases:[119] in the 61 published case histories of diagnosed male hysteria, there are only two instances of an adult man crying.[120]

A number of times, Charcot acknowledges the emotional differences between the disorder in the two sexes. He asserts, for instance, that male victims of hysterical illness display a greater degree of "symptomatological fixity" than female patients, meaning that the physical manifestations of their hysterias tend to be stable and persistent, whereas in women they are capricious and short-lived.[121] Mood and personality often differ as well: "The hysterical men of the working class who . . . fill the hospital wards of Paris today," he generalizes in 1888, "are almost always somber, melancholic, depressed, and discouraged people. . . . We should not expect to find in the male that morbid *brio* frequent in reality in the female."[122] Charcot in effect limits his account of male hysteria to the most "objective," externalized aspects of the disorder, while ignoring or downplaying symptoms we would today call psychoneurotic. And by emphasizing the stability and tenacity of symptoms in males, he avoids a connection with the historical image of the flighty, emotionally theatrical female hysteric.

In his descriptions of the hysterical attack in women, Charcot devotes roughly equal time to the four stages of the fit. Of these stages, the third phase of *attitudes passionnelles* is the most revealing psychologically—a long and breathless performance during which patients reenact in words and actions emotionally painful scenes from their past. The Salpêtrian literature on female hysteria extensively documents this aspect of the attack: fear, ecstasy, surprise, pleasure, and religious enthusiasm are depicted at length in the volumes of the *Iconographie photographique*. Not so with masculine hysteria. In male patients, the range of emotions that Charcot reports in this third stage is noticeably more restricted, tending decidedly toward the darker, depressive end of the spectrum. One medical observer remarked aptly in 1885 that

> the characteristics of the attack in him [the male patient] present, as is usual, some differences from what is observed in the female. In the latter, there is a happy phase and a sad phase in the passional period, whereas in the male all the sentiments are sad and somber. Everything in him has a terrifying character,

which is moreover the standard psychical condition in these patients, whereas the contrary is found in the female.[123]

Charcot, in other words, effectively drained the hysteria diagnosis of its affective content; in his descriptions, the most physically extroverted aspects of the disorder predominate over subjective states of mind and emotion. It may well have been because he formulated such a narrowly neurologized model of hysteria that Charcot was able to apply the hysteria concept to members of his own sex with apparent ease and that the male medical profession of his time, after centuries of defensive rejection of the notion, was willing to accept the idea with relatively little reluctance.

For several millennia, hysteria, *la maladie de la matrice,* had been seen as a pathology of femininity whose diagnosis served as a kind of medical metaphor for everything that male observers found mysterious or unmanageable in the opposite sex. Working in the liberal political and cultural environment of France during the late 1870s and 1880s, the premier theoretician of hysteria in Europe formulated a full-blown theory of the disorder in the male sex. At the apogee of his career, Charcot devoted fifteen years to a scientific investigation of the topic, illustrating his ideas with scores of clinical histories and advancing his views with the full weight of his professional authority. The extent of his writings on the topic, the places where he published those writings, the polemical energy he invested in them, and the significance his contemporaries gave to these cases indicate the importance that the subject held for him and for his age.

At one time or another, Charcot located virtually the entire range of physical behaviors from past conceptualizations of female hysteria in men. The sensation of *globus hystericus* in the throat, which the ancients believed resulted from the pressure of a mobile womb on other organs of the body cavity, appeared regularly in Charcot's male patients. The anesthesias and hyperesthesias that occurred so copiously in Charcot's male hysterics were scientized versions of the *stigmati diaboli* found by Catholic demonology in women witches. For generations the hysterical attack had been interpreted synecdochically, as a sort of bodily symbolism for childbirth, the female orgasm, and feminine nature in general. In the late nineteenth century, Charcot described the attack frequently in men. Moreover, in the ultimate equation of the two sexes, he even attributed hysterical pain in the female organ believed to most differentiate men from women—the ovaries—directly to men. Taken together, these are signal departures in the history of medicine.

In the final analysis, Charcot's selective equalization of the hysteria diagnosis bears a highly ambiguous relation to the socio-sexual system of the time. In the *Iconographie photographique* of the 1870s, Charcot and his students created some of the most gender-stereotyped images in nineteenth-century science, and they did so specifically through the medical representation of hysteria in women. However, a decade later, under altered historical conditions, Charcot's "hysterization of men's bodies" challenged the gender-differentiated psychologies of the time and implicitly transgressed conventional gender roles of masculine and feminine.[124] The means and methods for interpreting the two sexes in hospitals, in doctors' offices, and in outpatient clinics—literally the ways in which physicians envisioned men and women to be sick—were here drawing closer together. At the same time, however, in order to formulate such a theory Charcot felt the need to rigorously de-emotionalize and de-sexualize the diagnosis. To the same end, he chose systematically to limit his application of the hysteria label to groups of individuals whose social and occupational identities were notably different from his own. Although Charcot wrote more on—and more explicitly about—hysteria in men than any other figure in European medicine, his working conception of the disorder was still modified by gender and class in many subtle and historically significant ways.[125] In important respects, the provocation at the core of his published work on the subject remained unexplored.

# CHAPTER 4

# Male Hysteria at the Fin de Siècle

FROM TODAY'S VIEWPOINT, the 1880s and 1890s, both in Britain and on the European continent, seem heroic and superhuman, "an accumulation of steam, cast-iron, and self-confidence."[1] Europe's imperial reach, encompassing nearly the entirety of the African continent, south Asia, and several island areas, was at its greatest. The spread of modern, mechanized, industrialized economies effectively created the first global economic network. Western civilization had gained an unprecedented degree of mastery over the natural environment. The new ideologies of race science, eugenics, and Social Darwinism posited the manifest superiority of the European West, especially its Anglo-Saxon middle classes, over all other peoples of the world. Britain, Germany, France, and increasingly the United States far surpassed the rest of the world in their wealth, technological sophistication, and military prowess. A succession of extravagant world's fairs and expositions mounted in these countries showcased their unprecedented achievements. Except for a few curmudgeonly intellectuals like Friedrich Nietzsche,

Westerners believed universally that science and medicine were in the vanguard of civilization's astonishing progress.

Running beneath the oversized self-congratulatory optimism of the late nineteenth century, however, were darker currents. The fin-de-siècle concept connotes decadence, decline, degeneration, and death. Dire self-diagnoses of the age—of which Max Nordau's *Degeneration* (1893) and Gustave Le Bon's *Crowd Psychology* (1895) were only the best-selling examples—likened the time to the late Roman Empire and the biblical fall. For many contemporaries, particularly cultural traditionalists and social conservatives, signs of the age's dreadful downward tendencies were everywhere. Religious faith, which had provided moral discipline and underpinned European civilization, was rapidly waning in the current era of materialism and scientism. Cities were ballooning uncontrollably—by 1900 greater London, Paris, and Vienna, respectively, had populations of 6.5, 3, and 2 million—and they fostered crime, prostitution, vagabondage, disease, and drug addiction. Organizing into newly legalized trade unions and fired up by Marxist and socialist ideologies, working-class people across Europe were growing politically restless during the late 1800s. Scores of workers' strikes and the perpetual threat of class revolution marked the period. So did anarchism, which peaked in the mid-1890s with a series of high-profile assassinations—the terrorism of its day. The rates of suicide, alcoholism, and insanity—what the French sociologist Émile Durkheim termed the "social pathologies" of the day—also seemed to be skyrocketing.[2] Urban sexual violence was on the rise, too, as illustrated graphically by the case of Jack the Ripper, who terrorized London's East End in 1888. It was little wonder that huge numbers of Europeans welcomed the outbreak of hostilities in August 1914: war, they imagined mistakenly, would end the orgy of self-indulgence and destructive domestic squabbling of the preceding decades and restore a sense of national purpose and patriotism.

People hoped that war would also revive and reinvigorate the masculine virtues. In the 1870s and 1880s, feminism had emerged as a mass political movement with large numbers of organizations, marches, petitions, publications, and congresses across Europe. The drive for women's legal, political, economic, and educational equality finally entered middle-class consciousness. In Britain, although the militant suffrage movement did not form until a generation later, the Married Women's Property Act of 1882 and the Guardianship of Infants Act of 1886 markedly improved women's legal status. In 1897 local and provincial suffrage groups across Britain united to form the National Union of Women's Suffrage Societies, under the able leadership of Millicent Garrett Fawcett. Women in significant numbers throughout the English-speaking world began entering white-collar sectors of the economy.[3] Similarly, French feminism, which had exploded fitfully with every revolutionary upheaval since 1789 but then had been suppressed, emerged as a powerful, permanent wave during France's third republican regime. French feminist journalism flourished. The Camille Sée Law of 1880 mandated secular secondary schooling for girls across the country, and as part of the anti-clerical campaigns of the 1880s, the Naquet Law of 1884 effectively relegalized divorce in Catholic France.[4]

From the 1860s onward, France and Switzerland, followed by Scandinavia, the Low Countries, Italy, Spain, and then Germany and Austria, began to admit women into their universities for undergraduate education. The universities in Scotland and several English regional medical schools (although not Oxford and Cambridge) were accepting women by 1890.[5] During the 1880s, substantial numbers of women also began to enter medical schools in Paris, Nancy, Lyon, and Montpellier, and in 1886 the first two French women were granted medical internships or hospital residencies. By the turn of the century, 340 women were enrolled in medical schools across France.[6]

Fin-de-siècle feminism obviously challenged directly the ideology of separate spheres. Novels and plays proliferated about "the new woman" *(femme nouvelle),* who was economically productive, domestically independent, intellectually curious, politically engaged, and sexually assertive.[7] Avant-garde male authors like Ibsen, Shaw, Butler, Gissing, and Strindberg further challenged the system of marriage and patriarchy. Needless to say, anti-modernists of all sorts opposed women's emancipation, with anti-suffragism emerging as an angry, organized counter-movement. These opponents, who composed the overwhelming majority of middle-class men in Europe, feared female promiscuity, the decline of the family, and the loss of male prerogatives in public and private. Despite the fact that actual feminist legislative gains in the decades after 1870 were modest, fin-de-siècle anti-feminist rhetoric reached tones that were near-hysterical.[8] Women's efforts to gain undergraduate admission to Oxford and Cambridge were met with rallies and riots. Depictions of women as depraved, diseased, and devouring, remarkable for their overt misogyny, crop up ubiquitously in the art and literature of the period.[9]

At the same time, male homosexuality achieved greater public visibility than ever before. What looks in retrospect like rudimentary male gay subcultures began to form in several European cities during the last two decades of the nineteenth century.[10] In Paris, Berlin, London, Amsterdam, and St. Petersburg, an increasing number of venues—cafés, cabarets, restaurants, and salons—with a predominantly gay clientele were publicized during these years, and the sexual geography of these cities, including meeting grounds for men in parks, quays, and bath facilities, became common knowledge.[11] Coined a generation earlier, the terms "homosexuality" and "homosexual" became popular in the 1890s. The 1885 Labouchere Amendment to the British criminal code and Paragraph 175 of the German Reich penal code, which made all public and private sex acts between men illegal, had the paradoxical effect of highlighting homosexuality. For the first time, several brave voices—Symonds, Carpenter, Shaw, and Ellis in Britain, Ulrichs in Germany, Raffalovitch in France—expressed enlightened defenses of same-sex sexuality, urging greater tolerance and a liberalization of criminal codes—the beginnings, in effect, of a homosexual rights movement.[12]

At the same time, a steady stream of arrests for acts of "gross public indecency" by "pederasts" and "inverts" reinforced the middle-class equation of crime and male homosexuality. The tabloid presses across late Victorian Europe published sensational accounts of homosexual activities, including the Germiny affair of 1876–1877, involving a lawyer from a distinguished family arrested in a public urinal along the Champs-Élysées; the Cleveland Street Scandal of 1889–1890, which brought to public attention the world of high-class rent boys in West End London; Oscar Wilde's prosecution in 1895; and the Eulenberg affair of 1907–1908, concerning the purported homosexuality of the German chancellor and members of the Kaiser's circle.[13] Against this background, the Boy Scouts, leagues for "social purity," and campaigns to reform boys' public schools were launched as strategies for maintaining healthy, heterosexual masculinity.[14]

Ratcheting up the level of social anxiety still higher was "the venereal peril." Estimates today cite as much as 13 to 15 percent of the adult male population of Paris as being infected with the pox, and up to one-third of the population of municipal asylums at the century's turn as victims of "general paralysis of the insane," or spinal and cerebral syphilis.[15] "Civilization has become syphilization," quipped the German-Austrian psychiatrist Krafft-Ebing. "Everybody is more or less infected with it" reads Gustave Flaubert's laconic entry in his *Dictionary of Received Ideas*.[16] Because its contraction was deemed shameful, its incubation period was so long, its advanced forms were so horrific, and there was no cure, dread of the disease was high among anyone with a wayward youth or a promiscuous partner. Terror at contracting the disease was so great in this pre-antibiotic age that "syphilophobia," or pathological anxiety about syphilis, appeared in the medical textbooks of the day as a cause of nervous and mental breakdown.[17] Furthermore, the venereal peril spread just as Louis Pasteur's new germ theory of contagion was gaining scientific acceptance and popular familiarity. Fears of life-threatening diseases carried by mysterious, microscopic agents were irrational but real and widespread.[18]

Although the phrase "crisis of masculinity" has been overused by scholars in recent years,[19] there can be little doubt that a strong feeling emerged in the last two decades of the nineteenth century that traditional notions of manhood and womanhood were under siege. The sentiment was especially strong among middle- and upper-middle-class heterosexual males in the cities, suburbs, and large towns. The 1880s and 1890s were a time of "sexual anarchy," in the words of the novelist George Gissing, when all the laws that governed sexual identity and behavior seemed to be breaking down. Male public personalities as different as Theodore Roosevelt, Émile Zola, and Rudyard Kipling warned repeatedly of the dangers of effeminization. The new rhetoric of force and energy that emerged in Europe from 1900 onward and pointed toward World War I was motivated in part by a perceived softening of masculinity.[20]

France occupied a rather special position in this scenario. During the penultimate decades of the nineteenth century, men in Britain, Germany, Italy, and the United States were engaged in great national exertions that permitted them, individually and collectively, to perform their masculine duties and identities routinely. Britain's global empire was a crucible for forging "imperial masculinities."[21] In the generation after unification, Wilhelmian Germany was absorbed in expanding its industrial and military might.[22] So, to some extent, was post-unification Italy. And Americans were still killing off Indians on the western frontier and beginning to make their first fateful entrance onto the world stage with imperialist claims in the Caribbean and South Pacific. In all four nations, the historical warrior ideal of masculinity remained viable.

In contrast, France during the fin de siècle lacked a powerful project to serve as a proving ground for national manhood. The Third Republic, France's first sustained and successful experiment in democracy, owed its existence to the country's swift, catastrophic defeat by the Prussians, who in turn used the French humiliation on the battlefield to achieve their long-sought national unification. Throughout the 1870–1914 period, the German annexation of the formerly French territories of Alsace and Lorraine was often characterized as a dismemberment or castration of the French nation. Not surprisingly, the French imperial drive during the 1880s and 1890s in North Africa, Madagascar, and Indochina was widely regarded as compensation for France's military and territorial losses at home. Making matters worse, in a number of embarrassing confrontations with other colonial powers (for example, the first and second Fashoda crises), France was forced to back down. With the army trounced, the Napoleonic heritage in tatters, and the Bourbon and Orleanist royal lines dying out, there were reasons to doubt French manhood in the 1870s and beyond.

Reinforcing the nation's military and geopolitical anxieties were demographic concerns. Today, we would call the population stable, but to nervous guardians of the national welfare, the French birth rate in the late nineteenth century was alarmingly low, especially in contrast to the explosive growth of France's newly powerful neighbor beyond the Rhine.[23] Who in the future would achieve the imagined military revenge on the German Empire? The Dreyfus Affair, the most divisive event in the domestic history of the early Third Republic, further inflamed these concerns. "Republican manhood," with its emphasis on courage, honor, and justice, eventually prevailed; but once it became clear that the real traitor was not the Alsatian Jew Alfred Dreyfus but Major Esterhazy, and that a long, dishonorable cover-up had taken place, the integrity of the French military was again in crisis for all the world to see.[24]

Social and cultural developments added still further to these insecurities. As many French people experienced it, traditional morality was under siege in the cultural wars of the early Third Republic. The nation's historic Catholic identity was being methodically dismantled by godless secular republicans. In the greatest literary saga of the age, Zola chronicled in his series of twenty novels the moral and biological degeneration of two interconnected French families. Alarmists, many of them anti-republican critics, pleaded for a national "regeneration." The school of literary decadence, which to uncomprehending cultural conservatives wallowed in excess of all sorts, was headquartered in Paris/Babylon.[25] The very term "fin de siècle," with its doomsday implications, was French. The city's café and boulevard culture catered to every appetite, and as Impressionist paintings, travel guides, journalistic exposés, and police reports recorded, commercial sex thrived in the French capital. It was no coincidence that the Marquis de Sade had been French and that venereology became a specialty of French physicians. Long-standing stereotypes about the French as a feminized nation endured. The new cultural figure of the Baudelairean dandy or *flâneur,* with his air of leisure and effeminacy, flourished in the parks, cafés, and boulevards of Baron Haussmann's new Paris. After his prison release in 1897 Oscar Wilde had repaired to France, where he was welcomed in several circles and where private homosexual conduct was not criminalized.[26]

In the outlook of many French people, these sources of social disintegration and moral disarray reinforced one another and expressed "a single degenerational syndrome:"[27] feminist women were less likely to marry and have children, thereby inhibiting population growth; an effeminate society bred sexual deviants, who also neither married nor reproduced; excessive drink encouraged sensuality, including commercial sex; prostitution spread syphilis, which in turn undermined male virility; and avant-garde painters, novelists, and playwrights celebrated disease, adultery, and prostitution in their work. By no means all French people saw their country in this light, but for many the fear of national enfeeblement, which was especially a fear about the degeneracy of French masculinity, was strong.[28] The picture of late-nineteenth-century France as a carefree, party-driven *belle époque* is in fact a postbellum idealization, constructed nostalgically after the carnage of World War I. Contemporaries perceived their age very differently. Had France deserved to lose the war in 1870? Did the French people have the collective will to remain a great nation? Was the French "race" dying out? Many French people pondered these questions a century ago with deep anxiety.

IN ONE EUROPEAN COUNTRY after another, fin-de-siècle medicine and science engaged these urgent social questions. But whereas medical commentators earlier in the century had used existing genres, such as the treatise on insanity written by asylum doctors, physicians during the period running from 1870 to the First World War worked at a time when new biomedical discourses were being created. Each of the "new knowledges" they deployed had its own methods, terminology, and classification, but they all operated to similar effect.

Evolutionary biology proved the most successful of the new sciences. Charles Darwin was the greatest life scientist of the nineteenth century, and in 1871 he finally applied his powerful new evolutionary paradigm to Homo sapiens.[29] In his appropriately titled *The Descent of Man,* Darwin takes for granted the natural and innate intellectual inferiority of women. Since men's minds and bodies are constantly being sharpened in the environmental struggle for survival, they are fitter in terms of adaptation. Furthermore, Darwin argues in his influential text that greater variability exists in the human male; and since variations of form and function fuel evolutionary change by natural selection, males in essence are the engine for humanity's marvelous achievements.[30] Darwin's ideas may have been revolutionary in the biological realm; but *The Descent of Man,* published in London against the backdrop of Mill's proto-feminist broadside *The Subjection of Women* (1869), simply reinforced traditional sexual difference. British evolution-oriented texts appearing in Darwin's wake—like George Romanes's "Mental Differences between Men and Women" (1887) and Harry Campbell's *Differences in the Nervous Organization of Man and Woman* (1891)—argued directly against the extension of the franchise and higher education to women on alleged medico-biological grounds.[31] Both British and continental Darwinians argued that the sexual division of labor was natural and inevitable.

Eugenics was another "new" discipline of the day that had gender implications. Founded by Darwin's cousin Francis Galton, who coined the term in 1883, eugenics sought to improve the human race through selective directed breeding. Galton and his followers brought a mass of pseudo-statistical data to bear on their social and cultural prescriptions. Race mingling between east and west or black and white, they contended, would dilute the vigor of the Anglo-Saxon races. Correspondingly, a woman's primary social duty lay in conventional motherhood. Feminist campaigns for higher education and economic independence would only hurt the nation, the eugenicists argued, and to tamper with domestic ideology was to court sociobiological disaster.

The most curious of the turn-of-the-century disciplines was criminal anthropology. This Italian contribution to the field applied French degeneration theory to criminals, prostitutes, mad people, and the poor, who it claimed could be identified by brain size, head shape, and facial features. Cesare Lombroso and Guglielmo Ferrero's *The Delinquent Woman, the Prostitute, and the Normal Woman* (1893) offers a compendium of cultural stereotypes of female deviance. One key idea in the text is that prostitutes are endowed with bodily and behavioral traits that are fundamentally masculine and that this female masculinity is itself pathological. Similarly, Scipio Sighele's *The New Woman* of 1898 applied bogus anthropometric measurements to women who were independent, assertive, or rebellious, claiming to discover in such women forms of degeneracy akin to crime, alcoholism, and epilepsy.[32]

Like evolutionary biology, endocrinology was another disciplinary innovation that has fared well scientifically in the twentieth century but that, in its early phase, was no less inflected with Victorian assumptions. Following the identification of the sex hormones around 1900, the Viennese physician and laboratory physiologist Eugen Steinach claimed that the male/female dichotomy was the most elemental distinction in the human species. He believed that masculinity and femininity suffused every cell, tissue, and organ in the body, as well as our psychic, behavioral, and corporeal selves. In Steinach's new biochemical construction of sexuality and gender identity, testosterone and estrogen mapped directly onto the two sexes—the chemical correlates to masculinity and femininity, as it were. For the early endocrinologists, anatomy and physiology dwindled in importance, and experience and the environment were irrelevant, but glandular secretions acting through the blood-stream became omnipotent.[33] Included in Steinach's laboratory work were experiments to "cure" male homosexuals through the surgical transplantation of monkey testicles. Male and female hormones, too, had their separate spheres.

Sexology was certainly the most sensationalistic of the new fin-de-siècle biomedical sciences. From the Berlin psychiatrist Karl Westphal's article on "contrary sexual instinct" in 1869 to the Zurich psychiatrist Auguste Forel's *The Sexual Question* in 1906, European physicians formulated a new scientistic vocabulary to account for a wide spectrum of sexual behaviors. As medical classifications, sadism, masochism, fetishism, exhibitionism, pedophilia, sexual inversion, transvestism, and hermaphroditism all came into existence during this formative period. In an intriguing process, fin-de-siècle physicians took over from clergy, moralists, philosophers, and jurists as the self-appointed experts on human sexuality, imparting the authority of science to their labels, judgments, and classifications. What had previously been sins, vices, or crimes were newly construed as sicknesses.

The first generation of European sexologists consistently reinforced conservative moral judgments about human sexuality. In their influential 1882 article on "inversion of the genital sense," Charcot and Magnan had interpreted same-sex attraction as a sign of hereditary degeneration. Other French sexological texts, such as

Paul Moreau's *Des aberrations du sens génésique* (1880) and Émile Laurent's *L'Amour morbide* (1891), equated homosexuality with feminized behavior and assumed that all homosexuals were sick, sterile, and unstable.[34] In Britain, Havelock Ellis's early, popular *Man and Woman: A Study of Human Secondary Sexual Characteristics* (1894) marshaled hundreds of pages of data about the emotional, physiological, intellectual, and even spiritual differences between men and women. And Richard von Krafft-Ebing, working in Vienna, became the leading figure in the medicalization and morbidification of sexuality during the fin-de-siècle era with his encyclopedic *Psychopathia Sexualis,* the first "textbook" of the sexual perversions.[35] It is no coincidence of chronology that the first would-be sciences of sexuality appeared when and where they did.[36] By pathologizing minority sexualities, sexologists across Europe sought to shore up traditional notions of "normal" femininity and masculinity in the face of challenges that were increasingly visible and vocal.

Darwinian evolutionary biology, Galtonian eugenics, Lombrosian criminal anthropology, LeBonian crowd psychology, Krafft-Ebing's sexology, and Steinach's endocrinology were all new intellectual technologies of power that worked to reinforce the gender rigidities of the day. But there is an insufficiently appreciated side to these sciences, an aspect that was certainly clear to many contemporaries. Specifically, Charcot-era science and medicine simultaneously bore a critical, deconstructive relation to the sex/gender system of its day. The new knowledges accomplished this work principally by probing gender differentiation—and with it the biology, psychology, and ontology of masculinity and femininity—in original and provocative ways that reflected back obliquely on Victorian/Wilhelminian sexual culture. Within avant-garde European medical circles during these years, questions of gender, sexual behavior, and sexual identity were intensively argued, investigated, problematized, theorized, and reconceptualized in ways that would have been unthinkable at the beginning of Victoria's reign fifty or so years earlier.

Examples abound: Thomas Henry Huxley, "Darwin's bulldog," opposed the hard, deterministic versions of social-evolutionary theory, rejecting in his well-known essay "Evolution and Ethics" (1893) the sociobiological arguments against workers' and women's rights.[37] The new science of embryology, to which Darwin had devoted a chapter in *Origin of the Species,* had discovered recently that mammalian females and males were indistinguishable in the early stages of intrauterine development; for the first several months of life, all human life possessed the elements of both sexes. The Berlin ear, nose, and throat doctor Wilhelm Fliess argued that all human beings were bisexual, with the dominant side of the brain representing the dominant gender and the other side the repressed gender. Throughout much of the medical literature on the sexes during the period from 1880 to 1910, there is less and less talk about special feminine and masculine "natures" and "constitutions." And there is a steady corresponding movement away from biological, degenerationist paradigms and toward causal models based on individual psychology and social environment. Even in the twelve successive editions of his *Psychopathia Sexualis* published between 1886 and 1903, Krafft-Ebing gradually abandoned his commitment to degenerationism as an explanation of homosexuality and increasingly conceptualized masochism, sadism, and fetishism as intensifications of normal sexual desires.[38]

For his part, Havelock Ellis established more explicitly than any European physicians of his generation that sexology was not fated to serve only reactionary and counter-feminist purposes. Ellis was part of a group of radical and socialist intellectuals who openly sought more liberal approaches to sexuality, marriage, and family life. His early, essentializing *Man and Woman* undergirded traditional sexual differences; but Ellis's later multi-volume *Studies in the Psychology of Sex* is a key work in "the modernization of sex."[39] In these studies, which appeared from 1897 through the first decade of the new century, Ellis rejected the idea that women lacked sexual desires and instincts, skewered traditional superstitions about masturbation, and argued for greater enlightenment about male and female homosexuality. He in fact coauthored the first volume of his series, titled *Sexual Inversion,* with John Addington Symonds, a self-identified homosexual man who included his own autobiographical case history in the book.

Even Steinach's work can be read in this dual light. The new endocrinological model of gender identity that emerged after 1900 on first glance seems solely to support the conceptual polarization of masculine (androgen) and feminine (estrogen). But, after isolating the chemical essence of male and female, Steinach goes on to insist time and again that there are no ideal types of either gender; real people are only approximations to "an imaginary ideal" of masculinity and femininity.[40] Moreover, Steinach's rather Frankensteinian laboratory experiments included surgically grafting the genital glands of one sex onto the opposite sex in nonhuman vertebrates and then observing changes in their bodies and mating behavior. His writings are replete with references to masculinized females, feminized males, and experimental hermaphrodites. For Steinach, in other words, "feminization" and "masculinization" are processes that by degrees can be induced, extracted, injected, and engineered.[41]

The gendered culture of science during the last quarter of the nineteenth century was in fact significantly different from what it had been earlier in the century. On the whole, fin-de-siècle medical commentaries on gender are more sophisticated theoretically and more diversified internally, positing many types, degrees, and processes of gender differentiation. If the leitmotifs of Victorian biomedical discourse were certainty and consensus, for late-nineteenth-century science they were diversity and ambiguity. Furthermore, questions of masculinity and femininity became a vehicle for exploring not just sexuality and gender, but also science, method, modernity, and selfhood in general. At the same time, the European fin-de-siècle medical world was shot through with inner tensions. This succession of symptomatic texts generated ideas, insights, and theories—but often later abandoned them. They pursued promising lines of inquiry that concluded by contradicting their own points of departure. And they made observations and formulated models with social and political implications that went unexplored and unrealized.

No scientifically informed author from this remarkable period captures these internal contradictions more glaringly than Otto Weininger. Like Krafft-Ebing, Steinach, and Freud, Weininger worked in Vienna, which in the 1890s took over from Paris the role of the most active center of scientific and cultural speculation about sexuality. In 1903, freshly graduated from the University of Vienna, where he took a wide assortment of courses in philosophy, psychology, anatomy, physiology, zoology, chemistry, and mathematics, Weininger published his notorious *Sex and Character (Geschlecht und Charakter)*.[42] At the time, he was 22 years old. In strict intellectual terms, Weininger's book is a work of stunning precocity that offers a feverish synthesis of ideas and language circulating in late-nineteenth-century Europe. Weininger was not a scientist or physician with an institutional affiliation—he was barely an adult— but he intended *Sex and Character* to be a scientific treatise. Aspiring to be the Nietzsche of sexual science, he described his entire treatise as a study of "the special problem of the polarity of genders."[43]

According to Weininger, there are "laws" of masculinity and femininity, just as there are laws of physics, and these establish unmistakably the inferiority and insignificance of women. Addressing directly "the woman question" of his day, Weininger attempts to demolish women's claims to equality, individuality, and even personhood. In his view, ability, intelligence, and accomplishment are by definition masculine components, and a female genius is a freak of nature.[44] He characterizes maleness as existence itself, the totality of all human qualities, while femininity corresponds conversely to metaphysical nothingness. Hysteria, to which Weininger devotes a full chapter, reveals woman's inner sexual essence. To this vehement misogyny the author adds many pungent comments about Jews and homosexuals—both of which he views as effeminate, problematic populations in Europe at the time. Weininger thus seems to be the quintessential "reactionary modernist," and his book a *locus classicus* of late Victorian scientific sexism and racism.[45]

Yet even Weininger's overheated harangue can be read on a second level.[46] Throughout his treatise, Weininger gropes for appropriate scientific and philosophical metaphors to discuss gender. He variously conceptualizes masculine and feminine as "principles," "conditions," "substances," and "plasmas." While centrally important in life, masculinity and femininity are nonetheless only abstractions, he insists. Male (M) and Female (F) represent sexualized archetypes of mind and body that no individual embodies completely. "Males and females are like two substances combined in different proportions, but with either element never wholly missing."[47] In fact, each person can possess up to 50 percent of the opposite sex while still retaining their gender identity, Weininger maintains, and a principal object of anthropological study should be to locate the appropriate place of an individual on the continuum between these gendered polarities. Dissenting from Krafft-

Ebing, Weininger maintains that homosexuality is not a vice, perversion, or disease but a form of "sexual intermediacy" composed
of equal quantities of masculine and feminine properties that explicitly lies between, rather than beyond or outside, the male/
female spectrum.[48]

Weininger was a secular Jew who attacked Judaism and then
converted to Protestantism, as well as a "repressed homosexual"
who critically assaulted women and feminism. Nevertheless, during the next two decades, some twenty-five reprintings of his *Sex
and Character* appeared in German. Weininger was better known
than Freud during the first decade of the twentieth century, both
in Vienna and in Europe generally. Many readers—including
middle-class heterosexual males—found Weininger's treatise, with
all of its tortured, pathological contradictions, highly resonant.

From Darwin to Ellis, from Charcot to Féré, from Krafft-Ebing
to Weininger, scientific and medical thinkers between 1870 and
1910 engaged questions of sexuality and gender identity. The body
of speculation they produced about male and female is theoretically bold and innovative—occasionally even brilliant—but it is
also laden with internal anxieties and inconsistencies. For these
reasons, fin-de-siècle biomedicine simultaneously sustained and
subverted the socio-sexual regime of the day.

THE MEDICAL LITERATURE on male hysteria written during the
1880s and 1890s expresses directly this same complex of qualities.
Charcot's work was enormously influential and inspired a voluminous body of writing in the principal European languages. The
rapid spread of medical interest in the subject was in part a reflection of the challenge of a new topic of clinical investigation.
Young French physicians in particular came to view the study of
hysteria in its male incarnations as a choice field for making a quick

contribution to a scientifically innovative and intellectually fashionable subject. The upsurge of interest also reflected Charcot's professional clout: he was at once a *chef de clinique* at the largest hospital in France, a charismatic lecturer at the Salpêtrière amphitheater, an examining member of the Paris Faculté de Médecine, and the founding editor of three medical journals. Each of these positions provided formats for the dissemination of his ideas.

The official registry of dissertations at the library of the Paris Medical Faculty cites sixteen dissertations on male hysteria written at this one school between 1875 and 1893.[49] One of these, Émile Batault's *Contribution à l'étude de l'hystérie chez l'homme* (1885), includes a bibliography of well over 150 items written in several languages.[50] The first two series of the American-produced *Index-Catalogue of the Library of the Surgeon-General's Office*, which conveniently began publication in 1880, contain entire separate sections for "Hysteria in the Male." Listing works published between 1875 and 1895, these sections record 24 dissertations or book-length monographs in several languages and 93 French-language articles. From 1870 to 1902, the total number of articles is 296.[51] The greatest concentration of medical publications about hysterical disorders in adult men appeared in the mid- to late 1880s. As the opening sentence of Augustin Berjon's 1886 dissertation on the topic states, "[Masculine] hysteria is the disorder that engages the medical world the most today."[52]

We can glimpse the actual process by which the new diagnosis entered the thinking and practice of European physicians. Charcot began publishing on masculine hysteria in 1882. By the late 1880s, many doctors were willing to acknowledge publicly what they came to regard as their own earlier misdiagnoses. Dr. Robert Marquézy of the Hôpital Broussais in Paris, for example, conceded in 1888 that many male patients whom he had previously diagnosed as alcoholics or as simulators had probably been hysterics.[53] Physicians from near and far wrote to Charcot concerning their most inscrutable male patients to ask the great clinician if these might be cases of hysteria. Occasionally, these sea changes in praxis became matters of public display. At a meeting of the Société Médicale des Hôpitaux held on November 27, 1885, Dr. Georges Debove of the Hôtel Dieu hospital in central Paris took the podium and, in an act of professional self-correction, admitted:

> On the subject of hysteria in men, I held an opinion in 1879 that today I renounce completely. At that time, I denied that hysteria could be a part of the cases I presented. I am now convinced that I was in complete error.[54]

Remarks like those of Debove no doubt pleased Charcot greatly. What he could not have anticipated was that the medical commentary on hysterical males would push the clinical exploration of the subject in several directions he had avoided. Once the official prohibition on the concept within French academic medicine had been lifted, physicians began to wonder out loud just how widespread hysterical disorders in adult men were, and what the correct ratio of male to female hysteria was. In the fall of 1881, an intern at the Bicêtre hospital in southeastern Paris reported 12 cases of male hysteria in the hospital infirmary.[55] Working at the Hôtel Dieu hospital in the shadow of Notre Dame Cathedral, Dr. Pierre Marie reported 25 instances of hysterical symptoms in men during the year 1888 alone.[56] Other medical facilities contributed their share: at the Hôpital Broussais, "26 cases of indisputable authenticity" were treated in a single year.[57] Around the same time, the Hôpital Saint-Antoine discovered five male hysterics in a ward for adult men. And in his thesis on the masculine varieties of hysteria, Dr.

Paul Michaut analyzed 11 cases present in one hospital during a two-month period in 1890.[58] French provincial hospitals joined in the process: on the basis of a four-year study of a 38-bed clinic in Bordeaux, Dr. Émile Bitot discovered 22 instances of male hysteria "in which the diagnosis seems to us indisputable."[59]

As the number of reported cases of hysterical illness in French medical facilities burgeoned during the 1880s, the projected statistical relation of the disorder between the two sexes tightened dramatically. Charcot, as we have seen, followed Briquet's estimation that hysteria occurred 20 times more often in women than in men. Radical at the time, this ratio was soon supplanted. In an extensive study of Berlin hospitals, the incidence of hysteria in over 11,000 patients worked out to a 1 to 10 ratio between the sexes.[60] In a survey that "singularly augments the level of frequency of masculine hysteria," the Dean of the Bordeaux medical faculty reported that of 100 arbitrarily chosen hysterical patients from his practice, 31 turned out to be men.[61] And by 1890, Georges Gilles de la Tourette, in his three-volume codification of Charcotian doctrine, asserted that "it seemed to us that we saw one hysterical man for every two or three women struck by the same disease."[62] Specialized studies of the disease found equal rates of individual symptoms in men and women.[63]

By the end of the 1880s, Charcot posed a question that would have been unthinkable earlier in European medicine: "Hysterical neurosis, is it really . . . as we have claimed up to this point, more frequent in women than in men?"[64] For an answer, he enlisted one of his closest associates. During August and December of 1888, Charcot's former student Pierre Marie gathered figures on differential rates of hysteria among adult men and women at the Hôtel-Dieu's outpatient clinic. Marie published his findings the following year in a dense, statistical three-page article in Le progrès médical.[65] Among patients at the hospital that he characterized as middle- or upper-class, Marie discovered a rough equivalency of hysterical symptoms between the two sexes. For patients from "the so-called inferior classes," which is to say the majority of patients at this municipal facility, the results were disproportionately in favor of males. Out of 704 cases manifesting hysterical symptoms in Marie's study over a period of 60 days, 525 patients were men and 179 were women! Among these males, Marie maintained, 25 suffered from "massive hysteria."[66] "This result," the author concedes, "is obviously entirely unexpected; convinced as I had been for a long time of the frequency of hysteria in men, I had no desire to maintain a proposition that seemed so paradoxical: *that hysteria is much more frequent in men than in women.*"[67]

Less than a decade after Charcot had endorsed the 1:20 ratio, a clinical study undertaken by a leading French neurologist and published in a high-profile journal contended that a class of illnesses that for centuries had been restricted to women in fact occurred in equal if not greater numbers in the opposite sex. At least two subsequent studies conducted in the 1880s corroborated Marie's startling findings.[68] By 1890, statistical disproportion, the single most conspicuous element previously separating constructions of male and female hysteria, had been removed in French avant-garde medical thinking.

As the male hysteria concept caught on, three new groups of patients were brought under its diagnostic purview, each of which occupied a special position in the French national imagination. First to appear was a spate of French-language dissertations on functional nervous disorders in children. In *Hystérie chez les jeunes garçons* (1884), Dr. Léon Casaubon discussed 23 cases of juvenile hysterics that he had culled from Paris hospitals.[69] The fullest study was published in 1888 by a Finnish medical student writing in French. Saluting Charcot in his introduction, Arthur Clopatt went on to present no fewer than 272 instances of childhood hysteria—

more than one-third of the cases in boys. The patients in Clopatt's study ranged in age from 18 months to mid-adolescence.[70] Another noteworthy text was Dr. Hélène Goldspiegel's *Contribution à l'étude de l'hystérie chez les enfants* (1888). The first woman to write a dissertation under Charcot's direction, Goldspiegel presented the stories of six "precocious hysterics" whom she encountered in 1888 at the children's ward of the Salpêtrière. Goldspiegel argued that hysteria could even be found in children from the very first year of life. She projected a ratio of one hysterical boy for every two hysterical girls.[71]

During the early 1890s, French physicians identified hysteria in a second new patient population as well—the peasantry. In Auguste Klein's pioneering 1880 study, 3 out of 57 hysterical patients issued from solid peasant stock.[72] Other medical authors had observed in passing that a certain patient was a farmer, sheep herder, or dairy worker.[73] These scattered cases, however, became the subject of systematic investigation in the writings of Dr. Firmin Terrien. The director of a private *maison de santé* in Nantes who also maintained a thriving medical practice in the Breton countryside, Terrien presented a grim message:

> The worker in the fields is no longer the happy man of earlier times. . . . The psychoneuroses [*psychonévroses*], far from being rarer among peasants, are rather on the increase. . . . It is impossible to deny that neuropaths are extremely common today among peasants. We find among them many hysterics and, based on my personal experience, more than in the towns.

Terrien proceeded to detail 31 cases of hysterical fits, tics, twitches, trembling, fainting, hiccups, paralyses, coughs, and contractures drawn from his country clientele. Twenty-two were men.[74]

Men in the military comprised the third and most sensitive category brought within hysteria's diagnostic orbit during the last decades of the century. French medical writing about "l'hystérique soldat" in this period included nearly thirty articles and a number of medical dissertations. In Klein's study, 11 out of 57 of his male patients for whom an occupation was cited, or a fifth of the total, were soldiers. In the same year Dr. Léopold Jannet, a doctor at the naval base in Rochefort, published a study describing hysterical symptoms in six sailors.[75] Several years later, a practitioner in Brussels wrote in an army sanitation journal that "male hysteria should in my humble opinion strongly interest the military doctor" and went on to explain that he had personally observed many cases of the malady in the Belgian army.[76] Another French investigation of nervous disorders among select classes and occupations, this one dating from 1885, concluded startlingly that "the profession furnishing the largest number of hysterics is the military."[77]

The most in-depth analysis appeared in 1886. Dr. Émile Duponchel of the Val-de-Grâce military medical hospital in Paris produced a long and controversial article in the *Revue de médecine,* bluntly entitled "Hysteria in the Army."[78] "Scarcely a year ago," Duponchel announces at the outset, "a title such as this would certainly have seemed improbable"; and today, he acknowledges, "there are people who still would be tempted to smile" at the idea. But, the author insists, "my colleagues who will look for hysteria in the army and among recruits will often find it. . . . In the general nosology [of diseases] in the army, hysteria occupies an important place which has not been suspected until the present."[79]

Duponchel then illustrates his unprecedented claim with six case histories drawn from his recent practice. These include the stories of "Antoine Br.," a 23-year-old infantryman who collapsed with fits, gagging, and skin anesthesias, and "Ric.," a Marseilles trumpeter in the sixth French regiment afflicted with convulsions and color-blindness. Most dramatic among Duponchel's cases is "Sing." A soldier in the 122nd infantry, Sing experienced bouts of deafness, an inability to urinate, creeping zones of insensibility in his right arm, and occasional violent convulsions. The young man's seizures were often preceded by "small suffocations" that could be instigated by applying pressure to the top of his head or the right side of his groin.[80] Duponchel concludes his 1886 study with reflections on practical questions of recruitment, discharge, and compensation. The entire "delicate matter" of nervous disorders among soldiers, he warns, has extremely serious implications for government policy.[81]

Each of these "new" patient groups in late-nineteenth-century French medicine had clear social and cultural associations. In the bourgeois family order, children, the fragile future of the French nation, were typically believed to be free of various stigmatizing pathologies that beset adults. Analogously, the Rousseauvian myth of the peasant, recently restated in Émile Zola's novels, envisioned the French peasantry as the source of national regeneration. And the discovery of rampant hysteria in the French armed forces emerged in the mid-1880s, just as hostile *revanchiste* sentiment directed against Germany was at its high point. French soldiers, supposedly the finest specimens of French republican manhood, could hardly be expected to defend *la patrie* in the inevitable future war if they were infected with hysteria. Despite these contexts and concerns, French doctors were undeterred in applying the diagnosis of male hysteria to these populations.

FIN-DE-SIÈCLE MEDICAL literature on masculine hysteria probed new clinical manifestations of the disorder as well. The case reports published around and after Charcot are typically more detailed biographically than Charcot's terse narratives, revealing a greater awareness of subjective, emotional factors in the lives of patients. The most conspicuous change in the symptomatological construction of these cases, however, concerns sexuality. In contrast to Charcot's studied silence on the subject, countless other case histories of male hysteria published in the 1880s and 1890s are filled with sexual observations and prescriptions that suggest the degree to which troubled sexuality was a component in the psychological suffering of men diagnosed with hysteria at this time.

Hysteria doctors in fact questioned male patients in depth about their sex lives. Physicians routinely inspected their patients' genitalia and recorded pelvic pain, undescended testicles, prostate problems, and irregularities of size or formation. They also noted what they regarded as excesses or eccentricities of sexual behavior. Among the 78 men in Klein's study, there were innumerable instances of impotence, testicular pain, "spermatorrhea," and pain with intercourse. One patient described "a sharp pain in the right side of the groin . . . accompanied by continual erections." Of another, Klein noted: "first attack following intercourse."[82] In the *Gazette des hôpitaux,* Dr. Moty reported in 1885 that a male hysteric in his care displayed anaphrodisia, or diminution of sexual desire. A second complained of "an irritable testicle," while a third reported "peculiar sensations in the sexual parts."[83] Three out of the five men discussed in Dr. Maricourt's dissertation were afflicted with "testicular anesthesias."[84] Likewise, a prominent member of the Montpellier medical community stated in 1892 that "genital asthenia," or progressive diminution of the sexual drive to the point of frigidity, is "a cardinal symptom" of hysteria in men.[85] Drs. Ingelrans and Brongniart of Lille described a hysterical patient who had forced himself to go to prostitutes in an effort to overcome his lethargy but was unable to perform because of "weak erections."[86]

Just as with the female cases in the *Iconographie photographique de la Salpêtrière (IPS)*, the male hysterical attack could be a highly eroticized performance. In the prestigious *Annales médico-psychologiques*, Dr. Fabre from the Vaucluse asylum in the outskirts of Paris gave the following account of his patient:

> The least contact in the pubic area provokes cries like those of a pig being slaughtered. . . . At the beginning [of the fit], pelvic movements back and forth similar to those during the act of coitus and that have been seen in the libidinous forms of hysteria. We have observed no erection, emission, or ejaculation. . . . When the seizure is terminated, the patient reports the sensation of a ball rising from the genital region to the throat.[87]

In many published cases, the concern with sexuality extends from the description of symptoms to the physical examination of patients and the prescription of treatments. Charcot isolated cases of "male ovarian hysteria." Accordingly, other French practitioners now followed suit: "It is natural," explained Klein, "to see if compression of the male ovary, the testicle, would not have an analogous action on the course of hysterical attacks in men."[88] Indeed, scores of male patients labeled hysterics—especially those with convulsions—were subjected to pressure from the male physician's hand to the testes or seminal gland.[89] Testicular compression sometimes caused a decrease in the severity of a hysterical attack. Not surprisingly, however, it more often than not elicited from patients a sharply negative reaction. Writing in the popular *Union médicale* in 1883, Dr. Sevestre reported another kind of response:

> Examining the stomach and testes, we confirmed a phenomenon that is interesting in light of what exists in the female hys-

teric. The abdomen is supple and easily depressed. . . . Pressure
on the left testicle causes either a sharp pain or the peculiar sensation of a sort of voluptuous suffering [*une sorte de souffrance
voluptueuse*] producing a very distinctive facial expression.[90]

In several instances, medical staff provoked exhausting artificial seizures through the manual manipulation of genital hysterogenic
zones in their male patients. Two Bordeaux doctors reported that

the only hysterogenic zone noted in 'G.' occupies the testicle
and the tract of the spermatic cord almost as far as the groin on
the right side. The skin of the scrotum on this side is extremely
sensitive, and when you pinch it strongly you produce exactly the same effects as if you compress the testicle itself or the
cord, i.e., the development or the arrest of the attack as the case
may be.[91]

Some of the lengthiest case histories in fin-de-siècle French
medicine present quite extravagant clinical portraits. The story of
"Louis V." during the mid-1880s is especially valuable because at
least six different doctors recorded it, including Théodule Ribot,
France's first professor of experimental psychology at the Sorbonne,
and Henri Legrand du Saulle, chief physician at the Paris Police
Prefecture.[92]

"Louis V."—a barely concealed pseudonym for Louis Vivé—had
in young manhood been a sailor in the French navy. During his
military service he had served an 18-month prison term for petty
theft. One day when he was working in the prison quarry, a snake
lunged at him and nearly bit him on the left forearm. Terrified by
the incident, Louis V. soon afterwards began to lapse into uncontrollable fits of shaking. Fearing insanity, his local doctor transferred

him to the Bicêtre hospital outside Paris. Upon admission, Louis V. complained of intermittent seizures and paralysis of the fingers and forearm on the left side, where the snake had nearly bitten him. Then, during the autumn of 1883, Louis V. entered a period of especially creative symptom formation. From day to day, he suffered variously from stomach cramps, bouts of nausea, "a capricious appetite," loud gagging, spitting blood, and cold sweats. In late January of 1884, hospital doctors detected labored breathing and color-blindness that moved between the left and right eyes. On January 26, they observed contractures of the extremities as well as partial deafness.[93]

Suspecting hysteria, Dr. Jules Voisin transferred Louis V. to Charcot's neurology clinic at the Salpêtrière. Charcot personally performed further tests on the patient and discovered a still more florid set of symptoms, including "neuromuscular hyperexcitability" in the trunk of the body and three hysterogenic zones—in his eyelids, testes, and left Achilles tendon. A month later, Salpêtrière doctors recorded loss of the sense of smell in the right nostril and taste on the left side of the tongue.[94] Dr. Quinqueton stated that the patient "believes he has been chained to his bed by the orders of Charcot. He is furious at him, threatens to kill him, and talks of suicide. . . ."[95] Dr. Berjon commented further on the patient's "erotic dispositions": "He has wanton cravings [*il y a du satyriasis*], often accompanied by nocturnal emissions."[96]

During his seizures, Louis V. often displayed the stylized positions that, as one doctor noted, "are so often found in our female hysterics."[97] In the course of his *grandes mouvements,* his eyelids fluttered, and he flew into ventral and lateral arch positions. Several times, he broke his wooden bed and required physical restraint by the staff.[98] During his *période des attitudes passionnelles,* the patient experienced "terrifying hallucinations" of snakes. "He screams out and tears at his clothes. His facial features are distorted. We calm him down by assuring him that we have killed the snake," reads another account.[99] During one attack "a voluptuous phase" occurred, characterized by "erotic ideas," "vulgar gestures," and "rhythmic pelvic projections." A night nurse confirmed that during one such episode the patient achieved ejaculation.[100]

During his spectacular hospital stay, Louis V. also became the subject of much experimental testing. Staff members charted his shifting anesthesias with electrical tests and by running needles across his body. Nurses administered purgatives, anti-spasmodics, stimulants, and vomatives. Doctors sometimes terminated the patient's attacks through the forced administration of chloroform or the "energetic compression of the left testicle."[101] His medical handlers also hypnotized Louis V. numerous times and thereby manipulated his symptoms experimentally. Dr. Voisin branded the patient "a man seized with burning hysteria, convulsive and nonconvulsive, with extremely multiple symptoms."[102] In March 1885, after stealing money from an employee at a Paris hospital and disguising himself as a nurse, the patient escaped from the hospital. At this point, he vanishes from the medical-historical record.

French physicians a century ago perceived Louis Vivé as exceptional. He was not, however, wholly unique, and several similarly flamboyant cases came out of the French medical world during these years.[103] Charcot's case histories are centered on a sequence of chiefly neurological symptoms occurring in relatively narrow sociological categories of patients who had had physical accidents. In contrast, the writings produced by Charcot's contemporaries, as exemplified by Louis Vivé's saga, consist of more detailed and individualized case reports. They hystericized a wider population of adult men and presented an enlarged repertoire of symptoms and behaviors, including sexual behaviors and psychological states formerly reserved for female hysteria. Moreover, the projected gap in the statistical occurrence of hysteria between the sexes narrowed greatly in these studies. All of these changes worked in the same direction: they involved ever closer equivalences of the medical models of male and female hysteria. With Louis Vivé and a small circle of patients like him, the theatricalization of the disorder also came to incorporate men. In their descriptive drama, in the medical attention lavished on them, and in their cultural celebrity, these cases of *grandes hystériques masculines* rivaled their contemporary female counterparts. On point after point, French medical models of male and female hysteria were converging in the late nineteenth century.

By the mid-1880s, the School of the Salpêtrière was associated internationally with research on the functional nervous disorders in men. In a Paris dissertation completed in 1890, Dr. Jacques Roubinovitch observed that once the question of "hystérie virile" had been "a regrettable medical lacuna" in our knowledge. "But in the last twenty years," Roubinovitch continued, "a reaction . . . has completely changed the state of the question, and everyone today, with rare exceptions, believes in male hysteria, which has become the subject of a considerable volume of scientific literature in France and abroad."[104] In May 1891, Charcot acknowledged that "thanks to the work of the French school . . . masculine hysteria has taken an important place in the clinical medicine of Parisian hospitals where they have learned to recognize this type of illness."[105] Hysteria in the male sex, it would seem, had finally received its due.

OR HAD IT? It would be easy, as well as tidy from an interpretive and ideological perspective, to end our analysis at this point: submerged for centuries in ignorance, the European scientific community suddenly and unanimously became enlightened about a forbidden subject through systematic and dispassionate clinical investigation. But the full story is more complicated. If we probe deeper, we find within European medicine of the late nineteenth century a strong counter-current of resistance to the idea and the reality of masculine hysterical neurosis. It is not difficult to surmise why. The new writing on male neurotic vulnerability made doctors nervous. The medical literature of Charcot's time suggested the error of generations, if not millennia, of past Western medicine. The notion that men were as susceptible as women to hysterical pathology ran counter to prevailing patriarchal ideals and seemed to entail the need for a substantially revised understanding of masculine human nature. The implications of this idea called into question the accuracy and adequacy of the entire separate-spheres doctrine. Indeed, the male hysteria project opened up an extremely sensitive area—the idea of a component of mental and emotional femininity in the male psyche itself. Many physicians in late Victorian Europe, including the very authors of the medical literature reviewed above, did not welcome these possibilities. As a result, they responded with notable ambivalence to the implications of their own work.

On closer inspection, the medical discourse of male hysteria during the 1880s and 1890s repeatedly exhibits a set of rhetorical and interpretive strategies of resistance. These techniques of avoidance operated in one of two ways: *strategies of definition* manipulated the clinical content of the hysteria diagnosis—its projected nature, causes, and symptoms—toward a certain end, while *strategies of deployment* controlled when, how often, and to whom the diagnosis was applied.

"Until the present time," observed Briquet in 1859, "we saw little hysteria in men because we did not want to see it."[106] The first indication that this cultivated myopia persisted into the Charcot years comes from the pedagogical literature of the day. Given the volume of writing on the subject, we would expect male hysteria to have entered quickly into medical textbooks, dictionaries, and encyclopedias. But this was not the case. In the sources that represent the official codification of medical knowledge at the time, the topic is almost entirely absent. The second edition of the *Traité des névroses* (1883) by Drs. Alexandre Axenfeld and Henri Huchard, which claimed to reflect the cutting edge of the field, discusses many aspects of Charcot's work but never mentions male hysteria.[107] Dr. William Gowers, arguably the most distinguished British neurologist of his time, included a discerning 40-page discussion of hysteria in his highly influential *Manual of Diseases of the Nervous System* (1888; reprinted in 1893), yet neither edition of Gowers' classic text discusses hysteria in men.[108] In the standard American neurology textbooks by Horatio Wood, William Hammond, and Charles Dana, there is next to no discussion of hysterical symptoms in male populations, even though these works include substantial presentations on hysteria.[109] Two widely consulted Anglo-American medical manuals at the turn of the century, *Allbutt's System of Medicine* (1898) and *Saunder's Medical Hand Atlas* (1901), include only a single phrase on the subject and the *Lehrbuch der Nervenkrankheiten* of Dr. Hermann Oppenheim does not discuss it.[110]

Other works of medical reference were more explicit in their opposition. One of the longest entries in the *Nouveau dictionnaire de médecine et de chirurgie pratiques* of 1884 is dedicated to hysteria. In it, Dr. Gustave Bernutz concedes at the outset that "hysteria exists incontestably in men," but follows with a disclaimer: "The proportion of one out of twenty given by Briquet is certainly much too high; one out of a hundred, which gives us approximately ten cases of male hysteria for every one thousand female cases . . . still ap-

pears too much to me and exaggerated by the exceptional public-
ity given to unprecedented cases."[111] Bernutz later comments that
he has personally encountered only a single true case of hysteria in
a man, and he proceeds in his 120-page exposition to discuss the
disorder as an exclusively female malady. In the same spirit, Charles
Berger asks rhetorically in his *Principes élémentaires de la neurologie
clinique* of 1886, "Is it true that men have been hysterical? We are
inclined to believe that this malady is . . . a sad attribute of the feminine sex," he answers. "We do not deny that a very small number
of men have experienced the sensation of a ball rising in the throat;
but is this sufficient to qualify as an hysterical attack?"[112] In his
pungent and opinionated book entitled *Les hystériques* (1883),
Henri Legrand du Saulle, the senior physician at the Paris Police
Prefecture, affirmed that "hysteria is a malady of the feminine sex
par excellence. . . . This is a fact no one would try to dispute."[113]

In 1880, the eccentric medical dissertation of the naval doctor
Léopold Jannet went one step further, or rather backward.[114] Jannet
contended that Hippocrates and his followers had gotten it right
after all: "difficulties of genital function dominate the etiology of
hysteria." Concerning the disease in men, he stated that "masculine
hysteria . . . is so rare . . . that we military doctors have many other
fish to fry [*nous avons bien d'autres chats à fouetter*]."[115] Jannet was not
alone in his attempt to revive ancient Greco-Roman teachings in
the era of Charcot.[116] Remarkably, in French, British, German, and
American gynecology of the 1880s and 1890s the uterine model of
hysteria remained medical dogma, and citations of Charcot's work
in late-nineteenth-century gynecological texts are strictly limited
to his work on female hysteria.[117]

In the long nonhistory of male hysteria, simply ignoring the
subject had always been the easiest and most common technique of
resistance. As one late-twentieth-century critic commented, it was

as if through the ages there had been "a sort of unconscious complicity between male patients and male doctors to avoid the infamous and disgraceful diagnosis."[118] This tactic was particularly widespread in late Victorian Britain, perhaps because the prevailing code of middle-class masculinity was most stringent there. While French physicians flooded the medical world with books, dissertations, and articles on masculine hysteria, only a single book-length work, and no dissertations, by a British doctor or medical student appeared during the entire last two decades of the nineteenth century.[119] "Little or no attempt has . . . been made in this country to organize any collective investigation on this subject," complained one Edinburgh physician a year after Charcot's death.[120] Writing in 1892 in the *Dictionary of Psychological Medicine,* Dr. Horatio Donkin admitted that whereas male hysteria had been explored extensively by "the Paris neurologists" as a topic of scientific inquiry, "it has certainly been passed over too lightly by many English writers."[121]

Other authors developed subtler maneuvers that allowed them to support a medical idea perceived as avant-garde while at the same time distancing themselves from it. One linguistic strategy was to deploy alternative, less derogatory diagnoses for the clinical data brought to light by the Salpêtrians. In 1884, for instance, Dr. Audiffrent concluded that "the theory we have just given of hysteria does not allow us to say that this disease can exist in men. The cases of hysteria that have supposedly been verified in men are only cases of hypochondria and melancholia."[122] Five years later, in the new 1,500-page *Dictionnaire de médecine et de thérapeutique,* Dr. Eugène Bouchut equivocated similarly. Citing Landouzy for support, Bouchut writes that "men sometimes experience convulsive attacks similar to those in hysteria with the sensation of the *boule de cou,* but this is rare and these convulsions are nothing more than modified epilepsy."[123] In general, there was a much greater willingness in the late-nineteenth-century medical literature on hysteria to postulate an undiscovered organic basis for a case if the patient was male rather than female. A particularly clear British example is Dr. John S. Bristowe's "Hysteria and Its Counterfeit Presentments," published in the *Lancet* in 1885. Bristowe offers a series of studies in differential diagnosis in which he judges all the male cases to be other organic illnesses (anemia, epilepsy, tuberculosis, and hypertrophy of the esophagus), whereas the cases involving women retain their status as hysteria.[124] It is not uncommon in the late-nineteenth-century case-historical literature to encounter a male patient with, say, fits, a facial tic, and hysterogenic points who gets diagnosed as an obscure case of tertiary syphilis, multiple sclerosis, or tubercular meningitis. Dr. Fabre of Marseille, presumably with a straight face, proposed that many cases of so-called male hysteria were misdiagnosed dyspepsia.[125]

A related terminological tactic was to use hybrid diagnostic categories. In the late-nineteenth-century literature on masculine hysteria, diagnoses like "hystero-epilepsy," "hystero-neuropathy," and "traumatic hystero-neurasthenia" appear far more frequently with male than with female patients. In other cases, usage of the hysteria label is limited to the adjectival form, referring to specific symptom formations but never to a patient himself. A case of fainting, heart palpitations, or gastrointestinal pain might prove to be hysterical, but the patient himself was not so labeled.[126] In still other instances, doctors put the noun "hysteria" in quotation marks throughout their discussion of male patients.[127] Sometimes, they created new diagnostic language altogether. By accounting for hysterical symptoms in abstruse, scientistic language, physicians both displayed their prowess as men of specialized learning and avoided a pejorative label. Among fin-de-siècle surrogates for the hysteria diagnosis when applied specifically to men were such cumbersome neologisms as "neurospasmia," "neuropalia," "spasmodic encephalitis," and "acute cerebro-pneumogastric neuropathy"—little more than exercises in "diagnostic camouflage."[128]

A second category of strategy—the strategies of deployment rather than definition—involved whom the diagnosis was applied to. Charcot's was a theory of traumatic hysteria in males of the laboring class. In the entire French-language literature on male hysteria from the late 1800s, only two medical authors entertained a different social epidemiology of the disease.[129] The overwhelming majority of patients in the printed literature of the time had working-class parents, possessed little formal education, and earned a living with their hands as artisans or manual laborers. In Pierre Marie's study at the Hôtel Dieu, as we saw, the high ratio of male hysterics held true for "the so-called inferior classes" of society.[130] Similarly, based on an examination of two dozen patients from the Hôpital Broussais, Dr. Alexandre Souques concluded that hysteria in men was far more prevalent than had previously been suspected, but he quickly qualified the point: "If this deduction is true for the lower classes of society, it can hardly be applied to the comfortable, wealthy classes."[131] Cases drawn from private practices with well-off paying clients are conspicuously absent from the published literature on masculine hysterical disorders in this period. This glaring social exclusivity of the male hysteria diagnosis again served to distance middle-class male diagnosticians, and their readers, from an unpleasant behavioral reality in their midst.

Another group of individuals to whom French physicians enthusiastically affixed the hysteria label was characterized by sexual identity and gender traits. Earlier we saw Charcot's categorical views about hysteria, effeminacy, and homosexuality. "As Professor Charcot has shown a number of times in his magisterial lessons, we must permanently break with the idea that hysteria in a man is necessarily accompanied by a degree of feminism," insisted Dr. Paul Michaut in 1890.[132] Nevertheless, after the requisite genuflection before the master, many medical writers proceeded to re-introduce the lingering specter of gender indeterminacy.

Occasionally, French physicians lodged the unqualified accusation that male hysterics were homosexual. Several of Klein's patients, for instance, were described as displaying in their lives "a perversion of the moral and genital sense," which was sexologists' jargon for homosexuality.[133] More commonly, the charge was less direct but still transparent. In his 1886 study of hysterical breakdown in the French army, Duponchel observed that one hysterical soldier "carries with him cosmetic supplies, perfume, and obscene pictures."[134] Dr. Léopold Jannet described among his patients a 35-five-year old male hysteric named "Daugl.," who, "as his friends put it, 'is cold toward the opposite sex.'"[135] A detailed study conducted in 1891 by Drs. Paul Bourneville and Paul Sollier presented the case of 18-year-old Luçien Hir., who was plagued by fits. Concerning the patient's intimate behavior, Bourneville and Sollier wrote: "no masturbation; no sexual relations; he does not seek the companionship of young girls; however he touches and gladly embraces a male friend."[136] The previous year, one of Charcot's dissertation students related the story of a 21-year-old hysteria patient at the Salpêtrière labeled "a genital invert." The author wrote knowingly that the patient during his teen years had suffered from "uncontrollable erections when around certain of his male friends."[137]

In still other cases, an account of blatantly stereotyped dress or mannerisms served to convey the same meaning. Thus, Dr. Quinqueton claimed in 1886 that

certain men (the hysterical ones) clearly have a large number of characteristics belonging to the female sex. They are, in effect, men with narrow waists, a slender and shapely build, slightly developed breasts, no beard, fine silky hair, pale and soft skin. . . . Moreover, these men usually have underdeveloped genitals. The expression on their face is timid and gentle; their eyes, always lowered, are bright and languid, and their voice is soft, high-pitched, and affected like that of a woman.[138]

Dr. Colin contended in the same vein that the majority of men with hysteria "were close to women in character and inclination."[139] And Dr. Fabre, writing in the *Annales médico-psychologiques,* again surpassed his colleagues with his description of one middle-aged male patient:

Despite his very virile external appearance, Monsieur X likes to be dominated. . . . His genital organs are poorly developed. He cries and laughs easily according to circumstances and . . . emotions have a great effect on him. . . . His hips and pelvis are rounded. . . . We will find that individuals suffering from this neurosis provide certain physical and moral features that separate them from the biological sex to which they belong and push them, so to speak, toward a new sex defined above all by sexual neutrality and an exaggerated emotional impressionability.[140]

Thus, despite Charcot's innovative work, the male victim of hysteria in the late-nineteenth-century French medical imagination was still frequently envisioned as an effeminate heterosexual, an overt homosexual, or a physical or emotional hermaphrodite.[141]

The search for signs of perceived effeminacy in male patients with hysteria sometimes went to comical extremes. In 1888, Dr. Robert Marquézy described a 52-year-old patient named "Joseph

G." from the Hôpital Broussais in Paris who was married and in physically hearty condition. Nonetheless, Marquézy wrote that during his patient's childhood, his tastes "were those of a girl; he never left his mother and tended to all the housework with her."[142] Dr. Collineau likewise surmised that the early manifestations of hysteria in a 17-year-old boy included writing verse, reading novels, and listening to music.[143] And in his encyclopedia entry on hysteria, Dr. Bernutz cites a male patient who had "liv[ed] almost constantly with his highly hysterical mother."[144]

The effort to police hysteria's field of application assumed other forms, too. Doctors in the provinces routinely claimed that it was only in the overheated capital city where hysterical French men were found.[145] Using a parallel ploy, British physicians claimed that while sturdy Anglo-Saxon men were virtually immune from hysteria, the impressionable Latin races might well be inclined to the disease.[146] Far more serious for Charcot and his colleagues were accusations of this sort originating from France's despised foreign neighbor *outre-Rhin*. Unlikely as it may seem, the medical debate over male hysteria became entangled in the Franco-German cultural rivalry of the late nineteenth century.

Beginning in 1887, a number of articles in the central European medical press made the provocative accusation that male hysteria, if it existed at all, occurred only in France, as a sort of specialized national neurosis. In this view, French men were simply more *hystérisable* than their counterparts elsewhere in Europe—which, in the context of the time, meant that they were weaker, less virile, and more susceptible to degeneration. A few younger German neurologists and psychiatrists accepted Charcot's ideas on male hysteria,[147] but a vocal majority of German doctors rejected them.[148] A doctor from Leipzig, for instance, was said to dismiss the notion of hysteria in men as the concoction of a single, self-involved French physician. "A doctor can often contribute to the spread of hysteria and make an epidemic of it," he counseled his students. "In particular, do not waste much time on hysteria in men. Leave hysteria to women and children."[149]

In post-1870/71 France, these remarks struck a nerve, and the Parisian medical establishment reacted at once. In mid-November, 1887, *Le progrès médical* published the starkly titled "L'Hystérie en Allemagne [Hysteria in Germany]."[150] The unsigned article's appearance in the official organ of the Salpêtrière School left little doubt as to its provenance, and Pierre Marie later identified himself as the author. Marie did not mince words: the denial by German physicians of male hysteria reflected a "fit of scientific inhibition [*cet accès de pudeur scientifique*]" combined with "another curious sentiment, namely, racial arrogance."[151] Attempting to divide the German medical community, Marie observed that there are "a number of [German] doctors, better educated and certainly more open-minded, who have no difficulty declaring that hysteria . . . exists in Germany as elsewhere."[152] A month later Dr. Adolph Strümpell, the eminent director of a nerve clinic in Erlangen, decried the intrusion of petty nationalism into science: "It is regrettable that the great advances Charcot has made in the understanding of hysteria have still not become a standard part of the knowledge of German physicians." "Male hysteria," Strümpell added pointedly, "appears in our country exactly as it does in France and, most likely, in all other countries."[153]

With the exception of Mendel's and Strümpell's remarks, however, evidence for the widespread clinical reality of masculine hysteria continued to come almost exclusively from France. For this reason, doctors in Paris were elated when on March 11, 1889, two German physicians presented in a prominent German medical journal a case of hysteria in—unexpectedly—a Prussian soldier.

Written by Drs. Andrée and Knoblauch, the article appeared in the *Berliner klinische Wochenschrift* and described a case from a military hospital at Karlsruhe near the Alsatian border.[154] In his hospital lecture of March 19, 1889, Charcot himself commented wryly that "we see, then, that male hysteria is not, as we have heard from time to time, the exclusive product of French nationality. . . . Here we have a German soldier who is hysterical, and I am convinced that we could find similar cases in all the armies of the world."[155] Two months later, Georges Gilles de la Tourette, Charcot's most faithful follower, chimed in with "L'Hystérie dans l'armée allemande [Hysteria in the German Army]." The Karlsruhe case, Gilles de la Tourette maintained, "is the best response we can make to those German writers who doubt the existence of hysteria in men." He included in his article something that was absent from other medical writings on the topic: drawings, seven in total, of the soldier-patient, nude, in the throes of a full hysterical attack.[156] Here the medical culture wars over male hysteria remained, until a generation later when the topic resurfaced in the European literature on shell shock.

Fin-de-siècle French writing on masculine hysteria also contains many provocative comments regarding foreigners, including African, African-American, Arab, and eastern European Jewish men. In 1885, the *Gazette des hôpitaux* published the case of a hysterical soldier housed at a French military hospital in Constantinople. The primary significance of the case, the author stated, was "the sex and race of the patient." "We know," Dr. Moty continued confidently, "that the nervousness [*névrosisme*] of Arab men is much more pronounced than that of Europeans."[157] Two years later, in the prestigious *Archives de neurologie,* Dr. Lucas-Championnière reported that in his clinical experience African and south Asian men were more inclined to hysterical breakdown. In Algeria, where the food was

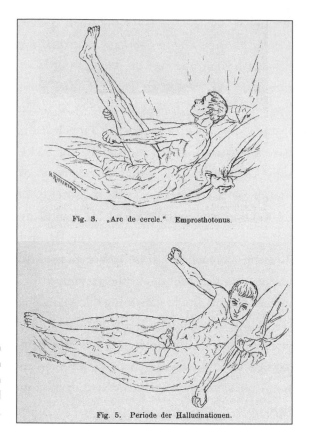

Fig. 3. „Arc de cercle." Emprosthotonus.

Fig. 5. Periode der Hallucinationen.

Drawings of a hysterical Prussian soldier from a German medical article in 1889.

spicy, Lucas-Championnière explained, hysterical anesthesias were "infinitely more common than in us."[158] Without citing particulars, he surmised further that certain Islamic religious rituals marked by wanton emotionalism fostered hysterical tendencies in Algerian boys from a young age. He also believed that Chinese and Mongolian men had "a nervous system much more emotive than ours" and thus a greater proclivity to hysteria than Europeans.[159]

Other French physicians applied similar analyses to other ethnopsychiatric subjects. In 1888, a short article on hysteria in black adult men appeared in a New York medical journal. The author, Dr. Ray of Washington, D.C., claimed to have made the remarkable retrospective discovery that hysteria had been extremely common among American slaves of the antebellum South. Ray informed readers that "the disease in all its forms is certainly very common now in the negro. Their low form of intelligence and emotional nature are both favorable to the disease." He illustrated these observations with two cases drawn from his recent practice. Ray's short article was quickly translated in the French journal *L'Encéphale*, where it appeared with an approving introductory commentary by the editor.[160] Dr. Rebourgeon, who practiced medicine in coastal Brazil, provided a similar Eurocentric account. Hysterical symptoms among the native men of the Amazon River basin, Rebourgeon claimed, were "extraordinarily frequent." "All forms of it are present, from the common convulsion to the great hysterical attack."[161]

No ethnic or national group was exempt from this line of accusation. Back in Paris, Dr. Collineau in 1887 published the first study of male hysteria from what purported to be a global anthropological perspective. Without any firsthand observations, Collineau speculated that rates of hysterical illness were high among Alaskan Eskimo men; that "seven-tenths" of the population of Greenland was gripped by the disease; and that the affliction was endemic among "the miserable Fuegians."[162] The lowest rates of hysteria, he added consolingly, were in "the temperate zones of the globe"— that is, western Europe.[163] In the same vein, British physicians, while reluctant to acknowledge hysterical neuroses among their own countrymen, were much less inhibited about applying the diagnosis to their far-flung colonial populations.[164]

European medical writing of the late nineteenth century also includes many statements about male hysterics who are Jewish. These comments chiefly concern what was widely regarded as the inordinate susceptibility of Jews to nervous and neurological infirmities. In his opening lecture of the *Leçons du mardi* in the fall of 1888, Charcot claimed that during a recent trip to a Jewish ghetto in Morocco he had observed every imaginable manifestation of neuropathology.[165] The following year, he related the story of a 23-year-old Hungarian Jewish man who suffered a paralyzed arm and partial loss of the sense of taste. Charcot pronounced the symptoms hysterical, adding that the patient, as a Jew, was "already especially predisposed to hysterical neurosis."[166] Two years earlier, Pierre Marie had pointed out facetiously that the same German universities that disparaged Charcot's work on hysteria were full of Jewish intellectuals, or "those predisposed par excellence" to the malady.[167] And Dr. Fulgence Raymond, the eventual successor to Charcot's chair on the Paris Medical Faculty, observed that "feminine and masculine hysteria is rather common in Warsaw. Hysterical men [there] are almost all Jews."[168]

Interestingly, the patients described in many of these passages are not only Jewish but non-French—specifically, Germans, Russians, eastern Europeans, North Africans—and, with only a few exceptions, they are adult men. The most complete coupling of the themes of male hysteria and the foreign-born Jew in nineteenth-century French medical discourse appears in an intriguing text by Dr. Henry Meige. One of Charcot's youngest pupils, Meige completed a dissertation in 1893, which he published serially in the *Nouvelle iconographie de la Salpêtrière.*[169] His topic was "the wandering Jew" as viewed from the perspective of contemporary medicine. In Meige's analysis, one of the wandering Jew's current incarnations was as a kind of medical vagabond, a full-time patient moving restlessly and relentlessly from hospital to hospital in search of a cure for his constant, ill-defined complaints.[170] Meige presents in vivid detail the stories of four such patients who in the course of their medical peregrinations journeyed to Paris to consult the

Salpêtrière master. The wandering Jews of the present age, Meige maintains, are actually "traveling neuropaths [*les névropathes voyageurs*]" who suffer from a bizarre "ambulatory neurosis." This rare compulsion, as he sees it, produces an obsessive drive to traverse large swaths of territory with no apparent aim or end. Two of these wanderers Meige describes as "frankly hysterical."[171] Four out of the five case histories involve men, and all five have German, Russian, Turkish, Hungarian, or Polish backgrounds. For each of his patients, Meige provides kinds of information that are notably absent from other published male hysteria cases of the day—the full and accurate name of the patient (rather than a pseudonym or truncated name), substantial biographical information, and full facial photographs.

In the centuries-long history of the non-recognition of male hysteria, the simple technique of denial was the most successful in suppressing the idea from the shared awareness of the male scientific establishment. During the later 1800s, however, largely because of the effects of Charcot's work, European physicians found it necessary to deploy an additional array of defensive procedures. These evasions, as we have seen, included a variety of tactics: acknowledging but then dismissing the male variant of the disorder as statistically negligible; using alternative, technical-sounding terminology to diagnose male patients; ascribing speculative organic etiologies to male (but not female) cases; camouflaging the diagnosis with less derogatory, more technical language; restricting the rubric to supposedly effeminate or homosexual men; applying the diagnosis only to males from certain cities, cultures, or nations; and illustrating the diagnosis with cases drawn from socially, ethnically, or racially stigmatized populations. These operations were feats of collective rationalization designed to deal with a discovery that was at once intellectually unavoidable, psychologically unsettling, and socially subversive. Taken together, these patterns of resistance kept a new and promising line of clinical inquiry from challenging the prevailing model of middle-class masculinity and the Victorian-Edwardian sex/gender system that it underpinned. Like so much Western biomedical commentary about gender in the late nineteenth century, the discourse on male hysteria from this era is fraught with evasions, tensions, and contradictions.

IN THE RICH gallery of fin-de-siècle hysterical males compiled so copiously by Charcot's colleagues, one figure conspicuously fails to appear: the white, Christian, middle-class, professional, heterosexual male. For this specimen, we must consult the novels, poems, plays, letters, and autobiographies of the age, where he appears in abundance.[172] It is not the madwoman in the attic of mid-Victorian times but the nervous man in the parlor who becomes the emblematic personality of this later generation. The neurotic susceptibility of these fictional characters is not an incidental feature but rather lies close to the core of their self-identities and their place in the social cosmos. Furthermore, to a far greater degree than earlier in the century, fin-de-siècle male nervousness was medicalized. Many creative writers of this generation read widely in the fields of medicine, psychology, and philosophy. Their mid-century "nervous precursors" were Flaubert, Baudelaire, Poe, and Goncharov. These writers formally assign the diagnoses of hysteria, nerve prostration, and sexual neurasthenia to large numbers of their male protagonists. Vague, quasi-clinical nervous symptoms of all sorts—exhaustion, insomnia, ennui, hypersensitivity—also proliferate in the fiction of the age. In many cases, it turns out, these nerve-related ailments marked the lives of both the authors and their fictional creations.

Late-nineteenth-century medicalized literary nervousness became a powerful form of critical commentary on middle-class Victorian masculinity and, beyond that, an implicit challenge to the entire polarized world of "man with the head and woman with the heart."[173] The work of the New Woman novelists directly critiqued conservative patriarchal ideology, including its medical stigmatizing of women.[174] Their novels centered on the need for new visions of femininity rather than masculinity, and thus they did not necessarily feature neuroticized males. Three other intertwining literary strands of the period, however, did address masculinity directly, and their leading characters could easily have been drawn from the medical case histories of the day.

First, the literature of French decadence peaked in the mid-1880s, at precisely the same time as medical interest in male hysteria was at its height.[175] The novels of J.-K. Huysmans, Catulle Mendès, Rémy de Gourmont, Rachilde, Joseph Péladan, Jean Lorrain, and Octave Mirbeau are full of adult men plagued by apathy and exhaustion to the verge of sterility. Fits—variously called epileptic, hysterical, and syphilitic—beset their characters. In Huysmans' novel *Against Nature* (1884), the "bible of French decadence," the Duc des Esseintes cultivates his tainted nervous heredity as a source of social eccentricity and sensory gratification. No stranger himself to nervous hypochondria, Huysmans had read Axenfeld and Huchard's *Traité des névroses* and Eugène Bouchut's *Nouveaux éléments de pathologie générale,* both recently out in new editions, for guidance in constructing his decadent hero.[176]

A gendered reading of the French decadent school also brings to light the large number of androgynes, hermaphrodites, transvestites, lesbians, and homosexuals in its novels and paintings. The literature of decadence is filled with mannish women and effeminate men, precisely the types of characters that Lombroso was classifying as degenerate criminals at the time, but here represented as the heroes of modernity. Degeneration meant degendering for these authors, and the feminization of the modern male in particular became a favored decadent theme.[177] In Anatole Baju's founding statement of the journal *Le Décadent* in 1886, "Man becomes more refined, more feminine, more divine."[178] And in a key scene of *Against Nature,* Des Esseintes stages a lavish dinner to mourn the death of his own virility, from too much sex, sensation, and excessive living. Like their fictional creations, Huysmans and his admirers developed dandified personae in high-society Paris and London, with the intention of shocking conservative, conformist sensibilities. Such decadent gender-bending was a deliberate rejection of the middle-class, Catholic, heterosexual, family-centered social regime, with its rigid assigning of male and female roles. Taking notice, the medical profession responded in character, by pathologizing the decadent movement itself.[179]

The British fin-de-siècle counterpart to French literary decadence was the aesthetic movement of Pater, Rossetti, Swinburne, Morris, Beardsley, and Wilde. In Britain, too, many artists and writers were advocating greater sensuality in life, a more artistic sensibility, and the cult of male friendship. Walter Pater's influential study *The Renaissance* (1873) and his novel *Marius the Epicurean* (1885) hold up purely artistic figures—Botticelli, Leonardo, Michelangelo—as models for emulation, rather than the humorless moral patriarchs of Victorian times. Beardsley's playful, virtuosic drawings are replete with swooning hermaphrodites and homoerotic innuendo. And Wilde, in his plays, novels, criticism, and aphorisms (as well as in his responses to the bench at trial), used wit and irony to lampoon patriarchy's conventions about marriage, the family, and sexuality.[180] Opponents of aestheticism understood that this rarefied program was dangerous both culturally and ideologically: it implied not just a bohemian pose but an alternative, possibly deviant, construction of masculinity, one that emphasized poetry, feeling, and cleverness over prose, respectability, and earnestness.[181]

A second relevant body of work during the closing decades of the century is the tradition of literary homosexuality, which began to form at the same time as the modern "medicalization" of the homosexual. The "love that dares not speak its name" in fact spoke up like never before in the late 1800s. Charles Baudelaire's *Les fleurs du mal* (1857), which the poet first intended to title *Les Lesbiennes,* and Walt Whitman's *Leaves of Grass* (1855), with its Calamus section, were the inspirational precursors of this tradition. The continuum of homosocial/homoerotic/homosexual literature flourished in Victorian and Edwardian Oxbridge.[182] Male gay autobiography also emerged in the late nineteenth century.[183] Rimbaud's *Season in Hell* (1873) includes many poems about his troubled relationship with fellow Symbolist poet Paul Verlaine, and among the decadents, Huysmans, Lorrain, Mirbeau, and Péladan depict homosexual scenes. A huge amount of homoerotic verse appeared during the age of Wilde.[184] In the traditions of Winckelmann and Pater, the adulation of classical civilization, with its uninhibited homoeroticism, was widespread. John Addington Symonds's two pioneering pamphlets, *A Problem in Greek Ethics* (1883) and *A Problem in Modern Ethics* (1891), were overt emancipationist statements. Heterosexual avant-garde literary intellectuals, too, like Shaw and Zola, spoke up with candor and enlightenment on the subject. Literary historians today emphasize that self-consciously homosexual writers occupied not just a notable but a central position in the literary avant garde of the late nineteenth and early twentieth century.[185] By definition, this emerging literary tradition dissented from compulsory heterosexual masculinity.

The third fin-de-siècle tradition of anti-Victorian writing that carried powerful meanings about gender is the literature of generational revolt. This was especially a British phenomenon, although other national cultures engaged the theme as well, as shown by Turgenev's *Fathers and Sons* (1862) and Strindberg's *The Son of a Servant* (1886).Victorianists have long noted that generational strife, and in particular father/son clashes, mark the literature of late-nineteenth and early-twentieth-century Britain. Interestingly enough, the textual prototype was Mill's *Autobiography* of 1873. Thomas Hardy published *Jude the Obscure* in 1895, the same year as Wilde's trial. In the novel, the stonemason Jude Fawley, who lacks a biological father, rejects with bitterness his teacher Richard Phillotson after a period of formative influence. Samuel Butler completed *The Way of All Flesh* in 1885, but, like Mill's autobiography, the book was published after the author's death, in 1903, to protect Butler's family. The novel depicts the young Ernest Pontifex's struggle to free himself from the stifling influences of his father, the parish vicar, and Dr. Skinner, the school director. Similarly, the best-known work in the literary tradition of filial rebellion, Edmund Gosse's *Father and Son* of 1907, relates the story of Gosse's efforts as a youth to separate himself from Philip Gosse, who was at once father, teacher, and fundamentalist. In Gosse's words, the book records "the struggle between two temperaments, two consciences, and almost two epochs"—and he might well have added between two visions of masculinity. Lytton Strachey's *Eminent Victorians* (1918), with its skewering of the Victorian age's heroes, caps the tradition at the end of the First World War.

These books by Mill, Hardy, Butler, Gosse, and Strachey appeared between 1873 and 1918, yet all of them dramatize emotional and psychological circumstances from the early and mid-Victorian period. In each work, young men in distress struggle to cast off the influence of overweening fathers, who have attempted to make their sons into replicas of themselves. The protagonists in each work specifically reject the teachings of such archetypes of Victorian patriarchal authority as clergymen, educators, schoolmasters, and imperialists. Viewed in gendered terms, these leading men of British letters were resisting the prevalent models of masculinity, whether their origins were Utilitarian/rationalist, as with Mill's and Matthew Arnold's fathers, or Calvinist/biblical, as with Thomas Carlyle and Charles Kingsley, or militarist/imperialist, as with Rudyard Kipling and Cecil Rhodes.

Needless to say, these rebellions against the strictures of Victorian manliness were fraught with stress, anxiety, and guilt. It could hardly have been otherwise. Like Mill with his nervous crisis of the mid-1820s, the literary protagonists of Hardy, Butler, Gosse, and Strachey—and quite often the authors themselves—endured their own hysterias, ranging from transient episodes of emotional breakdown to serious mental instability verging on madness. Moreover, in the cases of Flaubert, Symonds, Schnitzler, and Proust, the father-figures whom these literary hysterics repudiated were physicians. Among British male intellectuals, Ruskin, Spencer, Mill, Symonds, Gosse, Galton, Faraday, Lister, Sully, Benson, and Toynbee all suffered debilitating nervous maladies in the early years of their adulthood. Two reasons for their collapses were the struggle of young men with paternal authority and generalized anxiety about achieving the high standard of manliness expected by their families.[186]

Throughout these works of fiction, history, and autobiography, alternative versions of masculinity take shape. In the painful and protracted liberation from their stern, disapproving fathers, these literary men—like Mill, with his therapeutic discovery of Romantic poetry—became re-emotionalized. Wordsworth-like, they sought a reintegration of "manly intellect" and "feminine feeling." It was not just generational conflict that marked the British literary imagination of this period, but a quite specific trajectory of patriarchal upbringing, youthful rebellion, nervous collapse, emotional breakthrough, and mature feminized masculinity. If the rebellious daughters of late-nineteenth-century Europe took their struggle onto the streets, in the political form of history's first mass movement for suffrage, the revolt of the sons was set, more intimately and psychologically, inside the middle-class home.

To an impressive degree, the themes present in these three literary strands fuse in the life and literature of Marcel Proust, who seems the very prototype of turn-of-the-century literary neurasthenia. Proust's correspondence, literary criticism, early fiction, and final masterwork are saturated with the vocabulary of nervous dysfunction.[187] In each of these genres, Proust seems fascinated by the connections between psychological self-consciousness, artistic creativity, nervous vulnerability, and alternative sexuality. In his own life, Proust was a fragile, nervous, asthmatic child who clung to his mother. After her death in 1905, he spent two months in Boulogne-sur-Seine at the nerve clinic of Dr. Paul Sollier, a leading hysteria doctor in post–Charcot Paris.[188] As for Proust's father, Adrien Proust was Professor of Hygiene at the Paris Medical Faculty and the coauthor of a well-regarded manual on the preservation of nervous health.[189] Proust's reading from the 1890s onward included the writings of the leading nerve doctors of the day— Charcot, Ribot, Nordau, Janet, Dejerine, and Dubois—as well as his own father's work.

*In Search of Lost Time (À la recherche du temps perdu),* Proust's sprawling, multi-volume novel, appeared between 1913 and 1927. The narrator and central character is an aspiring but unproductive aesthete plagued by obsessions and a pathological lack of will power, who finally begins to write his great work only at the end of the story. The character Dr. Boulbon comments at one point that without nervous suffering there would be no great artists or scientists. Likewise, in the novel the nervous defects of Charlus and the emotional instability of the violinist Morel are inseparable from their artistic inclinations and activities. In Proust's world, the instincts, intuition, and ability necessary for cultural and intellectual creation of a high order seem inseparable from male nervous excitability and sensibility.[190]

Is it a coincidence that Proust—like Gosse, Wilde, Symonds, and Strachey—was gay and that his celebrated text features a spectrum of sexualities—the heterosexual Swann, the bisexual Odette, and the homosexual Charlus? Certainly as a writer, aesthete, decadent, homosexual, and neurasthenic, Proust stood well outside the conventional masculinities of his day. In fact, the major dichotomies of the age—Victorian/Modern, science/art, positivism/subjectivism, straight/gay, healthy/hysteric—all map directly onto Proust and his father. Adrien Proust's *Hygiène du neurasthénique* (1897) and Marcel Proust's *À la recherche du temps perdu* stand for alternative representations of male neurosis emerging a generation apart from the same family.[191] But whereas the physician-father produced a practical, moralizing medical manual, the literary son created a masterpiece of early European Modernism.[192]

To be sure, at the same time that the novelists discussed above were writing, other literary men of the time were championing traditional masculinities. The imperialist verse and fiction of Rudyard Kipling and the Catholic nationalist novels of Maurice Barrès reached much larger audiences than Huysmans, Hardy, Butler, and Gosse ever did. Adventure stories of empire, which projected male imperial power worldwide, were the most common reading among British boys and young men a hundred years ago.[193] The authors who challenged Victorian patriarchy were often personally uncertain and conflicted, and their biographies at times reveal that they were unable to free themselves fully from their own society's restrictive views.

Despite these qualifications, fundamental differences can be seen between the medical and literary representations of male neurosis during this period. As a professional culture, medicine remained far more masculine in its membership and masculinist in its profile. The two cultural fields enshrined the divergent ideals of objectivity and subjectivity. By the turn of the century a few medical intellectuals, such as Havelock Ellis and Magnus Hirschfeld, had begun to challenge directly the sex/gender system of the day. But the overwhelming majority of doctors during this period continued to defend the status quo energetically and to resist change. In contrast, New Woman novels, French decadent writing, the emerging gay literary tradition, and the British literature of filial rebellion were markedly more direct and powerful in their critiques. By the end of the long Victorian era and its Edwardian epilogue, these literary authors had mounted a full-throated assault on high Victorian masculinity. Moreover, they were far more imaginative than their medico-scientific contemporaries in conceiving alternative gender identities. In their fictional portrayals of the hystero-neurasthenic male, there is little evidence of the strategies of resistance that burden the medical texts of the 1880s and 1890s. Time and again, these poets, novelists, and autobiographers were able to hystericize both their characters and themselves. For them, male nervous vulnerability was an opportunity for self-exploration, not a cause for self-camouflage.

ONE FINAL SOURCE illuminates the relation between the scientific and the artistic traditions in Europe during the fin de siècle. The source is not textual but visual. French doctors during Charcot's

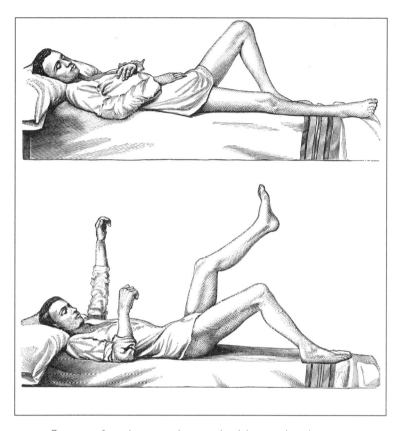

Drawings of a male patient diagnosed with hysterical catalepsy from *A Treatise on the Diseases of the Nervous System* (1891), written by the New York-based neurologist William A. Hammond.

generation, we know, liked to visualize female hysteria, and they did so over and over in dramatic detail. Brouillet's big painting (1887), Bourneville's glossy photographic volumes (1876–1880), and the line drawings in Paul Richer's *Études cliniques sur l'hystéro-épilepsie ou grande hystérie* (1885) successfully publicized the popular belle-époque image of the hysterical patient: a young adult female with her hair disheveled, head tossed back, limbs contorted, eyes rolling, body rigid and writhing erotically. In contrast, the medical literature on masculine hysteria is largely without illustrations. Proving the rule, the few exceptions consist of either photographs of foreign, ethnic male patients (as in Meige's dissertation) or characterless line drawings of stick figures. Certainly, there were no male counterparts to the extravagant, theatricalized renditions of Brouillet, Bourneville, and Richer.

Or were there? Such a source does in fact exist, but it has not previously been acknowledged or analyzed by medical historians. It consists of twelve black-and-white chronophotographs affixed to two pages of thin cardboard portraying an adult male patient in the throes of a full-fledged hysterical attack. In style and setting, the photographs resemble closely the hysterical women in the *Iconographie photographique de la Salpêtrière,* indicating that they too were taken at the studio of Dr. Albert Londe located in the new Service Photographique at the Salpêtrière. Handwritten notations at the top of the two pages read "Guinin," the patient's name, followed by "Salle no. 3" and "1885." At the bottom of the pages the identifying diagnosis, also in ink handwriting, reads "Attaque d'hystérie chez l'homme."

With these twelve images, the viewer finally sees the male hysterical body in full, uninhibited display: the patient, who appears to be in his late twenties or early thirties, is entirely nude. Londe's photographs capture him as he passes through the classic stages of the Charcotian attack, including the crucifix position and the lateral and ventral arched back movements. Viewed together, the consecutive positions call to mind the sequential snapshots of Eadweard Muybridge and Étienne-Jules Marey, which also date from the 1880s, of animals and people in motion—almost as if you could shuffle through the series to create a moving cartoon of a hysterical seizure. Squirming convulsively on a metal frame bed, the patient Guinin is surrounded by four male figures, all fully dressed, who stand at each post of the bed. Two of the figures appear to be male nurses with white aprons; another, dressed in a uniform with a leather cap, could be a policeman. No doctors and no women appear in the photographs. As the slender, well-built patient thrusts his pelvis upward and outward, the attendants gaze either at him or at the camera. The patient's face, buttocks, and penis are on full display. White sheets hang on the walls beside the bed.

By all indications, the patient in these striking photographs is the same man Charcot wrote about in his 1885 paper in *Le progrès médical,* which he later republished in the *Leçons sur les maladies du système nerveux.* In the later text, the case history of "Gui" is the third one in the two-part lecture "À propos de six cases de l'hystérie chez l'homme," which forms the eighteenth chapter of volume III of the *LMSN.*[194] This is also the lecture in which, more than any other of his writings, Charcot intended to establish programmatically the similarity of male and female hysteria, and it was Charcot's description of Gui's seizure that provided a model of the *grande attaque masculine.*

In the published case history, we learn that "Gui" was a 27-year-old locksmith who had fallen onto the street from a third-story balcony while working one day. Several months after the accident, Gui began having dizzy spells; his hands started to tremble; and he lost sensation over much of the right side of his body. In due course, he also had difficulties in speaking. His condition deteriorated, and eventually he began to lapse into "spasmodic seizures," which followed with textbook fidelity the stages of the Charcotian fit. Gui's convulsions were usually preceded by the sensation of a painful aura in his right testicle, which mounted upward through his abdominal and cardiac areas to the throat. He also manifested hysterogenic points in his scrotum and along "the spermatic cord almost as far as the groin on the right side," which upon digital

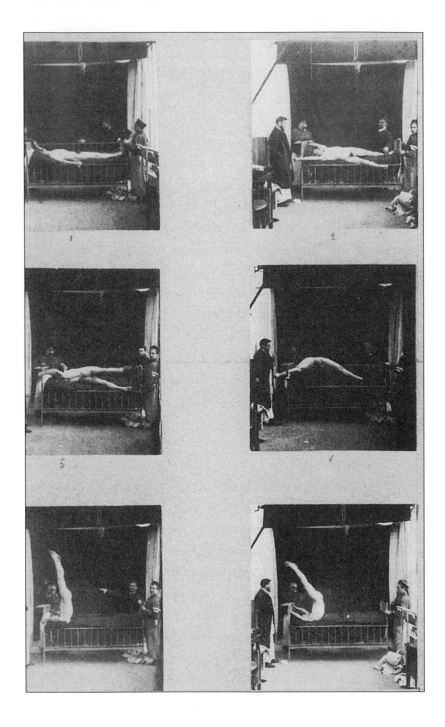

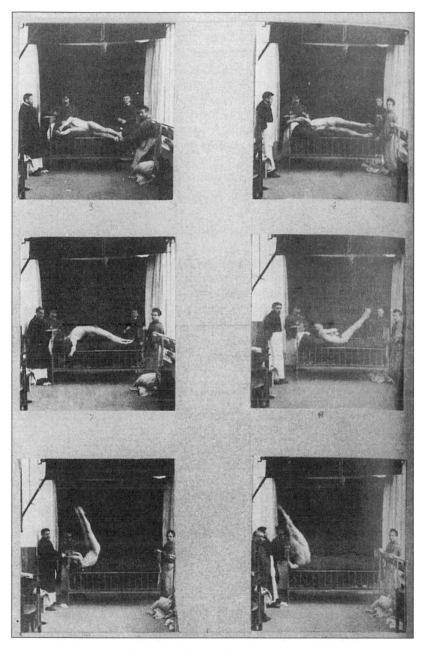

A two-page set of sequential photographs taken by Dr. Albert Londe at the Salpêtrière.

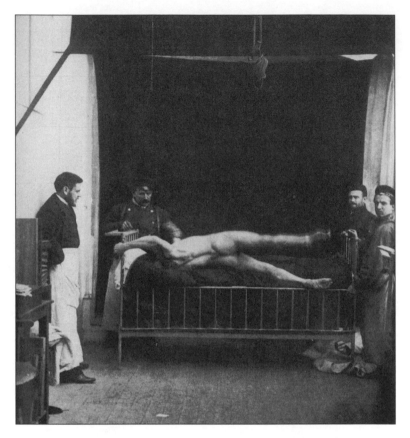

Close-up taken in 1885 at the photographic studio in Charcot's Paris hospital. The patient, named "Guinin," is in the throes of a classic hysterical attack.

stimulation could arouse or arrest an attack. Charcot presents the case as full-blown hysteria, commenting that "the attacks in Gui. yield nothing to those that we observe every day in our hystero-epileptics of the female sex." He obligingly adds that the hospital photographer Londe has captured the patient in images "that from the point of view of art . . . leave nothing to be desired."[195]

Despite their interest, quality, and drama, these photographs of male hysteria in pure form did not become part of the official

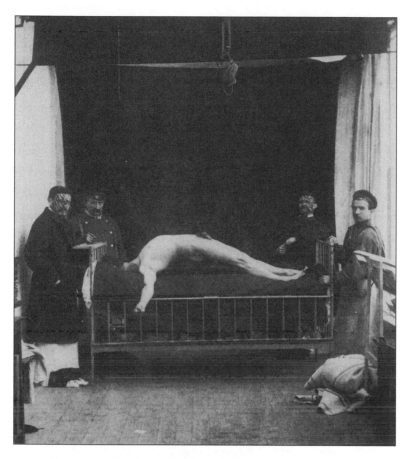

Guinin in another phase of the Charcot-style seizure.

archive of medical knowledge that was the Salpêtrière publishing industry. In 1887, when the first edition of the third volume
of Charcot's *Leçons sur les maladies du système nerveux* appeared,
the book did include five images of "Gui" derived from Londe's
work. But rather than displaying the photographs themselves, in all
their power, the images Charcot chose to print are lifeless black-
and-white engravings that omit the setting and the surrounding
personnel as well as the patient's facial features and genitalia.[196]

Likewise, although Bourneville's *Photographic Iconography* ceased publication in 1880, Londe's studio continued in full operation, but the images were never reproduced in the *Nouvelle iconographie de la Salpêtrière,* a successor series that began in 1888 and ran until 1918. Nor do they appear in Londe's several books on medical photography, or in Gilles de la Tourette's three authoritative volumes, or in any of the hundreds of publications on hysteria from the late nineteenth century. In fact, they were never reproduced in any printed medical text that I am aware of. For that matter, the photographs are not cited in French- or English-language scholarship on the iconography of hysteria, including Georges Didi-Huberman's 300-page study of the *IPS.*[197]

Londe's striking suite of images is known to us today because it was discovered in the private London studio of the twentieth-century British painter Francis Bacon. Soon after Bacon's death in 1992, and upon the settlement of the artist's estate, archivists and art historians began to sort through the contents of Bacon's famously chaotic studio at Reece Mews in South Kensington. Among the legendary mountains of clutter, they found a 20-page catalogue of a small exhibition staged in Paris at the Galerie Texbraun, an avant-garde photographic gallery on the rue Mazarine, in 1982.[198] Since the discovery of the catalogue, the photographs have been reproduced in a number of books about Bacon's art and the history of photography.[199]

The pamphlet catalogue includes in total about two dozen medical photographs from the Salpêtrière, representing hysteria and other neurological disorders. On the title page of the catalogue appear the names Hugues Autexier and François Braunschweig as well as the title of the exhibition, *De l'angoisse à l'extase. From Agony to Ecstasy* was also the title of a study of religious psychology by the

French psychologist Pierre Janet, which appeared in 1926; so it seems likely that Autexier and Braunschweig, who were Paris-based photography buyers and critics, assembled the collection of images, coordinated the exhibition, and printed the catalogue under Janet's well-known title. Bacon's copy is now housed in the Bacon Archive at Dublin City Gallery.[200] How Bacon acquired the pamphlet is easy to surmise: a lifelong Francophile, he considered Paris his second artistic home and visited often. In 1971–72, the Grand Palais in central Paris had staged a prestigious retrospective of Bacon's work.[201] Copies of the exhibition catalogue, which includes no publication date or ISBN, are rare today. How Autexier and Braunschweig obtained the photographs, and where the original chrono-photographic plates are today, if they still exist at all, is anyone's guess.

Surely there is more than one reason why Francis Bacon would have been attracted to these photographs. They are pictures of a young, good-looking naked man in vulnerable, quasi-coital positions, characteristics that the homosexual Bacon would have appreciated. But the artist was also no doubt struck by the expressive intensity of this modern medical inquisition. Londe's images in fact are highly reminiscent of Bacon's mature artistic style, which often features twisted and distorted male bodies confined in dark, box-like spaces in an atmosphere of fear, mystery, and violence. Like some of Bacon's best-known canvases, these images from the world of fin-de-siècle French medicine depict an adult man in an extreme psychological state, with blurred specters of the male body in painful motion. Some of the visual analogues between Charcot's theories, Londe's photographs, and Bacon's paintings are closer still: the crucifixion position, for instance, is one of the most recognizable poses of Charcot's convulsing hysterics, captured with "Gui" as

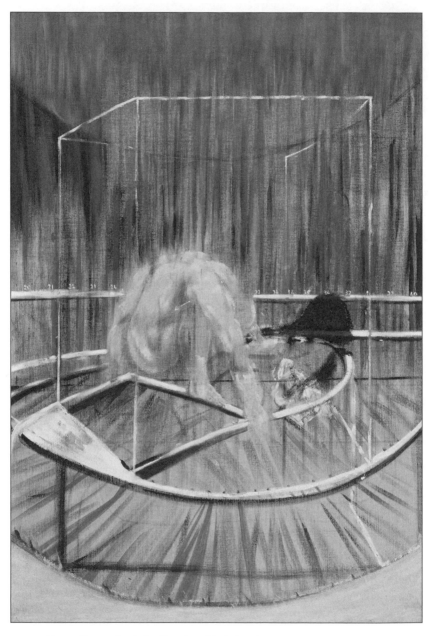

Francis Bacon, *Study for Crouching Nude* (1952).

well as the women patients in the *Iconographie photographique;* and some of Bacon's most arresting images take crucifixion as their subject.[202]

These photographs from the year 1885 are the most dramatic visualizations of male hysteria that I know of. Yet, in contrast to their female counterparts, they never entered the record of shared, permanent, cumulative knowledge that is the history of medicine. Their existence reveals unmistakably that the masculine medical gaze encountered male hysteria—naked, direct, convulsive—and systematically recorded and "objectified" that reality using the most up-to-date visual technologies. But the Salpêtrière physicians at the height of the heroic positivist era chose not to publicize this new knowledge, in either textual or iconographic forms, to the scientific world at large. It was, rather, three artists—two French photographers and an Anglo-Irish painter—who found sufficient meaning in these extraordinary images to acquire, preserve, and display them, and, beyond that, to draw inspiration from them in their own creative endeavors. It is through their efforts, not those of medical professionals, that these historic photographs have finally come to light.[203]

# CHAPTER 5

# Freud and the Origins of Psychoanalysis

FREUDIAN PSYCHOANALYSIS, the most influential set of psychological ideas in the twentieth century, began as a theory of and therapy for hysterical neurosis. Today Freud is associated with hysteria more closely than any other figure in medicine, so much so that some critics believe that with the lessening of the influence of psychoanalysis in the past few decades has come the disappearance of hysteria as a form of psychopathology. The role of psychoanalysis in the history of hysteria is in fact open to interpretation, and the place of hysteria in Freud's work has still not been fully reconstructed. In particular, Freud's engagement with the male hysteria concept represents an underappreciated element in the intellectual genesis of his system of ideas, a hitherto hidden genealogy of psychoanalytic thought. It is not a coincidence that Freudian psychology emerged during the twilight of the golden age of male hysteria in nineteenth-century France. Several themes that for generations had been only latent in the medical literature of masculine hysteria were for the first time theorized—and to great effect—by Freud during the closing years of the nineteenth and early years of the twentieth centuries.

FREUD'S HISTORIC ENCOUNTER with the great neurosis can be divided into four phases, running chronologically from 1885 to 1886, 1892 to 1896, 1896 to 1900, and 1900 to 1908. Stage one is the most explicit in its concern with male hysteria. During the autumn and winter months of 1885 and 1886, Freud traveled to Paris in order to study for several months at the Salpêtrière hospital and then returned to Vienna where he translated a book of Charcot's and delivered two lectures to medical audiences on what he had learned in the French capital.

By the summer of 1885, when he was twenty-nine, Freud had completed medical school as well as clinical residencies in several fields at the Vienna General Hospital, including work at Professor Theodor Meynert's psychiatric service. From 1882 to 1885, he had also worked in the physiological institute of Professor Ernst Brücke and in Meynert's Laboratory for Cerebral Anatomy. Abandoning a prospective career in laboratory research for financial reasons, Freud had decided to pursue a career in private practice, as a specialist in neuropathology. By the mid-1880s, he had numerous publications to his name that dealt with human and animal neuroanatomy and with the recently discovered drug cocaine. On the basis of these and other accomplishments, he had recently been appointed *Pivatdozent,* or Lecturer, at the University of Vienna. Since 1882, Freud had been engaged to be married to Martha Bernays, who lived outside of Hamburg in north Germany, some eight hours away by rail. In the summer of 1885, with his extensive medical education coming to an end and his independent professional career about to begin, he won an academic travel fellowship. Freud

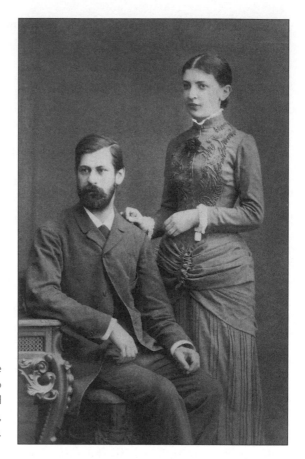

Freud, age 29, the year he left Vienna to study in Paris, seated beside his fiancée, Martha Bernays.

had been steeped in the Germanic tradition of materialist medicine, with special knowledge of "pathoanatomical psychiatry."[1] Not surprisingly, then, he looked outside the German-language medical world to apply his travel fellowship, and, as he later wrote in his autobiography of 1925, "in the distance shone the great name of Charcot."[2]

If Freud was at the beginning of his career in 1885, Charcot, fifty-nine years old, was at the zenith of his. By the mid-1880s, however, Charcot's medical thinking was at a decisive point: after decades of work using the proven techniques of pathological anatomy, he had become convinced that a class of maladies existed beyond the investigative reach of postmortem analysis and the microscope. Foremost among these ailments was hysteria. Still more controversially, Charcot had begun to use hypnosis with certain hysterical patients in order to artificially reproduce, induce, and remove their symptoms, a procedure that he believed established the ideogenic nature of the cases. Charcot's work, in other words, was taking a psychological turn just at the moment when Freud came to Paris. Nonscientific factors may also have contributed to the compatibility between Freud and Charcot: Charcot was a principled atheist and aggressive anti-clericalist, and his social circle included many Jewish friends and associates.

The city of Paris in the years 1885–1886 was the glittering cultural capital of Europe and home to its one large republican government. The cultural politics of the early Third Republic were playing out dramatically in favor of the anti-clerical republicans. The French legislature had recently passed laws to "laicize" public institutions, especially primary schools, and in 1884 the Naquet Law re-legalized divorce. Anti-German *revanchiste* sentiment, centered on the lost eastern provinces of Alsace and Lorraine, was at an all-time high, and in 1886 General Georges Boulanger was appointed Minister of War, launching Boulanger's alarming, if ill-fated, rise to right-wing power. The Dreyfus Affair was a decade away, but in 1886 the journalist Édouard Drumont published his poisonous book *Jewish France (La france juive)*, the most influential anti-Semitic diatribe in Europe before *Mein Kampf.*

Louis Pasteur's vaccination against rabies, a disease that terrorized the French countryside, was the most controversial event in French science during the mid-1880s. In the art world, the last exhibition of the Impressionist painters showcased Georges Seurat's stunning canvas *Sunday Afternoon on the Grand Jatte;* Auguste Rodin completed his voluptuous sculpture *The Kiss;* and Émile Zola's shocking proletarian novel *Germinal* was the literary *succès de scandale* of 1885–1886. Not surprisingly, these were eventful years in French psychology as well. A young and little-known provincial psychologist named Pierre Janet began to publish in the *Revue philosophique* case histories about a remarkable set of hysterical patients; the Sorbonne researcher Alfred Binet probed the unconscious in *The Psychology of Reasoning;* and the Nancy-based physician Hippolyte Bernheim codified his innovative ideas about the use of hypnosis in *Suggestive Therapeutics.*

Freud lived in Paris from October 13, 1885, to February 28, 1886, a total of about four and a half months. The major documents from this period of his life are the nearly daily letters he wrote to his fiancée Martha.[3] During his sojourn in belle époque Paris, Freud rented rooms in the Hôtel Brésil, located a block from the Jardin du Luxembourg, between the Sorbonne and the Panthéon. In his early letters from Paris, he mainly yearns for his fiancée, frets about his shortage of money, worries over his spoken French, and diagnoses himself as lazy. The sober young doctor does not seem to have appreciated, much less indulged in, the famous sensory delights of the city—drink, cuisine, cafés, cabarets, fashion, art, nightlife, or women. Outside of work, he made no French friends. Although he occasionally went to the theater, it was chiefly to brush up his French, and the experience gave him a headache. He never mentions the ravishing new face of Baron Haussmann's Paris. Nor does he discuss any of the political issues that roiled French life.

What did dazzle the young visitor from Vienna was Charcot. It is well known that Freud's stay in Paris was a pivotal moment in the prehistory of psychoanalysis, and that Freud idealized Charcot. Freud was impressed by everything about Charcot: his personality, his teaching methods, his relations with students (which, in their openness and equality, Freud experienced as distinctly French), his medical ideas, and his cultural taste. In a letter penned to Martha after his first month at the Salpêtrière, Freud rhapsodized:"I think I am changing a great deal. I will tell you in detail what is affecting me. Charcot, who is one of the greatest of physicians and a man whose common sense borders on genius, is simply wrecking all my aims and opinions." Freud goes on to liken Charcot to a revered French monument: "I sometimes come out of his lectures as from out of Notre Dame [Cathedral], with an entirely new idea about perfection."[4] Several years later, in his critical but admiring obituary of Charcot, Freud was still praising his teaching style: "As a teacher, Charcot was positively fascinating; each of his lectures was a little work of art in construction and composition; it was perfect in form, and so impressive that the words spoken resounded in one's ears and the subject demonstrated remained before one's eyes for the rest of the day."[5] Tellingly, images of creation and gestation recur in Freud's scattered remarks about Charcot. "Whether the seed [of Charcot's example] will ever bear fruit, I don't know," he wondered to Martha in late November, 1885, "but what I do know is that no other human being has ever affected me in the same way."[6]

What the older Charcot impregnated the younger Freud with during the winter of 1885–86 was the idea of male hysteria. Freud arrived in Paris intending to work in the Salpêtrière's pathology laboratory, on a study of cerebral paralyses in children. He found the project unchallenging, however, and by early December he had abandoned the microscope and workbench for the clinical investigation of the "functional nervous disorders" under Charcot's direction. "What impressed me most of all while I was with Charcot," Freud recalled in his autobiography, "were his latest investigations

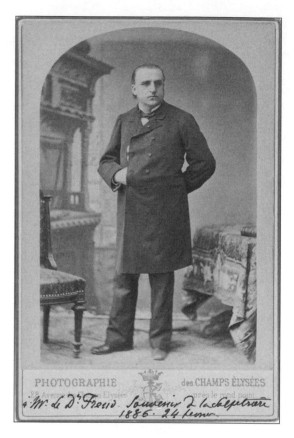

Photographic portrait of Charcot, in Napoleonic pose, inscribed by Charcot and given to Freud as a memento of his study trip to Paris.

upon hysteria, some of which were carried out under my own eyes."[7] Although it was an exaggeration, he claimed that Charcot earned "the fame of having been the first to explain hysteria."[8] By the middle years of the 1880s, several doctors were already beginning to question aspects of the Charcotian model of hysteria, but Freud embraced Charcot's teachings completely and uncritically. Especially compelling for him were Charcot's claim that hysteria was a genuine ailment and not the refuge of the malingerer, his categorical dismissal of genital etiologies of the malady, his establishment of the frequent occurrence of hysteria in men and its essential clinical equivalence with female hysteria, and his artificial production of hysterical paralyses and contractures using hypnotic suggestion.[9] In several cases that Freud found particularly suggestive, Charcot emphasized that the key causal factor in hysterical breakdown was the accumulation of traumatic experiences, which could be either physical or emotional in nature. All these points contrasted with what Freud regarded as the sterile, scientifically conservative approach to the neuroses taken by his professors back in Austria.

Male hysteria was front and center in Charcot's work during precisely the months Freud was in Paris. Charcot published cases of masculine hysteria between 1882 and 1893, but the greatest concentration of his publications on the topic occurred during the years 1885–1888. Included among these articles are "L'hystérie chez l'homme comparé à l'hystéric chez la femme," which appeared in the *Journal de la santé publique,* and the important two-part "Six Cases of Hysteria in Men," published in *Le progrès médical* in May 1885, in which Charcot presented to the world the case of "Gui." (Recall that Londe's photographs of "Gui" are dated 1885.) Several of Charcot's lectures delivered in the winter and spring of 1885–86 were later incorporated into the third volume of the *Leçons sur les maladies du système nerveux,* which Freud would translate.

Similarly, if we explore the Parisian medical press during these two years, male hysteria is everywhere. The Société Médicale des Hôpitaux was among the most active medical organizations in France. The records of the Society's weekly minutes, published in the *Gazette des hôpitaux,* reveal that at the meeting of November 15, 1885, Dr. Rendu presented a 28-year-old male patient with a hysterical brachial monoplegia. Two weeks later Dr. Debove, a Charcot protégé, offered a hysteria rediagnosis, cited above, of an earlier case of syphilis in a man. On December 11, 1885, Dr. Millard discussed a male case of left-sided hysterical hemianesthesia. And later that month Dr. Féréol presented two male patients, one an army veteran who had first developed hysterical seizures while a prisoner at Metz during the war fifteen years earlier.[10] Publications on hysteria in men likewise cascaded from the Parisian medical press during the months Freud was there.[11]

We know for certain that Freud occupied himself with male hysteria during his months in France. Charcot, Freud wrote after his return to Vienna, "began by reducing the connection of the neurosis with the genital system to its correct proportion, by demonstrating the unsuspected frequency of cases of male hysteria."[12] During his time at the Salpêtrière, Freud interacted regularly with Dr. Pierre Marie, Charcot's *chef de clinique* in 1885, who subsequently led the defense against German accusations that male hysteria occurred only west of the Rhine and who conducted the comparative study of male and female hysteria at the Hôtel Dieu. We can also assume that in his daily work at the hospital Freud visited all parts of Charcot's clinic for the nervous disorders, including the recently established Service des Hommes. In addition, Freud's work as Charcot's German translator engaged him in twenty clinical accounts of male hysteria, including the cases of Leon Brodsky, Francois X., Rig, Gil, Mark, Pin, Porcz, Charv, and Gui.[13] Upon completion of the translation, but before its publication in book form, Freud excerpted two chapters in a German medical periodical as a preview of the work; he chose the 23rd and 24th lectures, titled "On a Case of Hysterical Coxalgia in a Man, Resulting from an Accident."[14] In installments between 1892 and 1894, Freud also published a translation of another Charcot text concerning an additional 11 cases of male hysteria, most of them involving unnamed patients.[15] In all, between 1886 and 1893, Freud translated into his native language no fewer than 33 case histories of Charcot's dealing with hysteria in male subjects.

The most immediate consequence of this encounter between Freud and the French male hysteria tradition occurred when Freud returned to Vienna. Freud rather wistfully departed from Paris late in February, 1886, and after a stint in Berlin studying childhood diseases, he returned to Vienna and settled in, both professionally and personally. In April 1886 he opened a private medical practice, and on September 13, 1886, he finally married Martha Bernays. From the beginning, nervous disorders formed the mainstay of his fledgling clinical practice—"As a clinician I depend more than anything else on the study of hysteria," he conceded to Koller— and from this time onward, he treated both men and women.[16]

Soon after his return, Freud submitted to the University of Vienna an official document entitled "Report on My Studies in Paris and Berlin." The very first document in the first volume of the Standard Edition of Freud's complete English-language writings on psychology, the report offers an excellent sense of what Freud found most compelling during his Parisian interlude. He lavishes attention on Charcot and praises "the French school of neuropathology," which he quite undiplomatically presents as superior to its counterparts in the German lands.[17] Male hysteria crops up often in the report, and he cites Pierre Briquet twice. Freud notes that one topic particularly seized Charcot's attention: "The enormous practical importance of male hysteria (which is usually unrecognized) and particularly of the hysteria that follows upon trauma was illustrated by him from the case of a patient who for nearly three months formed the centerpoint of all Charcot's studies."[18] He brags that he spoke often and at length with Charcot about these clinical investigations. And he reports that "I had an

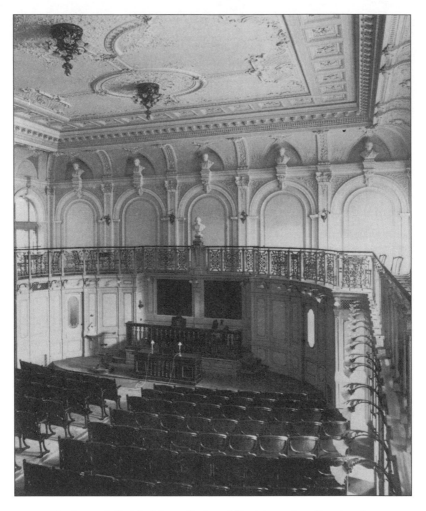

The lecture hall of the Vienna Society of Physicians, where Freud made his professional debut with a lecture on masculine hysteria on October 15, 1886.

opportunity of seeing a long series of patients, of examining them myself, and of hearing Charcot's opinions on them."[19]

Three months after completing the translation of Charcot's lectures, Freud went public with his new clinical interests by delivering a formal lecture to the Vienna Society of Physicians on the evening of October 15, 1886. The Gesellschaft der Ärzte in Wien was the most prestigious professional organization of its kind in the Austro-Hungarian capital, and a formal evening lecture in its white marble neo-Renaissance hall at the heart of the university in central Vienna would have been a significant event in a young doctor's career.[20] For his professional debut before the Viennese medical establishment, Freud, whether out of bravery or naiveté, chose to discuss—indeed, to champion—the idea of hysteria in the male sex. Titled simply "On Male Hysteria," his presentation focused on a single clinical example that Charcot had studied and Freud had observed while in Paris.[21]

The patient is an unnamed 18-year-old bricklayer's apprentice. The young man's defective heredity, according to Freud's presentation, includes an alcoholic father and a "nervous" sister. One day while at work, the patient fell several yards from a window onto the ground. He seemed uninjured at the time, but three days after the accident he began to feel scattered areas of anesthesia, both cutaneous and muscular, all over the left side of his body. His sense of hearing diminished, and he lost the perception of taste. In conversation, the patient was fretful and preoccupied with his health. After several weeks he began to experience generalized nervous fits, which then intensified, at times taking the form of a full-fledged, multi-stage hysterical attack. At his worst, Freud reports, the victim also manifested hysterogenic zones, on the left side of his chest and in his right testicle. At present, the patient was showing improvement with gradually returning sensation. His prognosis, Freud adds, is hopeful.

According to the secondhand reports of this lecture, Freud made several polemical points in the course of his descriptive narration: hysteria, he insisted at the podium, is not just a synonym for nervousness but is a discrete and delineable disease entity. The malady has a coherent clinical course. In most cases, patients aren't faking. Hysteria has nothing to do with the female reproductive organs, and the disorder in males is identical, symptomatologically and etiologically, to its better-publicized female form, although Freud qualified this by saying that in men, it is more often brought on by a physical trauma.

The summaries of the meeting all indicate that the audience's response to Freud's talk in 1886 was decidedly critical. Among the big names in attendance, some of them Freud's former professors, the internist Heinrich Bamberger announced that there was nothing new in Freud's presentation. The neurologist Moritz Rosenthal claimed that hysteria in men was widely known to exist, and that he himself had once published a case twenty years earlier. Meynert, who then occupied the Chair of Psychiatry at the University of Vienna, voiced his preference for an organic explanation of the described symptoms. Max Leidesdorf, another academic psychiatrist, proposed that "traumatic neurosis" rather than hysteria was a better diagnosis for the patient. There seem to have been few, if any, favorable comments from the audience. None of the respondents commented on what today we would probably judge to be the most clinically novel aspect of the case—that dual traumas of a mixed physical and emotional nature affected the patient over the years.

Most provocatively, Meynert, who was clearly irritated that his talented former student had been seduced by a professional rival and a Frenchman at that, scornfully challenged Freud to produce before the Society of Physicians a case akin to Charcot's but drawn from the hospitals of Vienna—a homegrown male hysteric, so to speak. This Freud did, but not without difficulty. According to him and other contemporaries, his efforts were blocked by senior university physicians at the Vienna General Hospital who, no doubt aware that this was risky professionally, chose not to give him access to their wards.[22] (Meynert and Freud in fact continued to cross swords until Meynert's death in 1892, but not without a deathbed conversion of sorts: in an eye-popping aside in *The Interpretation of Dreams* of 1900, Freud quotes Meynert as confessing to him during his final illness that "you know, I was always one of the clearest cases of male hysteria."[23] Regardless of whether it was true, factually or symbolically, the episode captures in miniature a fascinating dynamic: the masculine personification of positivistic science exerting himself to officially suppress the reality of hysteria that lurks just beneath the surface of his own sex.)

On November 24, 1886, five weeks after his earlier presentation, Freud did indeed bring before the Vienna Society of Physicians a fresh case of his own, one he had located from the private practice of a cooperative ophthalmologist. This time Freud published the lecture in the *Wiener medizinische Wochenschrift* under the title "Observation of a Severe Case of Hemi-Anaesthesia in a Hysterical Male."[24] The case involved a 29-year-old male engraver named "August P." Freud editorializes that this is "a very ordinary case of frequent occurrence, though one which may often be overlooked."[25] He highlights the patient's nervous ancestry and explains that three years earlier the patient had had a violent quarrel with his brother, in which he was nearly stabbed with a knife. Since then, August P. had developed increasingly debilitating symptoms. In order to demonstrate and demarcate the regions of sensory loss, Freud performed tests on the patient in front of his colleagues, which revealed several "hysterogenic zones," including one on the left side of the throat and one "along the course of the spermatic chord into the abdominal cavity to the area which in women is so often the site of 'ovaralgia.'"[26]

Most likely because the Society's schedule that November evening was crowded, there was no discussion of Freud's follow-up case. Freud, however, interpreted the silence as a sign of resistance to his ideas and as a personal snub. "This time I was applauded, but no further interest was taken in me," he complained with lingering bitterness in 1925. "The impression that the high authorities had rejected my innovations remained unshaken; and, with my hysteria in men and my production of hysterical paralyses by suggestion, I found myself forced into the opposition."[27]

Scholars have disagreed heatedly about the interpretation of these events.[28] Ultimately, what matters most is the subjective meaning of these experiences for Freud and their role in his subsequent intellectual biography. That Freud's half-year study at the Salpêtrière was a turning point in his career is well known.[29] More specifically, Freud's first publication on a psychological subject, his first two public presentations on psychopathology, and the first of his translations of other physicians' work all concerned hysteria in men. The first time Freud clashed with his professional elders—and therefore most likely the time when he began to realize the need to separate himself intellectually from the conservative medical majority of his day—also occurred in connection with his early study of hysterical males. Psychoanalysis originated as a theory and therapy of hysteria, the paradigmatic malady of fin-de-siècle Europe; but Freud's initial encounter with the neurosis began with his study of hysteria *in men*. Expounding the ideas and duplicating the observations of Charcot in the middle years of the 1880s, the future creator of psychoanalysis tentatively confronted for the first time the question of psychology and gender identity. Although Freud's first official pronouncements on the theme caused him much subjective distress, at a time when he was vulnerable both professionally and financially, he did not abandon the topic; rather, over the next two decades he continued to ponder the subject in various clinical arenas and theoretical incarnations.

DURING THE YEARS 1887 to 1896, Freud built up a steady medical practice, improved his financial standing, and, with Martha, reared six children. Intense and productive male relationships—at once personal, professional, and intellectual in nature—characterize this period, too, especially with Josef Breuer, a prominent family doctor specializing in internal medicine who was respected in Viennese scientific circles. By the late 1880s, Breuer had already communicated to the younger, appreciative Freud his story of the extraordinary patient whom they would later christen "Anna O.," the ur-patient of psychoanalysis. In effect, Breuer and his celebrated patient, Freud always acknowledged, co-discovered the cathartic treatment of the neuroses.[30] During the five years between 1887 and 1892, Freud published almost nothing. In light of the fundamental changes in his thinking about hysteria when he did begin writing again, however, it is clear that these were not fallow years intellectually but rather that Freud's ideas, like Charcot's latent traumas, were incubating.

Subsequently, between 1892 and 1897, Freud produced a highly impressive succession of publications that, taken together, propound the early psychoanalytic theory of the neuroses.[31] In comparison with his writings from the 1880s, what is most striking about this sequence of texts is the intellectual turn away from Charcot. One way to read the emergence of a specifically Freudian theory of hysteria in the 1890s, in fact, is as the story of Freud's growing distance from Salpêtrière orthodoxy.[32] As early as an 1888 entry on hysteria in a German medical dictionary, Freud departed from his former mentor: the article loyally restates Charcotian doctrine—with the significant exception of its long closing paragraph, in which Freud introduces Breuer's idea of hypnotically tracing the "psychical pre-history" of hysterical symptoms and exploring the "unconscious ideational life" of the patient.[33] Then, in editorializing footnotes to a second volume of Charcot's clinical lessons, published between 1892 and 1894, Freud pointedly and rather presumptuously dissented from key elements of Charcot's teachings in the very text he was translating. Although he preserved their collegiality in correspondence, Charcot, then in the final months of his life, was miffed.[34]

Coincidentally or not, Freud's major statements of independence appeared in the immediate wake of the most important event in a man's intellectual life, the death of his professional father-figures. Between 1892 and 1893, not only Charcot but Meynert and Brücke passed away. Accordingly, in the series of proto-psychoanalytic publications appearing between 1893 and 1897, Freud abandoned the French obsession with exhaustive symptom reportage and began to focus his writings intensively on questions of etiology. While preserving the Charcotian emphasis on the traumatic origins of many hysterias, he increasingly asserted the purely emotional nature of these traumas and located the causative events farther and farther back in the patient's psychological life.[35] As in avant-garde European psychiatry generally at this time, psychological causation progressively replaces material/somatic explanations, including central nervous system lesions. Even Charcot's hysterogenic zones, Freud now suggests, correspond with psychologically fraught parts of the patient's body. Furthermore, whereas the French school had tended to see hysterical patients as weak-willed and pathetic, Freud and Breuer in their jointly written *Studies on Hysteria* of 1895 praise their hysterical patients as exceptional individuals who share decisively in both the doctor's discoveries and the patient's recovery. In this second phase, Freud also explored new techniques of clinical inquiry, privileging listening more and more over seeing as a mode of investigation.

Most substantively, Freud's 1896 article on hysteria and heredity offers a full-blown critique of degenerationist theory, which after a half century of dominance in French mental medicine was finally under fire from several quarters. Freud knew that he had to sweep away once and for all a theory that Charcot had clung to until the very end. In Freud's writings, neuropathic heredity ceases to be the sole primary cause of neurosis and instead becomes little more than a possible precondition. Likewise, he permanently jettisons the French notion of a "famille névropathique," not least perhaps because it was often over-applied to patients who were Jewish.[36] In this same pivotal essay of 1896, the theme of sexuality appears more than in any of his previous publications: whereas Charcot had utterly marginalized the sexual, Freud reintroduced it here in the form of a passive, prepubertal sexual trauma. In the opening paragraph of the essay, he addressed his paper directly to "the disciples of Jean-Martin Charcot," and he published the article in a leading French neurology journal. Significantly, this is also the essay in which Freud first used the term "psycho-analysis."[37]

Taken together, Freud's writings of the 1890s offer a complicated structure of interlocking hypotheses. In these texts, hysteria becomes a purely psychological malady with elaborate quasi-physical symptoms. Hysterogenesis begins with the repression of traumatic memories. These memories are usually remote in the emotional past of the individual and are often (in years following, he would contend always) sexual in content. Because these remembrances are painful or unpleasant, they at times are unable to find conscious psychological expression. That is, the psychological energy associated with the experience and its memory fails to be adequately discharged in everyday mental life. Freud likens this lodged emotional energy to a parasite or foreign body in the psyche of the individual.

Freud maintains further that the negative emotional energy or "strangulated affect" associated with these memories is unconsciously converted into the somatic manifestations of hysteria. In this process of "hysterical conversion"—the core of Freud's new theory—physical functions alter in ways that unconsciously give expression to the repressed instinctual impulses. The actual causative event, he insists, can vary enormously, and under certain psychological circumstances, even a minor or seemingly innocuous experience can be heightened into a trauma. Such events, moreover, often accumulate in an individual's psychological life, forming a reinforcing chain of repressed traumas with later memories concealing earlier, more primal ones. In one of his most intriguing formulations, Freud hypothesizes that hysterical symptoms are not simply arbitrary and meaningless phenomena—which was Charcot's view—but rather complex symbolizations of repressed psychological experiences. These symptom-symbols represent invaluable clues to the hysteric's psychological history.

The new Freudian/Breuerian model of hysteria formulated in the mid-1890s entailed new ideas about therapy as well, which Freud outlines in the final, 50-page chapter of *Studies on Hysteria,* titled "The Psychotherapy of Hysteria." Because in his view hysteria is caused by strictly mental entities—ideas, emotions, desires in the life of the individual—the disorder is open to psychotherapeutic intervention. Drawing directly on Breuer's concept of psychological abreaction derived from the case of "Anna O.," Freud proposes that by bringing into the conscious mental life of the patient the past event that had created the hysterical repression, the symptom in question will vanish. That is, to introduce the experience into normal consciousness, and to express its underlying idea verbally, is to remove the symptom and work toward cure. Locating the past experience, however, often proves arduous: "Traveling backwards into the patient's past, step by step, and always guided by the organic train of symptoms and of memories and thoughts aroused," he explains, "I finally reached the starting-point of the pathological process."[38] As Freud explored these ideas, his consulting room technique evolved from physical massage, warm baths, and static electricity to the application of pressure on the temples and forehead, suggestive hypnotherapeutics, and finally to "free association."

Freud would later revise several key elements of his thinking about the psychoneuroses. Nevertheless, his work from these years represents a totally different type of writing and thinking about hysteria than we have encountered previously. Discarding both the Platonic/Hippocratic model of female reproductive determinism and the Morelian/Charcotian paradigm of defective nervous heredity seems to have opened up an entire field of fresh theoretical possibilities for Freud and his contemporaries. In his writings between 1887 and 1896, Freud eschews moral judgments about his patients in the pursuit of analytical understanding. He offers not scattered insights, in the manner of Willis, Sydenham, or Georget, but sets of interlocking concepts that point to an increasingly comprehensive model of the mind. In contrast to Briquet or Charcot, who constructed a single, unchanging account of hysterical illness, Freud's book and articles of the 1890s present hysteria as an ongoing scientific inquiry. Philosophically, his theorization of conversion places hysteria squarely at the center of mind/body interactions. And although the question of whether childhood psychological traumas underlying hysterical neuroses are "real" or "imaginary" would later be debated vehemently, the basic idea of

STUDIEN

ÜBER

HYSTERIE

VON

Dr. JOS. BREUER und Dr. SIGM. FREUD

IN WIEN.

Title page of *Studies on Hysteria,* co-authored by Freud and Josef Breuer. The first distinctly psychoanalytic book, it introduces the famous cases of Anna O. and Emmy von N.

LEIPZIG UND WIEN.
FRANZ DEUTICKE.
1895.

psycho-physical conversion remains embedded in current clinical psychiatry.[39]

"Literariness" is yet another innovative feature of Freud's writings from this period, particularly with the five case histories in *Studies on Hysteria,* which is often considered the first distinctly psychoanalytic book.[40] In places, Freud incorporates in these cases direct statements from his patients, or he reproduces dialogue between himself and the patient. By seeing both the patient's words about his or her condition and the therapist's ongoing observations, the reader of the cases gets a sense of the ongoing thought processes of both individuals. Running from 10 to 60 pages, the case histories in *Studies on Hysteria* are considerably longer than earlier nineteenth-century case reports. They give us believable, individualized characters, rather than the bloodless stick figures of earlier clinical portraits.[41] The short case history of "Katharina" in particular brims with metaphorical language (for example, a hysterical symptom is a pictographic script that gradually becomes legible; a psychological analysis is like excavating a lost city; cathartic psychotherapy is akin to surgery). "It still strikes me myself as strange," Freud commented in a much-quoted passage from the case of Fräulein Elisabeth von R., "that the case histories I write should read like short stories and that, as one might say, they lack the serious stamp of science. I must console myself with the reflection that the nature of the subject is evidently responsible for this, rather than any preference of my own. The fact is that . . . a detailed description of mental processes such as we are accustomed to find in the works of imaginative writers enables me, with the use of a few psychological formulas, to obtain at least some kind of insight into the course of that affection."[42]

Of the five illustrative case histories in *Studies on Hysteria,* all are female patients. These pseudonymous dramatis personae of early psychoanalysis—Fräulein Anna O., Frau Emmy von N., Miss Lucy R., Katharina, and Fräulein Elisabeth von R. are now celebrated.[43] In the text and in lengthy running footnotes, Freud introduces other patients—Frau Cäcilie M., Fräulein Mathilde H., Fräulein Rosalia H.—all of them female as well.[44] These clinical protagonists vary in age, class, occupation, and education, as well as in the nature of their affliction and length of treatment. But they are all women.

In "The Etiology of Hysteria" (1896), Freud reports that his ongoing findings are based on his work with eighteen patients, "comprising six men and twelve women." Likewise, in "Further Remarks on the Neuro-Psychoses of Defense" (1896) he states that "I have found this specific determinant of hysteria . . . in every case of hysteria (including two male cases) which I have analyzed."[45] In light of Charcot's work on male neurosis and Freud's own lecture to the Vienna Society of Physicians a decade earlier, as well as the fact that Freud's major twentieth-century case histories involve adult males, why does "this primal book of psychoanalysis" not include the cases of hysterical men?[46]

Viewed historically, what may well be most remarkable about the fin-de-siècle Freudian theory of hysteria, the most detailed and comprehensive ever to emerge from the Germanic medical world, is what it excludes: in the hundreds of pages that Freud published on the malady during these years, there are no references whatsoever to female anatomy and physiology. Freud's reintroduction of sexuality into the picture takes the form of an expanded *psycho-sexuality* that is gendered neither male nor female. Nor does Freud traffic in the well-worn notion of a "female temperament" or "constitution." Although all five case histories in *Studies on Hysteria* are about women, they are not presented as studies in femininity.[47] When gender does appear in his writings of 1888–1896, it operates in the form of socialization in boys and girls, which, Freud argues, causes a greater degree of internalized repression among females than males. Stated differently, gender in Freud's emerging theory is not primary and biological, metaphysical, existential, or temperamental, but rather secondary and sociological. The key theoretical components of the Freud/Breuer model of the neuroses—psychical affect, traumatic experience, repression into the unconscious, and remedial abreaction—are almost entirely ungendered.

This feature of the 1890s Freudian theory of hysteria reflects to a significant degree the enduring influence of Charcot and the

French school. Despite the fact of Charcot's death in 1893, Freud still peppered his publications with laudatory references to him. The first version of what became the *Preliminary Communication* of 1893, which Freud wrote without Breuer's assistance, opens: "All the modern advances made in the understanding and knowledge of hysteria are derived from the work of Charcot."[48] Moreover, Freud published two of the seven essays that he produced on hysteria in this period in French neurology journals.[49] A quarter of the books referenced in the bibliography of *Studies on Hysteria* are French-language studies, and Freud acknowledged that Bernheim, Liébeault, Delboeuf, and Janet were principal inspirations for his therapeutic ideas and practices—all indications that he remained engaged with the French hysteria tradition at this time.[50]

Freud built on and reworked Charcot's pioneering research on trauma in working-class male patients. Freud's innovations of the 1890s were to psychologize trauma fully, to sexualize past traumatic experiences, to push the traumatic events back into the early life of the patient, and to replace actual sexual events with unconscious ideas, wishes, and fantasies. This was a brilliant conceptual reformulation, but Freud never forgot his origins: "By uncovering the psychical mechanism of hysterical phenomenon we have taken a step forward along the path first traced so successfully by Charcot with his explanation and artificial imitation of hystero-traumatic paralyses," he wrote in 1893.[51] Most important was Charcot's programmatic insistence on rejecting gender as the universal and absolute determinant of nervous disease. Earlier, Freud had published a case and delivered a lecture about Charcot-style hysteria in male workers. Now, he recast the entire concept of male/female hysteria by constructing a full-blown, gender-neutral theory of neurosis.

And yet, the basic fact remains: by limiting their published cases in *Studies on Hysteria* to members of one sex, Freud and Breuer in effect reinforced the age-old perception that hysteria, including its fin-de-siècle incarnation, remained fundamentally a female malady.[52] Although their new *theory* of psychoanalytic hysteria was equally applicable to males and females, Freud and Breuer choose to illustrate it *clinically* with individuals from only one sex. There are a number of likely reasons why Freud and Breuer withheld their male cases. By the mid-1890s the existence of masculine hysteria had become much more widely accepted in German medical culture and required less emphasis. Meynert, with whom Freud had locked horns a decade earlier, was now dead and partially discredited. Stung by the reception of his 1886 lecture, Freud may well have wished to avoid a repeat battle on this belabored topic. He may also have thought that there was no need to argue for the non-gender-specificity of hysteria since he effectively incorporated the point into his larger theory of neurosis.

The role of Breuer is another factor. The coauthors of *Studies on Hysteria* tussled continually over the book's contents. Freud hagiographers have often tried to diminish Breuer's contribution by suggesting in effect that the good parts of the book are Freud's and the bad parts Breuer's. In fact, an unbiased reading of Breuer's long theoretical chapter proves that he was no slouch intellectually. On matters of gender, however, Breuer was extremely cautious. *Studies in Hysteria* was very long in preparation, with many delays, due largely to Breuer's resistance to publishing data he regarded as sensitive and ideas he found provocative. Significantly, in his write-up of the case, he chose not to report Anna O.'s alleged erotic and emotional attachment to him. Whereas Freud over time warmed to the role of intellectual revolutionary, Breuer was clearly not comfortable with the implications of their theories. He dissociated himself increasingly from Freud's later work, and in the business-like, one-paragraph preface that he penned for the second edition of the book in 1908, he seems to regret his involvement in the project altogether.[53] It can only be speculation, but if Freud had written *Studies on Hysteria* alone, the case history accounts might well have featured both women and men.

THERE IS ONE other reason why Freud failed to engage male neurosis in the 1890s, a much more personal reason. This brings us to the third and most complicated stage of his hysteria work, which runs from 1896 to 1900. These years are often regarded as the most intellectually creative in Freud's career—the fertile founding period of psychoanalysis. It was also a time in his life, the years between the ages of 40 and 44, of considerable mental and emotional turmoil.

Between the three 1896 articles on the neuroses and *The Interpretation of Dreams* in 1900, he published little on hysteria.[54] What Freud did produce during his early forties was a most remarkable set of unpublished documents, the letters to Wilhelm Fliess. Based in Berlin, Fliess had met Freud in the fall of 1887 during a visit to Vienna. Like Freud, he was a secular, assimilated Jew who was frustrated by and alienated from the medical orthodoxy of the day. In Freud's view, Fliess, unlike Breuer, was intellectually fearless and professionally iconoclastic. He was willing to speculate widely and wildly about all manner of scientific issues. In particular, his extravagant ideas about the relation between the nose and human sexual biology and between health and monthly periodicity, which today seem eccentric if not seriously misguided, received Freud's encouragement throughout the 1890s.[55] Fliess was the last in a series of male intellectual companions who were key to Freud's career during the late nineteenth century, after which time Freud sought obedient sons rather than inspiring fathers.

By 1895, Fliess had replaced Breuer as Freud's primary colleague and confidant. Separated by hundreds of miles, Fliess and Freud met whenever possible in various European cities for their "congresses," or several days of intense conversation, meetings that Freud eagerly anticipated and drew great sustenance from. Above all, the two men quickly developed an intimate writing relationship, which extended from 1887 to 1902 and generated hundreds of letters in both directions. Outside of his family, this was by far Freud's most important relationship during these crucial years.

Fliess's letters to Freud no longer exist, discarded by Freud after the termination of their passionate friendship. We therefore have only one side of a fifteen-year dialogue. Altogether, 301 letters *from* Freud *to* Fliess survive; an extensive selection of these was published by members of the Freud establishment in 1950/1954, and a complete, unexpurgated edition appeared in 1985.[56] In these epistolary exchanges, Freud shares with Fliess his ongoing ideas and theories about psychology, interspersed with family news, reports about his patients, arrangements for their next meeting, reactions to Fliess's letters, professional chitchat, and sundry observations about life. On several occasions Freud enclosed with the letters "drafts" or theoretical working papers that explore psychological issues over several pages. Scores of the letters deal with hysterical neurosis, and Draft L. is titled "The Architecture of Hysteria."[57]

Freud's letters and drafts are astonishing for their sheer intellectual energy and inventiveness. These texts are filled with spontaneous ideas, questions, observations, hypotheses, and theories—a case study in scientific creativity. They are driven, however, by more than simple curiosity. In the letters, Freud marshals observations, gropes for schemes of organization, postulates provisional theories, and reformulates a priori conclusions. In all of this "intellectual labor" there is a continual, at times obsessive, drive toward systematized knowledge about the human psyche. A striking number of

ideas and terms that today we label psychoanalytic appear embry-
onically in the letters and drafts—among them, unconscious feelings of guilt, stages of sexual development, the family romance, the
power of repressed feelings, mechanisms of dream production,
symptom formation, wish-fulfillment, auto-eroticism, reality testing, sibling rivalry, and psychological regression. Sprinkled through
the pages are also allusions to literary, artistic, and philosophical
subjects—to ancient Greek myths, Roman architecture, Dante,
Leonardo, Goethe, Burckhardt, Zola, and, above all, Shakespeare.

Part of the fascination and the integrity of these documents is
their revelation of the author's intellectual dead ends. Sometimes
the ideas come in a rush, with moments of sudden insight and ex-
citement, but these instances are often accompanied by periods of
paralysis or the realization that an earlier construction is unwork-
able. "I am alone in my mind, in which so much is stirring, for the
time being stirring itself into a muddle," Freud wrote to Fliess on
October 8, 1895.[58] Like Darwin's *Transmutation Notebooks* of the
1830s and 1840s and Marx's *Economic and Philosophical Manuscripts*
of 1844, the letters to Fliess are intellectual progress reports, not
intended for public consumption but discovered and printed posthumously, revising utterly the origins of the thinker's ideas.

Unlike Darwin and Marx, however, Freud was a medical psychologist, which meant that he confronted head on the question of
how the human mind can know itself. Distinctively, Freud decided
in the later 1890s that he would draw on the resources of introspection in his psychological system building. On October 23,
1896, Freud's 81-year-old father died, and although Freud had not
considered himself particularly attached emotionally to the man,
his father's death—like Mill's father's passing sixty years earlier—
unleashed a torrent of psychological reactions. Rather than suppressing these feelings as an interference with his work, Freud envi-

sioned his own mental behavior as a fertile field for psychological insight that could complement his clinical work with patients.

"The cherished centerpiece of psychoanalytic mythology," Freud's "self-analysis," as he himself called it, began in earnest sometime around the late spring of 1897 and continued until early in the new century.[59] Although there is much that we don't know about the process, Freud apparently during these years studied intensively and systematically his own dreams, memories, reactions, wishes, and emotions.[60] Clearly, introspection had long been used in psychological inquiry, and penetrating autobiography has a rich heritage from St. Augustine onward. Nevertheless, Freud's thoroughgoing exercise in self-scrutiny required great discipline and determination, and a number of its features were unique. Freud never fell into morose self-absorption but pursued his venture as a source of general psychological knowledge. He continually sought to synthesize ideas and information that originated in his personal self-examination with those from his clinical consultations, the two categories of observation continually fertilizing one another. There is in these letters an almost Socratic sense that self-understanding is a desirable, possibly indispensable, condition for a scientist and a philosopher of the mind.

In this third phase, then, Freud drew, simultaneously and symbiotically, on several sources: his continued reading in the scientific literature of the day; his clinical practice, centered on neurotic patients; his daily self-analysis; and the record of cultural, especially literary, history. Freud was surprisingly alert to the methodological relations among these different domains: on November 14, 1897, he speculated to Fliess about one of his painful dry spells: "My self-analysis is still interrupted. I have now seen why. I can only analyze myself with objectively acquired knowledge (as if I were a stranger); self-analysis is really impossible, otherwise there would be no illness."[61]

Freud chose not to conceal the autoanalytical inception of his new ideas.[62] Above all, *The Interpretation of Dreams,* which punctuates this third phase in 1900, contains scores of self-observations, including childhood memories, screen memories, parapraxes, and countless dreams of his own, which Freud interprets symbolically, like texts of fiction.[63] Freud himself, in the Preface to the second edition of *The Interpretation of Dreams* published in 1908, acknowledged the "subjective significance" of the landmark book, adding that it served as "a portion of my own self-analysis, my reaction to my father's death."[64] Goethe, one of Freud's favorite German authors, famously referred to his own lifework as "the fragment of a great confession." With Freud's early writings as well, autobiography, after a century's long eclipse, makes a dramatic reappearance in the medical history of hysteria.

Self-observation of course is not without its epistemological problems, and from its beginnings psychoanalysis has been bedeviled by the question of its scientific status. Literature, philosophy, and religion may employ self-confession, but not science, which throughout the nineteenth century placed tremendous emphasis, rhetorically and ideologically, on segregating the Object and the Subject of investigation. We cannot imagine Charcot in Paris, or Gowers in London, or Meynert in Vienna—the leading European hysteria doctors in the immediate pre-Freudian era—citing intimate autobiographical details in their scientific publications. Freud in the later 1890s, however, suggested that a theory of psychological functioning entails equally the resources of "introspective knowledge" and "objective knowledge."[65] In the process, he erased the cultural dichotomy between the scientific/objective/clinical and the literary/subjective/introspective idioms of inquiry in a way that had not been accomplished since the two cultures of art and science began to go their separate ways a hundred years earlier.

Freud's voluminous correspondence with Fliess is thus a cardinal document in Freud's psychological as well as intellectual biography. What becomes much more evident in the complete, unabridged edition of Freud's letters to Fliess is a flourishing nervous and mental symptomatology throughout this third period. Time and again, Freud reports to Fliess a train of his own symptoms: dizziness, dyspnea, migraines, aches and pains of all sorts, and one heart irregularity after another. "I have not been free of symptoms for as much as half a day," he confesses early in May, 1894, "and my mood and ability to work are really at a low ebb." His agonizing struggles to quit smoking provoked further outbreaks. Most likely in response to his father's passing, he developed "a death delirium," predicting that he would die in his early fifties of "a ruptured heart." "I feel aged, sluggish, not healthy," he gripes.[66]

Not surprisingly in light of his work at the time, Freud openly ponders the nature of his own symptoms. Speaking of himself in the third person, he writes at one point: "It is too distressing for a medical man who spends every hour of the day struggling to gain an understanding of the neuroses not to know whether he is suffering from a justifiable or a hypochondriacal mild depression." In private, his moods were often dark, self-tormented. He fears that his work is "rubbish," he frets that he will die in obscurity, he nurses a phobia of train travel, and he cycles through spells of doubt, elation, inhibition, and depression. In one letter, he seems close to collapse; in the next, he says that "things are fermenting inside me," and "I cannot convey to you any idea of the intellectual beauty of this work."[67]

As he grew closer to Fliess during the later 1890s, Freud discussed without inhibition his own daily psychological travails. The richest passages appear in the second half of 1897, just as Freud was beginning to reformulate his ideas about the role of sexual trauma in the etiology of psychopathology. On June 22, 1897, he concedes that "I have been through some kind of neurotic experience, curious states incomprehensible to [my patient] C.s, twilight thoughts, veiled doubts, with barely a ray of light here or there"—almost as if he were undergoing a mystical experience.[68] Two weeks later, he elaborates: "I still do not know what has been happening to me. Something from the deepest depths of my own neurosis set itself against any advance in the understanding of the neuroses."[69]

Freud in fact goes one step further. Over time, he inevitably realizes that many of his personal troubles are classic conversion symptoms.[70] On August 14, 1897, he writes to Fliess from Aussee, Italy, where Freud and his family are vacationing. He reports that he is "in a period of bad humor." His Mediterranean holiday is not preventing him from being "tormented by grave doubts about my theory of the neuroses" nor "diminishing the agitation in my head and feelings." He observes further that "my little hysteria, though greatly accentuated by my work, has resolved itself a bit further." Referring to his self-analysis, which he is continuing while on vacation, he acknowledges that "the chief patient I am preoccupied with is myself."[71] Similarly, in the fall of the same year, Freud, now back in Vienna, relates a rush of images from his recent dream life and expresses the hope that his analysis of these images will "succeed in resolving my own hysteria."[72] And once again, on August 31, 1898, before leaving Vienna with his wife for another trip to the Adriatic coast, he complains about his lack of motivation and the slow pace of his work. "The secret of this restlessness," he concludes, "is hysteria."[73] In the 1950s, as they frankly assessed the writ-

ten record from this period of Freud's life, the psychoanalytic estab-
lishmentarians Ernest Jones, James Strachey, and Max Schur could
only agree with Freud's autodiagnosis.[74]

However else the Freud/Fliess correspondence may be read, it is
also a most remarkable set of documents in the history of male hysteria. Of greatest significance is not the fact that Freud affixed the
hysteria label to himself but that his protracted neurotic episodes at
this time were so intimately bound up with his prodigious intellectual activities. Freud intended his private musings to Fliess to
remain wholly separate from his published work. But these dual
sources can now be read side by side, in reliable editions, as the expressions of a single, integrated mind. Taken together, Freud's writings of the 1890s give us the most original and wide-ranging set of
ideas about hysteria to date, as well as a strikingly vulnerable and
self-aware portrait of the masculine authorial self.

SINCE THE PUBLICATION of the complete Freud/Fliess letters in
the mid-1980s, a wave of scholarship has explored the possible ex-
periential sources of early Freudian theory.[75] This literature invariably asserts that Freud's hysteria patients of the 1890s were female,
as the published case histories would indicate. But this is a serious
error. In fact, *male* analysands played a fundamental role in the intellectual history of psychoanalysis during the penultimate years of
the century.[76] One male patient in particular was far and away the
most crucial patient for Freud's thinking during this creative neurotic phase.

Freud treated "Herr E." for five years, beginning a few months
after *Studies on Hysteria* appeared and terminating in mid-April,
1900, half a year after publication of *The Interpretation of Dreams*.
His therapy with Herr E., in other words, spans the years of Freud's
self-analysis, the Fliess friendship, and the formulation of key psy-

choanalytic concepts. It was the longest treatment that Freud undertook of a patient in the nineteenth century, and the only case he related continuously to Fliess. Freud never published the case, which is known to us today almost exclusively from the letters to Fliess. This fact probably explains why the case is not discussed, or even mentioned, in the major biographies of Freud or in the literature on Freud's case histories. Surprisingly, even the editorial notes in the full Freud/Fliess correspondence fail to note the significance of this paradigmatic patient.[77]

Some ten passages in Freud's letters to Fliess discuss Herr E. From these, we can piece together parts of a medical biography: the patient was a lawyer or judge, whose mother had died in his youth. As a child, his sexual curiosity had been aroused prematurely by his French nanny, Louise. He had suffered an anxiety attack associated with an insect at the age of ten. Among his adult neurotic symptoms were the fear of train travel, bouts of nervous sweating, a tendency to blush in public, fits of self-doubt, and a bizarre fear that he might assault someone sexually on the street or at the opera. We do not know how often Freud and Herr E. met, although Freud mentions daily encounters with some hysterical patients at this time.[78]

Most striking is Herr E.'s role in one after another of Freud's key theoretical formulations. In his first reference to the patient at the end of October, 1895, Freud already indicates that he expects to learn from Herr E.: "Fortunately for me . . . I have daily opportunities to be corrected or enlightened. My 'bashful' case . . . developed hysteria in his youth and later showed delusions of reference. His almost transparent history ought to clear up a few disputed points for me."[79] Two days later, Freud writes to Fliess again, more excitedly, about Herr E.: "One of the cases gave me what I expected (sexual shock—that is, infantile abuse in *male* hysteria!) and that at the same time a working through of the disputed material strength-

ened my confidence in the validity of my psychological constructions. Now I am really enjoying a moment of satisfaction."[80] The
so-called seduction theory of the neuroses, or the belief in an actual childhood sexual trauma, underpins Freud's early etiological
thought. Here we find that Herr E. provided confirmation of the
theory at the moment of its inception, which Freud experiences as
a gratifying insight.

Over the next half-decade, this same patient "corrected" and
"enlightened" Freud on other points, too. With his letter of May 2,
1897, Freud encloses Draft L, "The Architecture of Hysteria," in
which he excerpts a full paragraph of conversation with Herr E.
and interprets one of the patient's wish-fulfillment dreams.[81] In a
similar vein, on December 29, 1897, Freud offers "a little interpretation" of the patient's youthful anxiety attack. And on February
19, 1899, in the last year of their interaction, he analyzes at length
Herr E.'s tendency to blush and sweat at the theater, tracing the reaction back through different reinforcing experiences to the patient's early childhood.[82] These are fully psychoanalytic readings of
dreams, symptoms, and mental behaviors, performed by Freud for
the first time and on a male patient diagnosed as hysterical.

The most controversial revision of Freud's thinking during phase
three was "the abandonment of the seduction theory"—and here
again, Freud cites Herr E. illustratively. Freud's new theory emphasized the role of the child's own unconscious oedipal wishes and
fantasies in the origins of neurosis. In his letter of December 29,
1897, Freud hints that Herr E.'s childhood anxiety attack, which
the patient in adulthood still remembered, is relevant to his revised
theory.[83] Two years later, Freud claims he has struck gold with Herr
E.: "Buried deep beneath all his fantasies, we found a scene from
his primal period (before 22 months) which meets all the require-
ments [of the new theory] and in which all the remaining puzzles

converge," he reports, referring to the patient and himself collab-
oratively. "I can scarcely believe it yet." Two weeks later, there is
more confirmation:"In E.'s case, the second genuine scene is coming up after years of preparation; and it is one that may *perhaps* be
confirmed objectively by asking his elder sister. Behind it, a third,
long-suspected scene approaches." Here, too, Freud experiences his
clinical work with Herr E. as a breakthrough—so great a breakthrough, in fact, that he deploys a German archaeological metaphor
of special meaning to describe it: "It is as if Schliemann had once
more excavated Troy, which had hitherto been deemed a fable."[84]
Virtually all of Freud's references to Herr E. occur in conjunction
with the conception, revision, or illustration of significant theoretical advances.

In the last letter cited above, Freud reveals another sort of debt
to this extraordinary patient, too. Freud himself suffered from a fear
of train travel, and also, like Herr E., he believed that as a child his
libido had been aroused by his nursemaid. Furthermore, both men
worked in prestigious professions in the Hapsburg capital. Doctor
and patient, in fact, shared the same symptoms, diagnosis, and etiology, as well as nationality and professional status. As a consequence,
Freud seems not only to have sympathized with Herr E. but to
have identified with him psychobiographically.[85] Reflecting this
personal identification, and against the backdrop of his self-analysis,
Freud observes of Herr E. on December 21, 1899, that "he demonstrated the reality of my theory in my own case, providing me in a
surprising reversal with the solution, which I had overlooked, to
my former railroad phobia." He then adds:"For this piece of work
I even made him the present of a picture of Oedipus and the
Sphinx. . . . You will hear more about all of this at our next congress."[86]

In this remarkable letter, written during the very final days of the century, we learn that Herr E., alone among Freud's patients in the 1890s, had the power not only to verify, revise, and invalidate Freud's developing psychological ideas but also to elucidate one of Freud's own persistent neurotic symptoms. Four years into the treatment, the patient for all intents and purposes treats the doctor, successfully. Accordingly, the doctor appreciatively rewards the patient with a gift—rather than the other way around—in the form of a symbolically laden image of the classical/mythological figure whose name Freud later attached to one of the most essential new psychoanalytic concepts. This was a striking admixture of art, medicine, and autobiography indeed. "You can well imagine how important this one persistent patient has become to me," Freud comments to Fliess without exaggeration.[87]

In the spring of 1900, Freud composed for Fliess a final accounting of Herr E.'s treatment as their long therapy came to an end; it, too, reveals the striking combination of intellectual productivity and personal intimacy that marked the collaboration of doctor and patient:

E. at last concluded his career as a patient by coming to dinner at my house. His riddle is *almost* completely solved; he is in excellent shape, his personality entirely changed. At present a remnant of the symptoms is left. I am beginning to understand that the apparent endlessness of the treatment is something that occurs regularly and is connected with the transference [*Ubertragung*]. I hope that this remnant will not detract from the practical success. I could have continued the treatment, but I had the feeling that such prolongation is a compromise between illness and health that patients themselves desire, and the physician must therefore not accede to it. . . . I shall keep an eye on the

man. Since he had to suffer through all my technical and theoretical errors . . .[88]

Coincidentally or not, Freud ended his own analysis in the same
year when he finished treating Herr E. Thus, in the last several years
of the nineteenth century, three men—Freud, Fliess, and Herr E.—
presided over the birth of psychoanalysis. Two of the three Freud
formally diagnosed as hysterical, and the third, Fliess, effectively
served as caretaker to Freud's own neurosis.[89]

THIS IS NOT QUITE the full Freud/Fliess story. For decades, psychoanalytic historians lavished their attention on this singular relationship, mainly in order to reconstruct the intellectual interaction
between the two men. With the treasure trove of the complete, unabridged correspondence, however, the emotional and erotic dimensions of their alliance have also come into view.[90] From Ernest
Jones onward, biographers have acknowledged Freud's "really passionate relationship of dependence" with Fliess, certainly the most
intense male friendship of his life.[91] Brücke, Meynert, Charcot, and
Breuer were considerably older than Freud, and their relations with
him were variously avuncular and authoritarian; Fliess, in contrast,
was Freud's own age and was easy to talk to as an equal and confidant. He was also apparently charismatic and quite good looking.

Freud's side of their epistolary exchange is filled with expressions of admiration, affection, and at times desire: "I shall welcome
the summer if it brings what I have been longing for for years—
a few days with you without undue interruptions." "When I think
of the many weeks when I felt uncertain about my life, my need to
be with you again increases greatly." And "I cannot write entirely
without an audience, but do not at all mind writing only for you."[92]

Early on, Freud sent Fliess a photograph of himself, which Fliess had requested. Freud planned to name either of his two youngest children Wilhelm, after Fliess, had they been males. At the peak of their friendship around 1899, Freud wrote lengthy letters to Fliess every week. He dreamed about Fliess and idealized Fliess's scientific schemes. Throughout the latter half of the nineties, the two men met fairly often in Vienna, Berlin, or some other German or Austrian city for their "congresses." They stayed in the same hotel, often in fact in the same quarters, while their families remained at home.[93] Fliess's wife, Ida, apparently became jealous of her husband's time spent with Freud, and Freud expressed envy of Fliess's friendships with other men.[94] Not least, during these years Freud shared his neurotic sufferings, presumably one of the most private parts of his life, with Fliess and Fliess alone. Their friendship began to cool around 1900 and then flamed out in the summer of 1904—over a priority dispute about universal bisexuality.[95]

Freud never really got over their fifteen-year emotional and intellectual affair. In the spring of 1900, Freud attempted to explain his behavior to Fliess by acknowledging that "no one can replace for me the relationship with the friend that a special—possibly feminine—side demands."[96] The next year, as their relationship began to unravel, Freud observed more defensively that "I do not share your contempt for friendship between men, probably because I am to a high degree party to it. In my life, as you know, woman has never replaced the comrade, the friend." He then tried to elaborate by drawing on the example of an earlier friendship: "If Breuer's male inclination were not so odd, so timid, so contradictory . . . it would provide a nice example of the accomplishments into which the androphilic current in men can be sublimated."[97]

In 1910, reflecting back on the whole painful attachment, Freud responded with impressive candor to his Hungarian associate Sán-

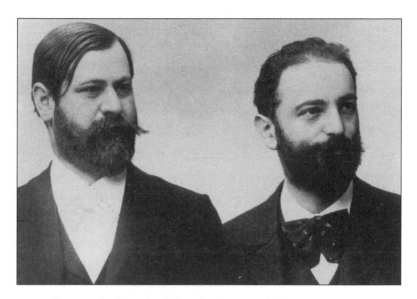

Photograph of Freud and Fliess, both sporting thick beards, in 1898, at the height of their friendship.

dor Ferenczi. Writing with clinical detachment and in the passive voice, he said that with the termination of his relationship with Fliess, "a piece of homosexual investment has been withdrawn and utilized for the enlargement of my ego." He assured Ferenczi that he had no further secrets to reveal: "I feel myself to be a match for anything and approve of the overcoming of my homosexuality, with the result being greater independence."[98] Still, two years later, when Freud fainted in a Munich hotel room, he connected the episode to an argument he had had with Fliess years earlier at the same location: "There is some piece of unruly homosexual feeling at the root of the matter," he confided self-analytically to a startled Ernest Jones.[99] In Freud's self-account, "the androphilic current in men" is something to be either "overcome," in a process of psychological self-mastery, or "sublimated" (a term Freud drew from Fliess) into higher cultural works. Freud never again experienced another Fliess-like relationship; but in his late middle years he identified with Leonardo da Vinci and wrote sympathetically of the Florentine painter's bisexuality. Michelangelo and Shakespeare, two male geniuses not afraid to express a "special, possibly feminine side" in their creative work, were likewise among the cultural figures he most admired.

Thus, during several of the most critical years in the early development of psychoanalysis, Freud was open on one front after another to interrogating the conventional gender polarities of his day. This process unfolded in his general psychological theory, in his self-analysis, and in his personal relationships. Not coincidentally, a parallel gendered phenomenon emerged during these years in the new psychological praxis that he invented. Charcot and Meynert had worked in masculinist epistemological modes that emphasized the objectifying medical gaze directed at an inert patient in a one-directional authoritarian relationship, which was then presented publicly in the objectivist rhetoric of materialist medical science. Freudian therapy is a wholly different enterprise. In the psychoanalytic "talking cure," the hysterical patient is introspective and confessional; the therapist/physician listens and empathizes; psychological subjectivities are central to the entire exercise; and written case histories make use of imaginative, novella-like narratives to capture individual consciousness over time. In Victorian science and medicine, these are all modalities of expression and apprehension regarded as "feminine."

FINALLY, IT IS interesting to look at Freud's publishing history during this third phase. Despite the remarkably rich role played by Freud's five-year encounter with Herr E., almost none of the clinical material about his star hysterical patient made its way into print. Given the length of the treatment, its theoretical importance, and

Freud's recurrent references to it in correspondence, this is a deeply puzzling omission. In March 1896, Freud reported to Fliess that he was planning to write a major treatise on the general psychology of the neuroses. The new study would incorporate all of his emerging ideas, he explained, free of Breuer's restraining influence. Surely, Herr E. would have figured prominently in such a work.

But Freud never wrote this book.[100] After the appearance of *The Interpretation of Dreams* at the end of 1899, the last book on hysteria that Freud did produce took as its subject the adolescent Dora. Freud's encounter with Herr E. had stretched across half a decade and for all intents and purposes was a success therapeutically. Dora's case, in contrast, lasted less than four months, ended in failure when the patient angrily terminated the treatment, and produced a text that became a preeminent statement of psychoanalytic misogyny. Why did Freud choose to write up the female rather than the male case? Was Herr E. too close to Freud personally and professionally, whereas Dora, like the women in *Studies on Hysteria,* represented "the sexual Other," whom he could more easily objectify?[101] Remarkably, the one diagnosed case of masculine hysterical neurosis that Freud published in his lifetime was the short 1886 presentation written after his return from Paris. Freud didn't just minimize the role of male hysteria in the origins of his psychology; he suppressed it.[102]

The other textual site of male hysteria during this period, the Freud/Fliess correspondence, has a quite different publishing history. In what must have been an act of violent willfulness, Freud at some point destroyed all the letters, presumably hundreds of them, that Fliess had written to him over the years. Fliess, however, preserved the 300 letters he received from his erstwhile correspondent. Soon after Fliess's death in 1928, his wife sold this stash to a Berlin-based bookseller, who, when the Nazis seized control of the

German government in January 1933, moved post-haste to Paris. The bookseller in turn offered the letters to Marie Bonaparte, who, in addition to being a wealthy enthusiast of psychoanalysis and a personal analysand of Freud's, was the Princess of Greece and Denmark. Bonaparte then brought the letters with her on a trip to Vienna. By this time, Freud was the renowned founder of an international movement, which he sought to control tightly, and he did not welcome this window onto his intimate past. Freud urged Bonaparte to burn the letters and offered to buy them from her, a possibility that Fliess's wife had specifically forbidden in the terms of her original sale. In consultation with Anna Freud, Bonaparte refused to act on Freud's request, the two women in effect defying the wishes of friend, mentor, author, and father.

The fascinating and dramatic story of how the letters survived the Nazi era reads like a plot summary of *The Maltese Falcon*.[103] Suffice it to say that after interludes in a Vienna safety deposit box and at the Danish Embassy in Paris, the precious cargo, like Freud himself, eventually made its way to the free English-speaking world. In 1950 and 1954 respectively, more than a decade after Freud's death, German and English editions of a sampling of the letters were published, but not without a final effort at censorship. Appearing under the title *Origins of Psychoanalysis,* this first printed version of Freud's letters to Fliess is replete with elisions and omissions. More than 130 letters were excluded altogether. Ernest Jones claimed that only "uninteresting details" had been deleted;[104] but a close, comparative reading of the 1950/1954 and the 1985 editions indicates that at least two types of information were consistently and deliberately struck out, namely, passages expressing Freud's endless neurotic agonizing and his crypto-homosexual attachment to Fliess. The resulting text presents the letters largely as documents in the early intellectual history of psychoanalysis.

The reason for these editorial excisions seems clear enough: psychoanalysis in the 1950s was at the height of its cultural influence and professional power. The official version of the founder's life portrayed Freud as a figure of enormous rationalist self-discipline and heroic masculine autonomy, which he may well have been. During at least one period in his life, however, the father of psychoanalysis had also been strikingly vulnerable, and however bound up these anxiety/neurotic difficulties may have been with his intellectual creativity, their revelation at that time was unacceptable. So countless passages were systematically edited out, and the knowledge of Freud's hysteria was kept private. Only in the mid-1980s, some ninety years after the letters were composed, was the early hysterical Freud made available to the world. How different our view of psychoanalytic history would be today if Marie Bonaparte and Anna Freud had failed to secure and preserve these singular documents or if Freud had succeeded in destroying them.

Past critics of this censorship have spoken of the cautious, protective motives of mid-century psychoanalytic insiders, but the history of hysteria suggests a larger framework for understanding the story. We have in fact encountered this pattern before: British Enlightenment nerve doctors wrote extensively about their nervous male patients, but their collective knowledge was forgotten in the following century. Charcot's students photographed the most extravagant male hysterical patients in their hospital wards, but then suppressed the images from publication. And Meynert railed against the idea of male hysteria, until his own private deathbed confession. In systematically studying his own psychological subjectivity and then attempting to convert that knowledge into formal psychological theory, Freud really did go where no medical man had gone before; but he was unable to follow through on the endeavor by going public with the insights that his extraordinary exertions had generated. For all his striking originality as a theoretician, Freud, too, contributed in this third phase to the long-running tradition of male European physicians who saw but concealed, who discovered and then tried to cover up, the knowledge of male neurosis.

THE FOURTH AND final phase of Freud's hysteria work forms a postscript to the earlier stages. After writing up the Dora case, Freud for all intents and purposes dropped hysteria as a subject of study. The major case histories that Freud published later in his career— Little Hans, the Wolf Man, the Schreber case, the Rat Man—involve male patients with non-hysterical psychopathologies whose analysis did not require him to confront the radical gender implications of his work on male hysteria, including a deconstructive analysis of masculinity itself.[105]

However, hysteria in Freud's twentieth-century career did not die but rather was reincarnated. After fifteen years of intensive study, several of the psychological issues that the great neurosis raised were transmuted conceptually by Freud into other lines of exploration. Although these later streams of Freudian thought do not carry the name "hysteria," they nonetheless bear unmistakable signs of their origins in the French hysteria research of the 1880s and 1890s and would in fact have been unthinkable for Freud without his long-standing engagement with hysteria and its masculine incarnations in particular.

Although Freud's entire later work exemplifies this stage, his *Three Essays on the Theory of Sexuality* of 1905 is the one really "revolutionary" medical text. Freud opens the work audaciously with a chapter on "the sexual perversions" which, he contends, illuminates both homosexuality and heterosexuality. Throughout the work, his tone is analytical and nonjudgmental. From the outset, he broadens the sense of the sexual to include *psycho*sexuality, or the entire complex of wishes, fantasies, and memories surrounding sexual acts, which he insists are crucial to human sexuality. He separates sexual desire from biological reproduction, and he introduces a basic distinction between the object and sexual activity. Freud hypothesizes that same-sex attraction is much more widespread than is generally believed, and that everyone is capable of making a homosexual object choice. He also introduces the provocative idea that children, far from being passive, sexless innocents, have a vivid, if diffuse and undifferentiated, erotic curiosity and a wide repertoire of erotically pleasurable activities. He goes on to argue that the parent–child relationship itself is often eroticized and that adult sexual object choice frequently has childhood determinants.[106] Many of Freud's shocked, if not uncomprehending, contemporaries refused to forgive him for these ideas, as have some subsequent readers right up to the present.

Pertinent to our story is the fact that nearly all of the new conceptual machinery that Freud constructs in *Three Essays on the Theory of Sexuality* is ungendered—a quite remarkable feat when viewed historically. In other words, the role of erotic fantasy, the reality of childhood sexuality, the capacity for same-sex response, the high level of sexual individuality, and the three stages of psychosexual development are all shared by male and female children and adults. This fact sets the Freudian model decisively apart from eighteenth- and nineteenth-century medical writing. Furthermore, two new lines of thinking in *Three Essays on the Theory of Sexuality* are quite specific theoretical extrapolations of themes that are latent in Freud's work on male hysteria.

Despite Freud's later substantive revisions of the *Three Essays* and the many long, complicating, revisionary footnotes added in later editions, the idea of universal psychosexual bisexuality remains fundamental in the work. "Without taking bisexuality into account I think it would scarcely be possible to arrive at an understanding of the sexual manifestations that are actually to be observed in men and women," Freud states.[107] Artists and philosophers of antiquity, German Romantic culture, Darwin, Von Haeckel, and Krafft-Ebing were all part of the background of European interest in the idea of a union of sexual orientations.[108] Reinforcing this cultural and scientific background were Freud's personal history and intellectual interests. It is surely no coincidence of chronology that Freud's particular model of universal psychosexual bisexuality emerged in the immediate post-Fliess period. In the Freudian theory of hysteria, elements of homosexuality are present in all male and female psychoneurotics; certainly Dora's 1905 "fragment of a case of hysteria" is pervaded with bisexuality. In *Three Essays on the Theory of Sexuality,* homosexuality is not a pathological departure from heterosexuality or the sign of a degenerating nervous system but a developmental variant on a preexisting bisexual disposition. In a short essay published in 1908 titled "Hysterical Fantasies and Their Relation to Bisexuality," Freud summarizes his clinical theory of hysteria. A capacity for both heterosexual and homosexual activity, he tellingly argues in that context, is especially prominent in hysterical neurosis.[109] The idea of universal psychosexual bisexuality, too, is notably non-gender-specific and owes something to the heritage of gender indeterminacy implicit in the whole French research tradition of masculine hysteria, which Freud was exposed to at an early and formative time of his career. Charcot's seed planted two decades earlier was continuing to germinate, in ways he could never have imagined.

FREUD'S HISTORIC twenty-year encounter with male hysteria was marked by both brilliance and ambivalence. Each phase of his engagement with the topic between 1885 and 1905 produced its insights, but these insights were conjoined with inhibitions. His interest in the subject was first sparked in belle-époque Paris during the winter of 1885–86, when the bedazzled young neurologist observed France's most famous physician in the wards of the Salpêtrière. The next autumn, in a Vienna medical lecture hall, he made his painful professional debut with a talk on the topic. His reflections on male hysteria then incubated during the later 1880s and early 1890s. During the second half of the 1890s, he cultivated the subject intensively, albeit privately—in his self-analysis, his treatment of Herr E., his reading of European literature, and the unprecedented collection of personal psychological *pensées* he addressed to Fliess. Finally, early in the twentieth century, under altered theoretical circumstances, he brought his thinking to a kind of fruition in foundational texts of psychoanalysis like *Three Essays on the Theory of Sexuality,* in which he bisexualizes the great neurosis. Ultimately, Freud's journey demonstrated how productive the study of this subject could be when an author dared to draw on all available resources, including listening closely and honestly to his own self.[110] It also illustrates how very difficult it would be for any male scientist of this era to transcend the inherited categories of masculinity and femininity and to break out of the historical "prison of gender."[111]

# Men and the Fictions of Medicine

IN THE WHOLE HISTORY of Western philosophy, no virtue has been valued more highly than self-knowledge. Two thousand years ago, the sun god Apollo's Oracle at Delphi urged its supplicants to "know thyself." Socrates famously condemned the unexamined life as not worth living, and Plato considered insight into the self the means to leading the good life. With the principle of *cogito ergo sum,* René Descartes theorized that through reflection on our consciousness we can know our own minds with greater certainty than we can know anything else. In a similar vein, Immanuel Kant claimed that self-deception—what he called "inner lies"—constitutes insincerity toward oneself, which he regarded as a contemptible assault on human dignity. And Jean-Paul Sartre advanced existentialist "authenticity" as the highest ideal in life. From the Greeks in the fourth century B.C. to Martin Heidegger in the mid-twentieth, the greatest philosophical thinkers in the Western tradition, all of them men, championed the well-examined life.

In modern times, science emerged in the European West as the most intellectually powerful and culturally prestigious instrument for depicting reality, generating knowledge, and pursuing truth. During the seventeenth, eighteenth, and nineteenth centuries, the sciences acquired immense explanatory power over an enormous array of subjects in the organic and inorganic world, often supplanting in influence earlier bodies of thought, such as mythology, religion, and metaphysics. Medicine, too, during these generations took on its distinctively modern form, heralding the dual methods of empirical investigation and rational critical analysis, and creating entire new anatomies, physiologies, and chemistries of the human body. The accumulation of vast bodies of factual information, the founding of great universities, institutes, hospitals, and laboratories, the organization of one specialized domain of disciplinary inquiry after another, the establishment of large professional networks of truth-seeking practitioners—all of these were historically unprecedented achievements. Together, men of science, medicine, technology, and industry also gained greater physical and intellectual mastery over "Mother Nature" during this 300-year span than in the entire previous history of humanity.

One European observer during science's high, heroic age, however, who had the irritating habit of seeing deeper than his contemporaries, remained unimpressed. For the better part of the 1880s, Friedrich Nietzsche inhabited the breathtaking alpine hideaway of Sils-Maria in the Swiss Engadine Valley, from which, Zeus-like, he cast his intellectual thunderbolts down upon an unsuspecting Europe. In 1887, Nietzsche prefaced his *On the Genealogy of Morals* with these skeptical words: "We are unknown to ourselves, we men of knowledge—and with good reason. We have never sought ourselves—how could it happen that we should ever *find* ourselves? . . . We are not 'men of knowledge' with respect to ourselves."[1] In the case of hysteria among men, past male knowledge makers, in the paradigmatically modern world of medicine, carefully cultivated an ignorance of themselves. They accomplished this feat cleverly and resourcefully but also unknowingly. From the early seventeenth to the early twentieth centuries, European medical men, with near unanimity, signally failed to constitute their own gender as a field of critical, systematized study. Scientific and medical elites over this long period described in celebratory tones the individual and group attainments of the male mind as a rational, mastering intelligence, often drawing negative contrasts with the mental profiles of women. However, they proved to be conspicuously incapable of taking masculine psychological subjectivity as an object of sustained, self-conscious investigation. The cumulative discourse on male hysteria can be seen as a micro-paradigm of an extended, but largely unsuccessful, attempt within Western medicine to achieve personal and collective self-knowledge of the male self.

WHEN WE LOOK at the full textual tradition of male hysteria, from Robert Burton in the 1620s to Freud in the 1890s, several patterns come into view. The ebb and flow of the discourse over these centuries clearly mirrors a larger cycle of gender polarization and liberalization. Those times and cultures in which people felt threatened—regardless of whether the nature of the threat was military, economic, religious, cultural, or sexual—experienced a greater need to rearticulate traditional gender identities, in contrast to the times perceived as ages of stability and security.[2] (Trotter's Napoleonic Britain and Weininger's fin-de-siècle Vienna are emblematic examples.) Accordingly, a society's capacity to accept the crossing of gender boundaries—and male hysteria is the quintessential gender-crossing diagnosis—waxes and wanes.

Over the long course of writing about hysteria, the forms and methods used by medical authors correspond more or less directly with the content of their work. Inside and outside of medicine, most of the authors who wrote productively about male neurosis in these centuries—my accounting includes Burton, Shakespeare, Mandeville, Hume, Cheyne, Johnson, Wordsworth, Mill, Flaubert, and Freud—drew on the resources of art and autobiography. Tellingly, those figures who did not—Sydenham, Georget, Charcot—construed hysteria somatically/neurologically rather than psychologically/emotionally. For most thinkers who were open at all to this line of investigation, literature and introspection were doubtless natural, even inevitable, allies in the systematized study of subjectivity, whereas the strict and exclusionary methodology of positivist science seemed insufficient to the task. Analogously, several of the most prominent and original characters in our story combined, in Wordsworthian terms, "manly intellect" and "feminine feeling" in their work. This is partly an instantiation of the familiar idea that a union of "male" and "female" sensibilities animates many of the most brilliant works of Western cultural history,[3] and partly an inevitable consequence of the dissolution of gender barriers involved in applying a historically feminine diagnosis to men.

The reasons for medicine's historic resistance to the idea of hysteria in members of its own sex are various. One reason is frankly epistemological: the question of whether it is possible for the human mind to know itself is one that has bedeviled the mental sciences, to say nothing of philosophy, through the ages. The subject of hysteria adds a gendered dimension to the classic dilemma of how to proceed intellectually when the subject and object of study—here, the male mind—are the same.

But if this epistemological conundrum had been enough to forestall inquiry, then the entire disciplines of psychology and psychiatry would never have come into being. A second reason for the denial of male hysteria, this one the most obvious, is political:

throughout the 1700s and 1800s, the critical construction of a civilized, respectable, and rational male subject was crucial to the ascent of middle-class politics and economics across much of Europe. Sustaining patriarchy, however, required both idealizing the virtues and denying the vulnerabilities of hegemonic bourgeois masculinity. Widespread medical recognition of rampant neurotic weakness in the male sex would obviously have undermined the image of a strong, mature, self-possessed species that in turn was entitled to master the rest of the world. When considered fully, male hysteria implied a reconfiguration of the structures of gender differentiation that were then underpinning society. So the homogeneously male medical community contrived to ignore an entire field of potential study. Although individual medical practitioners may have been unaware of this process, its social and cultural effects were active, dynamic, and purposive. Through accumulated acts of omission and commission, European medical commentary on male and female hysteria across three centuries contributed mightily to construct the dominant masculine identities that reinforced patriarchy. Although the model of masculine human nature that physicians advanced was fragile and ultimately untenable, it nonetheless operated successfully for quite a long time.

The bearded collectivity clad in black and white that formed the nineteenth-century "men of science" embodied a version of this rationalist self-representation that was especially stringent, almost a parody. In the period between the late Enlightenment culture of the nervous distempers and the advent of psychoanalysis, European hysteria doctors generated a deceptively coherent narrative of hysteria that sought to evade their own complicity in the subject. It is also most likely the gender politics of male hysteria that explains why medical professionals in the closing decades of the nineteenth century often resisted with particular virulence the admission of women into their world. In diagnostic theory as in the profession at large, the masculine was being infiltrated by the feminine.

The final reason for resistance to male hysteria, a psychological reason, is the most complex. The medical history of female hysteria is an account of how men in power have seen women—the story of a controlling, panoptic gaze of one sex onto the other. But the medical history of male neurosis differs: it is not a construction of the collective "others" of modern and early modern Europe (women, colonials, Jews, homosexuals, criminals); it is, rather, a discourse of the self. This distinction is all-important. To follow through on such a project requires an act of sustained, analytical self-reflexivity—a "turning of the male gaze inward"—and that endeavor is not only politically dangerous but psychologically fraught.[4] To be self-aware is itself "unmasculine." Moreover, for many hysteria doctors, this undertaking brought into the open the error and misogyny of millennia of past medical thought and practice. And to explore the possibility that hysteria was not a woman-only disorder risked uncovering the elements of mental and emotional "femininity" in the "male" psyche itself. In a related threat, just as the male medical gaze on female hysteria repeatedly produced a sexualized discourse, so the specter of male physicians gazing with passionate intensity on other adult men in intimate emotional distress suggested an unacceptable homoerotic intimacy. Fear, vanity, and the drive for power are the underlying sentiments operating in this story.[5]

Any one of these factors might have been overcome, but in convergence they proved insurmountable. By and large, the medical history of male hysteria in the years surveyed in this book is the story of lost opportunities, contradictory arguments, and half-formulated insights. Above all, it is the story of repeated and ritualized silences.[6] As a formal discourse, it is marked by the usual continuities and ruptures; but, in a striking parallel pattern, it is also troubled by countless omissions, resistances, and ambivalences. Throughout this long period, European medics lavished their descriptive powers and theoretical imagination on women suffering nervously, but those same professionals proved singularly incapable of conceiving themselves as cases.[7] As a consequence, male hysteria's considerable potential to deconstruct gender difference went almost entirely unrealized. From the early seventeenth to the early twentieth centuries, European medical science failed to achieve a cumulative, formalized, disciplinary discourse of emotional and nervous illness in males akin to what it created for women or for other pathologies in both sexes. This, I believe, is the true male malady—not the pains, twitches, and obsessions that accompany the human condition, but the chronic inability to reflect nonheroically, without evasion and self-deception, on oneself individually and collectively.

The "failed enterprise" that is the subject of this book did not, of course, end with the publication of Freud's *Three Essays on the Theory of Sexuality* in 1905.[8] There is an eventful twentieth-century sequel to this story, which features the battle trenches of Verdun and the Somme, the psychoanalytic diaspora, film noir of the 1950s, the successive editions of the *Diagnostic and Statistical Manual of Mental Disorders,* the advent of feminist psychologies, and the post-traumatic stress disorders (PTSD) experienced by Vietnam and Iraq veterans, among many other events. The specter of masses of emotionally incapacitated men during and after the First World War finally forced British and American physicians to confront in depth the reality of masculine hysterical neurosis.[9] But, in "the worst century there has ever been" in Western history, the well-known shell shock story was only the first in a train of man-made, world-historical catastrophes that marked the 1900s and produced a level of nervous and emotional collapse that could no longer be denied.[10] The new medico-psychological discourses of trauma created in response to twentieth-century wars, genocides, diseases, and disasters address men and women coextensively.

During these same decades, psychodynamic psychiatry, of which Freudian psychoanalysis was only one strand, developed and then spread out globally. Despite endless sectarian squabbling among their different schools, Freudian, Jungian, Adlerian, Kleinian, existentialist, and phenomenological psychiatrists all took the human psyche as an independent causal field. They strove to create new sciences of intrapsychic subjectivity, and together they educated generations of psychologically-minded mental health workers. As in psychoanalysis, their theories of human mental functioning were markedly less gendered than the psychologies they replaced and often addressed issues of masculinity and femininity. In a parallel development, Western psychiatry, beginning in the last third of the twentieth century, has increasingly withdrawn from the hysteria diagnosis itself, judging it to be a historical artifact that is as sexist, overgeneralized, and unscientific clinically as it is colorful historically. Today's successor categories to the great neurosis are free of ancient gender associations. No one claims that "somatization disorder," PTSD, "idiopathic pseudo-seizures," and "psychogenic pain disorder" are male or female maladies.

The decades from the 1960s onward in both Europe and America also witnessed one new social liberationist movement after another: the civil rights movement, the women's revolution, gay liberation, and so on. These waves of social reformism, advanced by hitherto marginalized groups, spawned comprehensive critiques of past structures of power, including the many historical ideologies of patriarchy. Within the Euro-American academy, whole new disciplines of inquiry and bodies of theory, such as gender studies, the history of the body, and queer theory, have arisen that take "the history of masculinities" as a field of critical, comparative scrutiny.

The synthesis of these developments—modern wars, trauma theory, psychodynamic psychiatry, human rights movements, academic gender studies—signals a fundamentally altered cultural environment for viewing and discussing gender in general, and masculinity in particular. In many Western cultures, a tremendous amount of observation that previously was excluded, repressed, or literally unthinkable has now become utterable.[11] Today, medicine no longer plays a commanding role in producing the dominant fictions of masculinity. The obstacles to masculine self-understanding have receded significantly, and in several cultural arenas men are exploring new kinds of discourse that can illuminate the past and present experience of masculinity. Still, it would be foolish to contend that the process is complete.

# NOTES

# INDEX

# NOTES

## Prologue

1. The similarity in scenes was intentional. In his stage instructions Sartre specifies a lecture hall "which is exactly like the one in the famous painting 'Une leçon clinique à la Salpêtrière.'" See Jean-Paul Sartre, *Le scénario Freud,* avec préface de J.-B. Pontalis (Paris: Éditions Gallimard, 1984), 53. On the painting itself, which now hangs in the Musée de l'Assistance Publique in Paris, see Nadine Simon-Dhouailly, *La leçon de Charcot—Voyage dans une toile* (Paris: Imprimerie Tardy Quercy, 1986), and J. L. Signoret, "Variété historique: *Une leçon clinique à la Salpêtrière* (1887) par André Brouillet," *Revue neurologique,* 139, no. 12 (1983), 687–701.

2. Michael Fleming and Roger Manvell provide a synopsis of the film in *Images of Madness: The Portrayal of Insanity in the Feature Film* (London and Toronto: Associated University Presses, 1985), 236–242. See also Michael Shortland's intelligent discussion in "Screen Memories: Towards a History of Psychiatry and Psychoanalysis in the Movies," *British Journal for the History of Science,* 20 (1987), 431–446.

3. The evolution of the scene within the screenplay is complicated. See *The Freud Scenario,* ed. J.-B. Pontalis, trans. Quintin Hoare (Chicago: University of Chicago Press, 1985), Editor's Preface, vii–x; First Version, Scene 11, 54–65; and Appendix A: The Synopsis, Scene 7, 511–512.

4. In two published case histories from the 1880s, Charcot contrasts male and female hysterical patients in front of medical audiences. See Jean-Martin Charcot, *Leçons sur les maladies du système nerveux* (1887), recueillies et publiées par M. M. Babinski, Bernard, Féré, Guinon, Marie and Gilles de la Tourette, in *Oeuvres complètes de J. M. Charcot,* 9 vols. (Paris: Bureaux du Progrès Médical, Delahaye & Lecrosnier, 1886–1893), vol. 3, lectures 7–8 and 18. Likewise, the theory of the transfer of hysterical symptoms, either from one side of the body to the other or from one patient to another by means of hypnosis, magnets, or metals, was formulated by French physicians in the Charcot circle during the

1880s. See Joseph Babinski, "Recherches servant à établir que certaines manifestations hystériques peuvent être transferées d'un sujet à un autre sous l'influence de l'aimant," *Le progrès médical,* 47 (November 20, 1886), 1010–1011.

5. Janet Oppenheim, *"Shattered Nerves": Doctors, Patients, and Depression in Victorian England* (New York and Oxford: Oxford University Press, 1991), chap. 5; Elizabeth Green Musselman, *Nervous Conditions: Science and the Body Politic in Early Industrial Britain* (Albany: State University of New York Press, 2006), chap. 1.

6. See Elaine Showalter, *The Female Malady: Women, Madness, and English Culture, 1830–1980* (New York: Pantheon, 1985), Introduction. Despite its title, to which I allude respectfully in this Prologue, Showalter's important book includes a chapter on World War One shell shock as a form of male hysteria.

## 1. Hysterick Women and Hypochondriack Men

1. Plato, *Timaeus,* 91-C, in *The Collected Dialogues of Plato,* 11th ed., Edith Hamilton and Huntington Cairns, eds. (Princeton: Princeton University Press, 1982), 1210.

2. Ilza Veith, *Hysteria: History of a Disease* (Chicago: University of Chicago Press, 1965), chap. 2; Étienne Trillat, *Histoire de l'hystérie* (Paris: Segher, 1986), chap. 1; Giuseppe Roccatagliata, *Isteria* (Rome: Il Pensiero Scientifico Editore, 1990), chaps. 3–5.

3. It should be noted that the very concept of "Hippocratic hysteria" has now been called into question in the able revisionist analyses of Helen King. See King, "Once Upon a Text: Hysteria from Hippocrates," in Sander L. Gilman, Helen King, Roy Porter, G. S. Rousseau, and Elaine Showalter, *Hysteria Beyond Freud* (Berkeley: University of California Press, 1993), 3–90; and King, *Hippocrates' Woman: Reading the Female Body in Ancient Greece* (London and New York: Routledge, 1998), chap. 11.

4. I use the term "Renaissance" in the comparatively broad sense that historians of science and medicine typically use, to denote the period from the mid-fifteenth to the early-seventeenth centuries. See Marie Boas's *The Scientific Renaissance, 1450–1630* (New York: Harper and Row, 1962).

5. On the "medicalization of divine madness," consult Roy Porter, *Mind-Forg'd Manacles: A History of Madness in England from the Restoration to the Regency* (New York: Viking Penguin, 1987), 79ff.

6. Edward Jorden, *A Briefe Discourse of a Disease Called the Suffocation of the Mother* (London: John Windet, 1603).

7. For the background to the case, read Michael MacDonald's introduction to *Witchcraft and Hysteria in Elizabethan London: Edward Jorden and the Mary Glover Case* (London and New York: Tavistock/Routledge, 1991).

8. Democritus Junior [Robert Burton], *The Anatomy of Melancholy, What It Is, with All the Kinds, Causes, Symptomes, Prognostickes and severall Cures of It* [1621], introduction by Holbrook Jackson (New York: Vintage Books, 1977).

9. Lawrence Babb, *Sanity in Bedlam: A Study of Robert Burton's Anatomy of Melancholy* (East Lansing: Michigan State University Press, 1959); Judith Kegan Gardiner, "Elizabethan Psychology and Burton's *Anatomy of Melancholy*," *Journal of the History of Ideas*, 38 (1977), 373–388.

10. Burton, *Anatomy of Melancholy*, Part One, 414–419.

11. Especially relevant is the section on "Love Melancholy" (Part Three, 40–257), a form of the affliction, Burton notes, that "turns a man into a woman." See Mark Breitenberg, *Anxious Masculinity in Early Modern England* (Cambridge: Cambridge University Press, 1996), chap. 1.

12. William Harvey, *Exercitationes de generatione animalium* (1651), trans. from Latin by Robert Willis as *Anatomical Exercises on the Generation of Animals*, in *The Works of William Harvey, M.D.* (London: Sydenham Society, 1847), 542.

13. Feminist psychoanalytic literary critics have made much of this stunning passage. See Coppélia Kahn, "The Absent Mother in *King Lear*," in Margaret W. Ferguson, Maureen Quilligan, and Nancy J. Vickers, eds., *Rewriting the Renaissance: The Discourses of Sexual Difference in Early Modern Europe* (Chicago: University of Chicago Press, 1986), 33–49; Juliet Mitchell, "From King Lear to Anna O. and Beyond: Some Speculative Theses on Hysteria and the Traditionless Self," *Yale Journal of Criticism*, 5 (Spring 1992), 91–107; and Kaara L. Peterson, "Historica Passio: Early Modern Medicine, King Lear, and Editorial Practice," *Shakespeare Quarterly*, 57 (Spring 2006), 1–22.

14. Hansruedi Isler, *Thomas Willis, 1621–1675, Doctor and Scientist,* trans. from the German (New York: Hafner, 1968); John D. Spillane, *The Doctrine of the Nerves: Chapters in the History of Neurology* (Oxford: Oxford University Press, 1981), chap. 3; Robert G. Frank Jr., "Thomas Willis and His Circle: Brain and Mind in Seventeenth-Century Medicine," in G. S. Rousseau, ed., *The Languages of Psyche: Mind and Body in Enlightenment Thought* (Berkeley: University of California Press, 1990), 107–146.

15. [Thomas Willis], *Dr. Willis's Practice of Physick, Being the Whole Works of That Renowned and Famous Physician,* trans. from the Latin by Samuel Pordage (London: T. Dring, C. Harper, and J. Leigh, 1684), 71.

16. Thomas Willis, *An Essay on the Pathology of the Brain and Nervous Stock in which Convulsive Diseases are Treated of*, trans. from the Latin by Samuel Pordage (London: Dring, Leigh, and Harper, 1684), 71.

17. Stanley W. Jackson, *Melancholia and Depression: From Hippocratic Times to Modern Times* (New Haven: Yale University Press, 1986), chap. 11; Ilza Veith, "On Hysterical and Hypochondriacal Afflictions," *Bulletin of the History of Medicine*, 30 (May 1956), 233–240.

18. *Dr. Willis's Practice of Physick*, 81–92.

19. Willis, *Pathologiae Cerebri et Nervosi Generis Specimen* (London: Jacobum Allestry, 1668), chap. 10, 68–80; Willis, *Essay on the Pathology of the Brain and Nervous Stock*, 68–69.

20. Willis, *Pathologiae Cerebri et Nervosi Generis Specimen*, 33, column 2, cited in Glafira Abricossoff, *L'Hystérie aux XVIIe et XVIIIe siècles: Étude historique* (Paris: G. Steinheil, 1897), 34.

21. *Epistolary Dissertation to Dr. Cole*, in *The Works of Thomas Sydenham*, 2 vols., trans. from Latin by R. G. Latham (London: Sydenham Society, 1848–1850), 2: 85.

22. Friedrich Hoffmann, *A System of the Practice of Medicine*, trans. from Latin by William Lewis, 2 vols. (London: J. Murray and J. Johnson, 1783), 2: 43–59.

23. I take the term "nervous culture" from George Rousseau, "'A Strange Pathology': Hysteria in the Early Modern World, 1500–1800," in *Hysteria Beyond Freud*, 165. My discussion of eighteenth-century Britain is profoundly indebted to the scholarship of Rousseau and Roy Porter. See G. S. Rousseau, "Towards a Semiotics of the Nerve: The Social History of Language in a New Key," in Peter Burke and Roy Porter, eds., *Language, Self, and Society: A Social History of Language* (Cambridge: Polity Press, 1991), 213–275; Rousseau, "Nerves, Spirits, and Fibres: Towards an Anthropology of Sensibility," in Rousseau, *Pre- and Post-Modern Discourses*, 3 vols., I: *Enlightenment Crossings* (Manchester and New York: Manchester University Press, 1991), 122–141; Rousseau, "Discourses of the Nerve," in Frederick Amrine and Robert S. Cohen, eds., *Literature and Science as Modes of Expression* (Dordrecht: Kluwer, 1989), 29–60; Rousseau, "'A Strange Pathology,'" in *Hysteria Beyond Freud*, 91–221; Rousseau, *Nervous Acts: Essays on Literature, Culture, and Sensibility* (New York: Palgrave, 2004); Roy Porter, *Mind-Forg'd Manacles*, chap. 2; Porter, "The Rage of Party: A Glorious Revolution in English Psychiatry?" *Medical History*, 29 (1983), 35–50; Porter, "'The Hunger of Imagination': Approaching Samuel Johnson's Melancholy," in W. F. Bynum, Roy Porter, and Michael Shepherd, eds., *The Anatomy of*

*Madness: Essays in the History of Psychiatry*, 3 vols. (London: Tavistock, 1985), 1: 63–88; Porter, "Bedlam and Parnassus: Mad People's Writing in Georgian England," in George Levine, ed., *One Culture: Essays in Science and Literature* (Madison: University of Wisconsin Press, 1987), 258–284; and Porter, *The Creation of the Modern World: The Untold Story of the British Enlightenment* (London and New York: W. W. Norton, 2000), chap. 12.

24. I use the term "Georgian" to designate the period of the reigns of the first three members of the house of Hanover, from the accession of George I in 1714 to the beginning of the regency of George IV in 1811. The term is roughly coterminous with Britain in the eighteenth century.

25. For vivid representations of "nervous man," see Robert Whytt, *Observations on the Nature, Causes, and Cure of those Disorders which have been Commonly called Nervous, Hypochondriac, or Hysteric*, 2nd ed. (Edinburgh and London: T. Becket, P. A. De Hondt, and J. Balfour, 1765), 13–84; and William Smith, *A Dissertation Upon the Nerves* (London: W. Owen, 1768), 143–183.

26. Spillane, *Doctrine of the Nerves*, chap. 4; Eric T. Carlson and Meribeth M. Simpson, "Models of the Nervous System in Eighteenth-Century Psychiatry," *Bulletin of the History of Medicine*, 43 (1969), 101–115.

27. Whytt, *Disorders Commonly Called Nervous, Hypochondriac, or Hysteric* (1765), 93.

28. Esther Fischer-Homberger, "Hypochondriasis of the Eighteenth Century—Neurosis of the Present Century," *Bulletin of the History of Medicine*, 46 (1972), 391–401.

29. R. S. Crane, "Suggestions Toward a Genealogy of the 'Man of Feeling,'" in *ELH: A Journal of English Literary History*, 1 (December 1934), 205–230.

30. Walter Francis Wright, *Sensibility in English Prose Fiction, 1760–1814: A Reinterpretation* (Urbana: University of Illinois Press, 1937); Northrop Frye, "Towards Defining an Age of Sensibility," *ELH*, 23 (June 1956), 144–152; Janet M. Todd, *Sensibility: An Introduction* (London: Methuen, 1986). On the medical underpinnings of the movement, see John Mullan, *Sentiment and Sociability: The Language of Feeling in the Eighteenth Century* (Oxford: Clarendon Press, 1988), chap. 5.

31. Henry Mackenzie, *The Man of Feeling*, ed. Brian Vickers (London: Oxford University Press, 1967).

32. Rebecca Gould, "Sterne's Sentimental Yorick as Male Hysteric," *Studies in English Literature, 1500–1900*, 36 (Summer 1996), 641–653.

33. See G. J. Barker-Benfield's *The Culture of Sensibility: Sex and Society in Eighteenth-Century Britain* (Chicago: University of Chicago Press, 1992), passim.
34. Markman Ellis, *The Politics of Sensibility: Race, Gender, and Commerce in the Sentimental Novel* (Cambridge: Cambridge University Press, 1996).
35. As Christopher Lawrence points out in "The Nervous System and Society in the Scottish Enlightenment," in Barry Barnes and Steven Shapin, eds., *Natural Order: Historical Studies of Scientific Culture* (Beverly Hills and London: Sage Publications, 1979), 19–40.
36. Rousseau, "'A Strange Pathology,'" in *Hysteria Beyond Freud*, 158, 164.
37. John Purcell, *A Treatise of Vapours, or Hysterick Fits, Containing an Analytical Proof of Its Causes, Mechanical Explanation of All Its Symptoms and Accidents, according to the newest and most Rational Principles* (London: Nicholas Cox, 1702); Bernard de Mandeville, *A Treatise of the Hypochondriack and Hysterick Passions* (London: Dryden Leach, W. Taylor, 1711); Sir John Midriff (pseud.), *Observations on the Spleen and Vapours: Containing Remarkable Cases of Persons of Both Sexes and all Ranks* (London: J. Roberts, 1721); William Stukeley, *Of the Spleen; Its Description and History, Uses and Diseases, Particularly the Vapors, with their Remedy* (London, printed for the author, 1723); Sir Richard Blackmore, *A Treatise of the Spleen and Vapours: or, Hypochondriacal and Hysterical Affections* (London: J. Pemberton, 1725); Nicholas Robinson, *A New System of the Spleen, Vapours, and Hypochondriack Melancholy: Wherein all the Decays of the Nerves, and Lowness of the Spirits, are mechanically Accounted for* (London: A. Bettesworth, W. Innys, and C. Rivington, 1729); George Cheyne, *The English Malady, or A Treatise of Nervous Diseases of all Kinds as Spleen, Vapours, Lowness of Spirits, Hypochondriacal, and Hysterical Distempers, Etc.* (London and Bath: G. Strahan and J. Leake, 1733); Sir Richard Manningham, *The Symptoms, Nature, Causes, and Cure of the Febricula, or Little Fever: commonly called the Nervous or Hysteric Fever, Vapours, Hypo, or Spleen* (London: T. Osborne, 1746); Charles Perry, *A Mechanical Account and Explication of the Hysteric Passion* (London: Shuckburgh, 1755); Robert Whytt, *Observations on the Nature, Causes, and Cure of those Disorders which have been commonly called Nervous, Hypochondriac, or Hysteric* (London and Edinburgh: T. Becket, P. A. De Hondt, and J. Balfour, 1765); Sir John Hill, *Hypochondriasis. A Practical Treatise on the Nature and Cure of that Disorder; Commonly called the Hyp or Hypo* (London, for the author, 1766); William Smith, *A Dissertation upon the Nerves* (London: W. Owen, 1768); Andrew Wilson, *Medical Researches: Being an Enquiry into the Nature and Origin of Hysterics in the Female Constitution, and into the Distinction between that Disease and Hypochondriac or Nervous Disorders* (London: S.

Hooper and Robson, 1776); William Perfect, *Cases of Insanity, the Epilepsy, Hypochondriacal Affection, Hysteric Passion, and Nervous Disorders, Successfully Treated* (Rochester: W. Gillman, 1779); James Makittrick Adair, *Essays on Fashionable Diseases* (London: T. P. Bateman, 1787); William Rowley, *A Treatise on Female, Nervous, Hysterical, Hypochondriacal, Bilious, Convulsive Diseases with Thoughts on Madness, Suicide, Etc.* (London: C. Nourse, T. Hookham, E. Newbery, 1788); John Reid, *Essays on Hypochondriasis and Other Nervous Affections* (London: Longman, Hurst, Rees, Orme, and Brown, 1816).

For a complete listing of titles in the major European languages, including scores of Latin dissertations on male hysteria, refer to Heinrich Laehr, *Die Literatur der Psychiatrie, Neurologie und Psychologie im XVIII. Jahrhundert*, 2nd ed. (Berlin: Reimer, 1895).

38. Blackmore, *Treatise of the Spleen and Vapours*, 31, 107.
39. Ibid., 107.
40. Robinson, *A New System of the Spleen*, 196–197.
41. Richard Browne, *Medicina Musica . . . To which is annex'd a New Essay on the Nature and Cure of the Spleen and Vapours* (London: John Cooke, 1729), chap. 4, 69–71.
42. Whytt, *Observations on . . . Disorders called Nervous, Hypochondriac, or Hysterical* (1765), 105.
43. Ibid., 212n, 215.
44. Wilson, *Medical Researches* (1776), chap. 1, 36–38.
45. Ibid., chap. 18, 174–183. See the similar statement in Thomas Dover, *The Ancient Physician's Legacy to His Country*, 2nd ed. (London: printed for the author, 1732), 59–60.
46. John Ferriar, *Medical Histories and Reflections*, 2 vols. (London: Cadell & Davies, 1795), 1: 37.
47. Ferriar, *Medical Histories and Reflections* (Warrington: printed by W. Eyres, for T. Cadell, London, 1792), 111–114. My thanks to Cath Quinn for bringing this passage to my attention.
48. John F. Sena, "Belinda's Hysteria: The Medical Context of *The Rape of the Lock*," in Christopher Fox, ed., *Psychology and Literature in the Eighteenth Century* (New York: AMS Press, 1987), 129–147.
49. Rousseau, "'A Strange Pathology,'" 152, 164.
50. See, for instance, the "Ode on the Spleen" that prefaces William Stukeley's 1723 treatise *Of the Spleen: Its Description and History.*
51. Margery Bailey, ed., *The HYPOCHONDRIACK*, 2 vols. (Stanford: Stanford University Press, 1920), esp. vol. 1, no. 5, and vol. 2, no. 63; Allan Ingram, *Boswell's Creative Gloom* (London: Macmillan, 1982); George E. Haggerty, "Boswell's Symptoms: *The Hypochondriack* In and

Out of Context," in Donald J. Newman, ed., *James Boswell: Psychological Interpretations* (New York: St. Martin's Press, 1995), chap. 6.

52. Cited in Irma S. Lustig and Frederick A. Pottle, eds., *Boswell: The English Experiment, 1785–1789* (New York: McGraw-Hill, 1986), 122. The editorial staff of the James Boswell papers at Yale kindly tracked down this citation for me.

53. Joseph Farington, *The Farington Diary*, ed. James Greig, 8 vols. (London: Hutchinson and Co., 1922–1928), 6: 100.

54. Letter from Edward Jenner to Dr. Alexander Marcet, dated March 5, 1822, in Genevieve Miller, ed., *Letters of Edward Jenner* (Baltimore: Johns Hopkins University Press, 1983), 109.

55. For the episode and its background, see Ernest Campbell Mossner, *The Life of David Hume*, 2nd ed. (Oxford: Clarendon Press, 1980), chaps. 6–7, as well as Roy Porter and Dorothy Porter, *In Sickness and in Health: The British Experience 1650–1850* (New York: B. Blackwell, 1988), 210–212.

56. Henri Ellenberger, "The Concept of 'Maladie Créatrice'" (1964), in Mark S. Micale, ed., *Beyond the Unconscious: Essays of Henri F. Ellenberger in the History of Psychiatry* (Princeton: Princeton University Press, 1993), chap. 13.

57. Quoted in Mossner, *Life of Hume*, 67.

58. The doctor in question was once believed to be Cheyne, but Hume's biographer believed the addressee was a different London practitioner, Dr. John Arbuthnot. See Ernest Mossner, "Hume's Epistle to Dr. Arbuthnot, 1734: The Biographical Significance," in *Huntington Library Quarterly*, 7 (1944), 135–152.

59. The extraordinary letter is reproduced in full in J.Y.T. Greig, *The Letters of David Hume* (Oxford: Clarendon Press, 1932), vol. 1, letter 3, written March or April 1734, 12–18, as well as at *http://serendip.brynmawr.edu/exchange/davidhume*.

60. Ibid.

61. Mossner, *Life of Hume*, 71, 85.

62. For the exceptions, see the entry on hysteria in Robert James, *A Medicinal Dictionary*, 3 vols. (London: T. Osborne, 1743–1745), vol. 2: 850–859; and John Leake, *Medical Instructions towards the Prevention, and Cure of Chronic or Slow Diseases Peculiar to Women, especially those proceeding from over-Delicacy of Habit called Nervous or Hysterical* (London: R. Baldwin, 1777), 218–273.

63. On medicine in Enlightenment ideology, see Peter Gay, "Enlightenment: Medicine and Cure," in *The Enlightenment: An Interpretation, 2*

vols. (New York: Alfred A. Knopf, 1967–1969), 2: *The Science of Freedom*, 12–23.

64. Burton, *Anatomy of Melancholy*, 615.

65. Blackmore, *Treatise of the Spleen and Vapours*, Preface, iv.

66. Joseph Raulin, *Traité des affections vaporeuses du sexe* (Paris: J.-T. Herissant, 1758), cited in Trillat, *Histoire de l'hystérie*, 71–72.

67. See Marie Mulvey Roberts and Roy Porter, eds., *Literature and Medicine during the Eighteenth Century* (London: Routledge, 1993), Introduction.

68. Gill Perry and Michael Rossington, eds., *Femininity and Masculinity in Eighteenth-Century Art and Culture* (Manchester: Manchester University Press, 1994), 9–12; Carolyn D. Williams, *Pope, Homer, and Manliness* (London: Routledge, 1993), 11–15, 27–53; Alan Sinfield, *The Wilde Century: Effeminacy, Oscar Wilde and the Queer Moment* (London: Cassell, 1994), chaps. 2, 3.

69. Philip Carter, *Men and the Emergence of Polite Society, Britain 1660–1800* (London: Pearson Education, 2001), chap. 4.

70. Bernard de Mandeville, *Treatise of the Hypochondriack and Hysterick Passions, vulgarly call'd the Hypo in Men and Vapours in Women* (London: Dryden Leach, W. Taylor, 1711). The treatise was reissued in 1715, and a second, extensively revised edition (cited in note 71 below) appeared in 1730.

71. *A Treatise of the Hypochondriack and Hysterick Diseases. In Three Dialogues*, 2nd enl. ed. (London: J. Tonson, 1730), 3–30.

72. Ibid., 29.

73. Ibid., 83–224.

74. Ibid., 106, 208–212, 216.

75. Ibid., 272–279.

76. Ibid., 238–249.

77. Ibid., 112–113, 118–119, 216–218.

78. George Cheyne, *The English Malady: or, A Treatise of Nervous Diseases of All Kinds as Spleen, Vapours, Lowness of Spirits, Hypochondriacal, and Hysterical Distempers, Etc.* (London and Bath: G. Strahan and J. Leake, 1733).

79. See Roy Porter's introduction to *George Cheyne: The English Malady (1733)* (London: Tavistock/Routledge, 1991), ix–li, as well as G. S. Rousseau, "Mysticism and Millenarianism: 'Immortal Dr. Cheyne,'" in Ingrid Merkel and Allen G. Debus, eds., *Hermeticism and the Renaissance* (Washington, D.C.: Folger Shakespeare Library, 1988), chap. 10; and Lester S. King, "George Cheyne, Mirror of Eighteenth-Century Medicine," *Bulletin of the History of Medicine*, 48 (1974), 517–539.

80. Cheyne, *English Malady*, 267–370.

81. Ibid., 267.
82. Ibid., 269.
83. Ibid., 307–324.
84. Ibid., 325–364.
85. Ibid., Preface ii, 329, 333, 344.
86. See ibid., 335.
87. Ibid., 346–347.
88. Gloria Sybil Gross, *This Invisible Riot of the Mind: Samuel Johnson's Psychological Theory* (Philadelphia: University of Pennsylvania Press, 1992); John Wiltshire, *Samuel Johnson in the Medical World: The Doctor and the Patient* (Cambridge and New York: Cambridge University Press, 1991); and Porter, "'Hunger of Imagination': Approaching Samuel Johnson's Melancholy," in *Anatomy of Madness*, 63–88.
89. [James Boswell], *Boswell's Life of Johnson*, ed. George Birkbeck Hill, revised and enlarged by L. F. Powell, 6 vols. (Oxford: Clarendon Press, 1934), 1: 63, 64.
90. For a concise account of the case and its many interpretations, see Wiltshire, *Samuel Johnson in the Medical World*, 11–63.
91. Cited in ibid., 118.
92. *Boswell's Life of Johnson*, 3: 152.
93. Margaret P. Boddy, "Burton in the Eighteenth Century," *Notes and Queries*, 167 (August 1934), 206–208; Porter, "The Hunger of Imagination," in *Anatomy of Madness*, vol. I: 81.
94. The biography, which first appeared in *Gentleman's Magazine*, 12 (1742), 633–635, is reprinted with scholarly commentary in Lawrence C. McHenry, "Samuel Johnson's 'The Life of Dr. Sydenham,'" *Medical History*, 8 (1964), 181–187.
95. R. W. Chapman, ed., *The Letters of Samuel Johnson, with Mrs. Thrale's Genuine Letters to Him*, 3 vols. (Oxford: Clarendon Press, 1952), 2: letter 617, p. 290. Roy Porter kindly brought this letter to my attention.
96. Samuel Johnson, *History of Rasselas: Prince of Abyssinia*, ed. George Birkbeck Hill (Oxford: Clarendon Press, 1954).
97. The story of Rasselas is related in chaps. 40–44 and 46.
98. On the possible influence of Mandeville's treatise on this aspect of Johnson's novel, see Wiltshire, *Samuel Johnson in the Medical World*, 188.
99. Richard B. Hovey, "Dr. Samuel Johnson, Psychiatrist," *Modern Language Quarterly*, 15 (1954), 321–355; Kathleen M. Grange, "Dr. Samuel Johnson's Account of a Schizophrenic Illness in *Rasselas* (1759)," *Medical History*, 6 (April 1962), 162–168; Wiltshire, *Samuel Johnson in the Medical World*, chap. 5.

100. Porter, *Mind-Forg'd Manacles,* 58.

101. John Mullan emphasizes these differences in "Hypochondria and Hysteria: Sensibility and the Physicians," *The Eighteenth Century: Theory and Interpretation,* 25 (Spring 1984), 141–174.

102. The fact that European literary culture of the late Enlightenment gave rise to three figures of the highest order who were centrally concerned with the representation of male emotional distress further bears out this interpretation. Like Johnson, Goethe and Jean-Jacques Rousseau were suffering and self-dissecting males who depicted characters with these same traits in both their fictional and autobiographical writings. Johnson and Goethe also combined deep literary and scientific learning; all three men are regarded today as forerunners of psychological modernism.

## 2. The Great Victorian Eclipse

1. Mona Ozouf, *Women's Words: Essay on French Singularity,* trans. from the French by Jane Marie Todd (Chicago and London: University of Chicago Press, 1997), ix–xxii and 229–283; Joan Wallach Scott, *Only Paradoxes to Offer: French Feminists and the Rights of Man* (Cambridge, Mass.: Harvard University Press, 1996), chaps. 1, 2.

2. Dena Goodman, *The Republic of Letters: A Cultural History of the French Enlightenment* (Ithaca: Cornell University Press, 1994), passim; Goodman, "Policing Society: Women as Political Actors in Enlightenment Discourse," in Hans Erich Bödeker and Lieselotte Steinbrügge, eds., *Conceptualising Woman in Enlightenment Thought / Conceptualiser la femme dans la pensée des Lumières* (Berlin: Arno Spitz, 2001), 129–141.

3. Dominique Godineau, "Daughters of Liberty and Revolutionary Citizens," and Elisabeth G. Sledziewski, "The French Revolution as the Turning Point," in Geneviève Fraisse and Michelle Perrot, eds., *Emerging Feminism from Revolution to World War,* vol. 4: *A History of Women in the West,* Georges Duby and Michelle Perrot, gen. eds. (Cambridge, Mass.: Harvard University Press, 1993), chaps. 1, 2.

4. Linda Colley, *Britons: Forging the Nation, 1707–1837* (New Haven: Yale University Press, 1992), 252.

5. The 1804 Code pronounced husbands the official head and master of the family, declared women legally incompetent, restricted the conditions for divorce, outlawed paternity suits, instituted skewed adultery laws for men and women, prohibited women from receiving an inheritance without their husband's consent, and required a wife to secure her husband's permission to take up employment outside the home.

6. Yvonne Knibiehler, "Les médecins et la 'nature féminine' au temps du code civil," *Annales: Économies. Sociétés. Civilisations,* 31 (July–August 1976), 824–845; Michel Gourevitch, "La psychiatrie sous l'Empire," *Histoire des sciences médicales,* 23 (1989), 27–32.

7. Don Herzog, *Poisoning the Minds of the Lower Orders* (Princeton: Princeton University Press, 1998).

8. Isser Woloch, *The New Regime: Transformations of the French Civic Order, 1789–1820s* (New York: W. W. Norton, 1994), chaps. 1–3, pp. 427–434.

9. Ian C. Bradley, *The Call to Seriousness: The Evangelical Impact on the Victorians* (London: Jonathan Cape, 1976); Leonore Davidoff and Catherine Hall, *Family Fortunes: Men and Women of the English Middle Class, 1780–1850* (1987), 2nd ed. rev. (London and New York: Routledge, 2002), 76–106; G. J. Barker-Benfield, *The Culture of Sensibility: Sex and Society in Eighteenth-Century Britain* (Chicago: University of Chicago Press, 1992), 65–77, 266–279.

10. Bradley, *Call to Seriousness* (1976), 15. Davidoff and Hall note that "evangelical manhood, with its stress on self-sacrifice and influence, came dangerously close to embracing 'feminine' qualities . . . In late eighteenth-century local records, we find Evangelical 'tender-hearted' men moved to tears by Waverley novels or by the first sight of Norwich Cathedral." *Family Fortunes* [2002], 111.

11. Walter E. Houghton, *The Victorian Frame of Mind, 1830–1870* (New Haven: Yale University Press, 1957), chaps. 7, 10; Boyd Hilton, *The Age of Atonement: The Influence of Evangelicalism on Social and Economic Thought, 1795–1865* (Oxford and New York: Clarendon Press, 1988); Herbert Schlossberg, *The Silent Revolution and the Making of Victorian England* (Columbus: Ohio State University Press, 2000), esp. chaps. 3, 6, 7, 9.

12. John Tosh, *A Man's Place: Masculinity and the Middle-Class Home in Victorian England* (New Haven and London: Yale University Press, 1999), 5, 36–39.

13. Nancy F. Cott, "Passionlessness: An Interpretation of Victorian Sexual Ideology, 1790–1850," *Signs: A Journal of Women in Culture and Society,* 4 (Winter 1978), 219–236.

14. Norman Vance, *The Sinews of the Spirit: The Ideal of Christian Manliness in Victorian Literature and Religious Thought* (Cambridge and New York: Cambridge University Press, 1985).

15. Peter N. Sterns, *Be a Man! Males in Modern Society* (1979), 2nd ed. (New York: Holmes & Meier, 1990), 40.

16. Adeline Daumard, *Les bourgeois et la bourgeoisie en France depuis 1815*

(Paris: Aubier, 1987), 70–75; Davidoff and Hall, *Family Fortunes* (2002), 195–315; Barbara Caine and Glenda Sluga, *Gendering European History, 1780–1920* (London and New York: Leicester University Press, 2000), chap. 2.

17. Stearns, *Be A Man!* (1990), chap. 3.

18. Janet Oppenheim, *"Shattered Nerves": Doctors, Patients and Depression in Victorian England* (New York and Oxford: Oxford University Press, 1991), 149.

19. Tosh, *A Man's Place,* 5.

20. I am paraphrasing here from Oppenheim, *"Shattered Nerves"* (1990), 141, and from Davidoff and Hall, *Family Fortunes* (2002), 180–192, 450–454.

21. Peter Gay, *The Bourgeois Experience: Victoria to Freud,* 5 vols. (New York: Oxford University Press, 1984–1998), vol. 1: *Education of the Senses* (1984), and vol. 2: *The Tender Passion* (1986); M. Jeanne Peterson, *Family, Love, and Work in the Lives of Victorian Gentlewomen* (Bloomington: Indiana University Press, 1989); Michael Mason, *The Making of Victorian Sexual Attitudes* (Oxford: Oxford University Press, 1994); Anne Summers, "Common Sense about Separate Spheres," in Summers, *Female Lives, Moral States: Women, Religion and Public Life in Britain, 1800–1930* (Newbury, Berks.: Threshold Press, 2000), 5–26.

22. Harry Cocks, "Abominable Crimes: Sodomy Trials in English Law and Culture, 1830–1889," Ph.D. diss., University of Manchester, 1998, chap. 1.

23. James A. Mangan and James Walvin, eds., *Manliness and Morality: Middle-Class Masculinity in Britain and America, 1800–1940* (Manchester: Manchester University Press, 1987); Mark C. Carnes and Clyde Griffen, eds., *Meanings for Manhood: Constructions of Masculinity in Victorian America* (Chicago and London: University of Chicago Press, 1990); Michael Roper and John Tosh, eds., *Manful Assertions: Masculinities in Britain since 1800* (London and New York: Routledge, 1991).

24. Mary Poovey, *Uneven Developments: The Ideological Work of Gender in Mid-Victorian England* (London: Virago Press, 1988), chap. 1; Davidoff and Hall, *Family Fortunes* (2002), chaps. 4, 5.

25. Diderot and D'Alembert, *Encyclopédie, ou Dictionnaire raisonné des sciences, des arts et des métiers,* 17 vols. (Paris: Briasson, 1751–1765), "Hystérique," VIII: 420; "Vapeurs," XVI: 836–837.

26. F. J. Gall, *On the Functions of the Brain and Each of Its Parts* [1825], trans. from the French by Winslow Lewis, Jr., 6 vols. (Boston: Marsh, Capen & Lyon, 1835), III: 158, 189–200.

27. John Reid's *Essays on Insanity, Hypochondriasis, and Other Nervous Affections* (London: Longman, Hurst, Rees, Orme, and Brown, 1816) is an interesting transitional text.

28. Marcel Gauchet and Gladys Swain, *La pratique de l'esprit humain: l'institution asilaire et la révolution démocratique* (Paris: Éditions Gallimard, 1980), 369–484; Jan Ellen Goldstein, "French Psychiatry in Social and Political Context: The Formation of a New Profession, 1820–1860," Ph.D. diss., Columbia University, 1978, chaps. 1 and 4.

29. Robert Baker, Dorothy Porter, and Roy Porter, eds., *The Codification of Medical Morality: Historical and Philosophical Studies of the Formalization of Western Medical Morality in the Eighteenth and Nineteenth Centuries* (Dordrecht: Kluwer Academic Publishers, 1993), 1: 1–14.

30. See also Janet Beizer, *Ventriloquized Bodies: Narratives of Hysteria in Nineteenth-Century France* (Ithaca and London: Cornell University Press, 1994), 53.

31. Philippe Pinel, *Nosographie philosophique, ou la méthode de l'analyse appliquée à la médecine,* 2 vols. (Paris: Maradan, An VI [1798]), II: 48–50.

32. Pinel, *Nosographie philosophique,* 4th ed., 3 vols. (Paris: J. A. Brosson, 1810), III: 279–286.

33. Ibid., 283, 285.

34. Pinel and Bricheteau, "Névrose" [1819], in Adelon et al., *Dictionnaire des sciences médicales,* 60 vols. (Paris: C. L. F. Panckoucke, 1812–1822), XXXV: [557–581], 562.

35. Biographical information on Louyer-Villermay and other French doctors in this chapter is drawn from: Georges Daremberg, *Les grands médecins du XIXe siècle* (Paris: Masson et Cie, 1907); René Semelaigne, *Les pionniers de la psychiatrie française avant et après Pinel,* 2 vols. (Paris: J.-B. Baillière, 1930–1932); Maurice Genty, ed., *Index biographique des membres, des associés et des correspondants de l'Académie de Médecine de 1820 à 1970,* 2nd rev. ed. (Paris: Doin, 1972); Françoise Huguet, *Les professeurs de la Faculté de Médecine de Paris: Dictionnaire biographiques, 1794–1939* (Paris: Institut national de recherche pédagogique, 1991); and Pierre Larousse, ed., *Grand dictionnaire universel du XIXe siècle,* 17 vols. (Paris: Administration du grand dictionnaire universel, 1865–1878). The official *éloge* for Louyer-Villermay, in the *Bulletin de l'Académie royale de médecine,* 2 (1837–1838), 322–325, alludes to his political allegiances.

36. Louyer-Villermay, "Dissertation sur l'hypochondrie" (Medical dissertation, University of Paris, 1802), vol. 7: no. 74, 195 pp. In book form, he changed the title to *Recherches historiques et médicales sur l'hypocondrie, isolée par l'observation et l'analyse de l'hystérie et de la mélancholie* (Paris: Méquignon, 1802).

37. Louyer-Villermay, *Traité des maladies nerveuses ou vapeurs, et particulière-ment de l'hystérie et de l'hypochondrie,* 2 vols. (Paris: Méquignon, 1816), I: 1–216; Louyer-Villermay, "Hystérie" [1818], in Adelon, *Dictionnaire des sciences médicales* (1812–1822), XXIII: 226–272.

38. The publication early in the new century of a French-language edition of the Hippocratic texts and of René Laennec's dissertation on Hippocratic medicine helped to fuel this revival of interest.

39. Louyer-Villermay, *Traité des maladies nerveuses ou vapeurs* (1816), I: 1.

40. Ibid., I: 7–8, 38, 41; Louyer-Villermay, "Hystérie," in *Dictionnaire des sciences médicales* (1818), 228; Louyer-Villermay, *Recherches historiques et médicales sur l'hypochondrie* (1802), 47.

41. Louyer-Villermay, *Traité des maladies nerveuses ou vapeurs* (1816), 1–53 passim.

42. Ibid., 37.

43. Louyer-Villermay, "Hystérie," in *Dictionnaire des science médicales* (1818), 231–234. Fittingly, Louyer-Villermay a year later contributed the article "Nymphomanie" to the same medical dictionary.

44. Louyer-Villermay, *Traité des maladies nerveuses ou vapeurs* (1816), I: 32 34; Louyer-Villermay, "Hystérie," in *Dictionnaire des sciences médicales* (1818), 232.

45. Étienne Trillat, *Histoire de l'hystérie* (Paris: Seghers, 1986), 105.

46. Louyer-Villermay, "Hystérie," in *Dictionnaire des sciences médicales* (1818), 260.

47. Ibid., 244.

48. Briquet, *Traité clinique et thérapeutique de l'hystérie* (Paris: J. B. Baillière, 1859), 587.

49. Louyer-Villermay, "Hystérie," in *Dictionnaire des sciences médicales* (1818), 228. Translation from Beizer, *Ventriloquized Bodies* (1994), 35.

50. Technically, the first textual enunciation of the French neo-Hippocratic view was Georges-Louis Duvernoy's "Dissertation sur l'hystérie" (Medical dissertation, University of Paris, 1801), no. 27, 95 pp.

51. In his *Traité des affections vaporeuses du sexe* of 1758, for instance, Joseph Raulin had reproduced entire cases of "vaporous men" from Willis's writings.

52. Louyer-Villermay, *Traité des maladies nerveuses or vapeurs* (1816), I: 4–7, 9–10, 209.

53. Jacques Léonard, "La Restauration et la profession médicale," in Jean-Pierre Goubert, ed., *La médicalisation de la société française, 1770–1830* (Waterloo, Ontario: Historical Reflections Press, 1982), 69–81.

54. Georget, *De la physiologie du système nerveux et spécialement du cerveau. Recherches sur les maladies nerveuses en général et en particulier sur le siège, la*

*nature et le traitement de l'hystérie, de l'hypochondrie, de l'épilepsie et de l'asthme convulsif,* 2 vols. (Paris: J. B. Baillière, 1821), I: 238–302; Georget, "Hystérie," in Adelon et al., *Dictionnaire de médecine,* 21 vols. (Paris: Béchet, 1824), XI: 526–551.

55.  Georget, *De la physiologie du système nerveux* (1821), I: 239.
56.  Ibid., 243, 245.
57.  Ibid., 240, 260.
58.  Ibid., 243, 259.
59.  Ibid., 290.
60.  Georget, "Hystérie," in *Dictionnaire de médecine* (1824), XI: 545.
61.  Georget, *De la physiologie du système nerveux* (1821), 262–264.
62.  Georget, "Hystérie," in *Dictionnaire de médecine* (1824), XI: 535.
63.  Ibid., 544; Georget, *De la physiologie du système nerveux* (1821), I: 259–260.
64.  Ibid., 264; Georget, "Hystérie," in *Dictionnaire de médecine* (1824), XI: 532, 541–542.
65.  Georget, "Hypochondrie," in ibid., 490–516. To further emphasize the pairing, Georget published the two articles together under the title *De l'hypochondrie et de l'hystérie* (Paris: Rignoux, 1824).
66.  Trillat, *Histoire de l'hystérie* (1986), 108.
67.  See L. S. Jacyna in "Medical Science and Moral Science: The Cultural Relations of Physiology in Restoration France," *History of Science,* 25 (1987), 111–146, esp. 134–137.
68.  Jacques Postel, "Georget et Bayle: deux destins contraires," *Psychoanalyse à l'université,* 3 (1978), 445–463.
69.  Foville, "Hystérie," in Andral et al., *Dictionnaire de médecine et chirurgie pratiques,* 15 vols. (Paris: Méguignon-Marvis, J.-B. Baillière, 1833), X: 275–295.
70.  Ibid., 287.
71.  Ibid., 287, 288.
72.  Frédéric Dubois d'Amiens, *Histoire philosophique de l'hypochondrie et de l'hystérie* (Paris: De Deville Cavellin, 1833).
73.  Ibid., 412.
74.  Ibid., 22, 67, 22, 63.
75.  Ibid., 114, 438, 441.
76.  Ibid., 442.
77.  Ibid., 67.
78.  Julien-Joseph Virey, *De la femme, sous ses rapports physiologiques, moral et littéraire* (Paris: Crochard, 1825).
79.  Ibid., 172.
80.  Ibid., 177.

81.  Ibid., 176–177.
82.  Ibid., 105.
83.  Ibid., 130.
84.  Ibid., 112–115.
85.  Ibid., 341, translation from Evelyne Ender, *Sexing the Mind: Nineteenth-Century Fictions of Hysteria* (Ithaca: Cornell University Press, 1995), 43.
86.  Jean-Louis Brachet, *Traité complet de l'hypochondrie* (Lyon: Charles Savy Jeune, 1844); Brachet, *Traité de l'hystérie* (Paris: J. B. Baillère, 1847). Brachet had also previously published *Recherches de la nature et le siège de l'hystérie et de l'hypochondrie* in 1832.
87.  Brachet, *Recherches de la nature et le siège de l'hystérie* (1832), 177; Brachet, *Traité de l'hystérie* (1847), 343, 349.
88.  See especially the chapter "Études du physique et du moral de la femme" in ibid., 62–99, as well as the perceptive discussions by Beizer, *Ventriloquized Bodies,* 32–53, passim, and Ender, *Sexing the Mind* (1995), 57–65.
89.  Brachet, *Traité de l'hystérie* (1847), 72, 75.
90.  Ibid., 63. Translation from Ender, *Sexing the Mind* (1995), 32.
91.  Ibid., 67.
92.  Ibid., Avant-Propos, 1.
93.  Trillat in *Histoire de l'hystérie* (1986), 98–99; Ender, *Sexing the Mind* (1995), 35–36.
94.  Cited in Ender, *Sexing the Mind* (1995), 36.
95.  Brachet, *Traité de l'hystérie* (1847), 194, 206–208.
96.  Ibid., 190–195.
97.  Ibid., 207, 492.
98.  Ibid., 98.
99.  Landouzy, *Traité complet de l'hystérie* (Paris: J.-B. and G. Baillière, 1846).
100. Jean-Marie Bruttin, *Différentes théories sur l'hystérie dans la première moitié du XIXe siècle* (Zurich: Juris Druck, 1969), 22–32; Diana Faber, "Making Distinctions: The Contribution of Hector Landouzy to Differential Diagnosis in Relation to Hysteria and Epilepsy," *Journal of the History of the Neurosciences,* 9 (2000), 67–75.
101. Landouzy, *Traité complet de l'hystérie* (1846), 13–16, 160–161, 193–199, 344–345.
102. Bruttin, *Différentes théories sur l'hystérie* (1969), 32.
103. Landouzy, *Traité complet de l'hystérie* (1846), 174.
104. Ibid., 126–127, 164, 174.
105. Ibid., 223.
106. Ibid., 218.
107. Ibid., 377, 223.

108. See ibid., 377–381, where he lists the cases, and 218–224, where he argues them away.

109. See, for instance, the pro-male hysteria statements in L. J. F. Monnet, "Dissertation sur l'hystérie" (Medical diss., University of Paris, 1808), no. 116; M. H. Desterne, "De l'hystérie chez l'homme," *L'Union médicale,* 115 (September 1848), 455–457; and M. Taulier, "Observations de l'hystérie chez l'homme," *Gazette médicale de Lyon,* 6, 2 (February 1854), 39–41.

110. Cullen, *Nosology; or, A Systematic Arrangement of Diseases by Classes, Orders, Genera, and Species,* trans. from the Latin [1769] (Edinburgh: C. Stewart, 1800), 128–129; Cullen, *First Lines of the Practice of Physic,* new enlarged ed. (Edinburgh: C. Elliot, 1789), chap. 13, 93–106.

111. Cullen, *First Lines of the Practice of Physic,* 97–98.

112. Ibid., 102–103.

113. Ibid., 99, 98.

114. "Nymphomania," *Oxford English Dictionary,* 2nd ed. (Oxford: Clarendon Press, 1989), vol. X: 620.

115. Thomas Trotter, *An Essay, Medical, Philosophical, and Chemical, on Drunkenness and Its Effects on the Human Body* (London: T. N. Longman and O. Rees, 1804).

116. Biographical information on Trotter and other British medical figures in this chapter is drawn from William Macmichael, *Lives of British Physicians* (London: Murray, 1830); Jessica Bendiner and Elmer Bendiner, *Biographical Dictionary of Medicine* (New York: Facts on File, 1990); *The Medical Directory* (London: J. & A. Churchill, 1845– ); and Leslie Stephen, ed., *Dictionary of National Biography,* 63 vols. (London: Smith, Elder, 1885–1900). See also Ian Alexander Porter, "Thomas Trotter, M.D., Naval Physician," *Medical History,* 7 (1963), 155–164, and Roy Porter's introduction to Thomas Trotter, *An Essay, Medical, Philosophical, and Chemical, on Drunkenness* (1804) (New York: Routledge, 1988), ix–xl.

117. Trotter, *Medicina Nautica: An Essay on the Diseases of Seamen,* 2nd ed., 3 vols. (London: Longman, Hurst, Rees, and Orme, 1804), II: 28–29.

118. Ibid, III: 360–386. Quotation on 360–361.

119. Ibid., 361.

120. Trotter, *A View of the Nervous Temperament, Being a Practical Enquiry into the Increasing Prevalence, Prevention, and Treatment of those Diseases commonly called Nervous, Bilious, Stomach and Liver Complaints, Indigestion, Low Spirits, Gout, Etc.* (London: Longman, Hurst, Rees, and Orme, 1807).

121. Ibid., xvi–xvii.

122. Ibid., xi.

123. Peter Melville Logan, *Nerves and Narratives: A Cultural History of Hysteria in Nineteenth-Century British Prose* (Berkeley: University of California Press, 1997), chap. 1. Logan argues that it is specifically the middle-class virtues of routine, efficiency, and self-discipline that Trotter enshrines as signs of nervous health.

124. Trotter, *View of the Nervous Temperament* (1807), 52.

125. Ibid., 40–41.

126. See George Rousseau's sensitive account in "Trotter's Sea Weed Poems: The Drying Up of the Sea," in Kevin Cope and Serge Soupel, eds., *The Sea in the Eighteenth Century* (New York: AMS Press, forthcoming).

127. The three editions of Trotter's book appeared in 1807, 1808, and 1811, during the high point of the Napoleonic challenge, after which time the volume went out of print.

128. James Cowles Prichard, *Treatise on Diseases of the Nervous System* (London: Thomas and George Underwood, 1822), 148–181; John Mason Good, *Study of Medicine,* 4 vols. (London: Baldwin, Cradock, and Joy, 1822), III: 528–534; John Conolly, "Hysteria," in John Forbes, Alexander Tweedie, and John Conolly, eds., *The Cyclopedia of Practical Medicine,* 4 vols. (London: Sherwood, Gilbert and Piper, 1833–1835), II: 557–586.

129. Brodie, *Lectures Illustrative of Certain Local Nervous Affections* (London: Longman, Rees, Orme, Brown, Green, and Longman, 1837).

130. Ibid., 46.

131. Ibid., 37.

132. See, in contrast, Brodie's undated and posthumously published manuscript notes in which he discusses, briefly but openly, several cases of hysteria in adult male patients. Charles Hawkins, ed., *The Works of Sir Benjamin Collins Brodie,* 3 vols. (London: Longman, Green, Longman, Roberts, and Green, 1865), II: 661–665.

133. Edwin Clarke and L. S. Jacyna, *Nineteenth-Century Origins of Neuroscientific Concepts* (Berkeley: University of California Press, 1987), 141–147; Frederick E. James, "The Life and Work of Thomas Laycock, 1812–1876," Ph.D. diss., University of London, 1995; James, "Thomas Laycock, Psychiatry and Neurology," *History of Psychiatry,* 9 (1998), 491–502.

134. Laycock, "A Selection of Cases Presenting Aggravated and Irregular Forms of Hysteria, and an Analysis of Their Phenomena," *Edinburgh Medical and Surgical Journal,* vol. 49 (1838), 78–109, 436–461; vol. 50 (1838), 24–66, 302–356; vol. 52 (1839), 43–86; Laycock, *An Essay on Hysteria* (Philadelphia: Maswell, Barrington, and Haswell, 1840); Laycock, *A Treatise on the Nervous Diseases of Women; Comprising an Inquiry*

*into the Nature, Causes, and Treatment of Spinal and Hysterical Disorders* (London: Orme, Brown, Greene, Longmans, 1840).

135. Laycock, "Aggravated and Irregular Forms of Hysteria," *Edinburgh Medical and Surgical Journal,* 50 (1838), 302–303; Laycock, *Treatise on Nervous Diseases of Women* (1840), 5–9.

136. Laycock, "Aggravated and Irregular Forms of Hysteria," *Edinburgh Medical and Surgical Journal,* 52 (1839), 60.

137. Laycock, *Treatise on Nervous Diseases of Women* (1840), 14–75.

138. Ibid., 131–143.

139. Laycock, *Essay on Hysteria,* 69. See also Laycock, *Treatise on Nervous Diseases of Women* (1840), 115–125.

140. Laycock, *Essay on Hysteria,* 3–57.

141. Laycock, "Aggravated and Irregular Forms of Hysteria," *Edinburgh Surgical and Medical Journal,* 50 (1838), 317; Laycock, *Essay on Hysteria* (1840), 112.

142. Laycock, "Aggravated and Irregular Forms of Hysteria," *Edinburgh Surgical and Medical Journal,* 50 (1838), 319; Laycock, *Essay on Hysteria* (1840), 113.

143. See especially "The Mental and Corporeal Peculiarities of Woman," in Laycock, *Treatise on Nervous Diseases of Women* (1840), 76–84, which I take to be a locus classicus for the medical doctrine of separate spheres.

144. Laycock, *Essay on Hysteria* (1840), 102; Laycock, *Treatise on Nervous Diseases of Women* (1840), 82.

145. Anderson, *The Causes, Symptoms, and Treatment of Eccentric Nervous Affections* (London: Churchill, 1850), 65–111; Carter, *On the Pathology and Treatment of Hysteria* (London: John Churchill, 1853).

146. Robert Brudenell Carter, *Practical Treatise on Diseases of the Eye* (Philadelphia: Henry C. Lea, 1876); Robert Brudenell Carter and William Adams Frost, *Ophthalmic Surgery* (London: Cassell, 1887).

147. Ilza Veith, *Hysteria: The History of a Disease* (1965), 199–210.

148. Carter, *Pathology and Treatment of Hysteria* (1853), 33–34.

149. Ibid., 33.

150. Ibid.

151. Ibid., 152.

152. Alison Kane and Eric T. Carlson, "A Different Drummer: Robert B. Carter and Nineteenth-Century Hysteria," *Bulletin of the New York Academy of Medicine,* 58 (September 1982), 519–534.

153. Carter, *Pathology and Treatment of Hysteria* (1853), 35, 33.

154. Ibid., 33–34.

155. Ibid., 69.

156. Ibid., 111, 114.

157. P. Briquet, *Traité clinique et thérapeutique de l'hystérie* (Paris: J. B. Baillière, 1859). See also François M. Mai and Harold Merskey, "Briquet's *Treatise on Hysteria:* A Synopsis and Commentary," *Archives of General Psychiatry,* 37 (December 1980), 1401–1405; and François M. Mai and Harold Merskey, "Briquet's Concept of Hysteria: An Historical Perspective," *Canadian Journal of Psychiatry,* 26 (February 1981), 57–63.

158. Briquet, *Traité clinique et thérapeutique de l'hystérie* (1859), 599–604. See also p. 3.

159. This summary of Briquet's book draws on Micale, *Approaching Hysteria: Disease and Its Interpretations* (Princeton: Princeton University Press, 1995), 50–53.

160. Briquet, *Traité clinique et thérapeutique de l'hystérie* (1859), 4.

161. Ibid., 11–51.

162. Ibid., Preface, v.

163. Ibid., 33.

164. Ibid., 38–40.

165. Ibid., 41–45.

166. Ibid., 36.

167. Ibid., 15–32.

168. Ibid., 50.

169. Ibid., 48, 49, 51.

170. Ibid., 36, 37.

171. Ibid., 100. As Nicole Edelman points out, Briquet never produced a 700-page treatise on these "male pathologies." See Edelman, "Représentation de la maladie et construction de la différence des sexes. Des maladies de femmes aux maladies nerveuses, l'hystérie comme exemple," *Romantisme: Revue du dix-neuvième siècle,* 110 (2000), 86.

172. Briquet, *Traité clinique et thérapeutique de l'hystérie* (1859), 101. My italics.

173. B. A. Morel, *Traité des maladies mentales* (Paris: Victor Masson, 1860); Alexandre Axenfeld, *Des névroses* (Paris: Germer Baillière, 1864); Jacques-Joseph Moreau (de Tours), *Traité pratique de la folie névropathique (vulgo hystérique)* (Paris: Germer Baillière, 1869), 163–170.

174. C. P. Snow, *The Two Cultures* (1959), Canto Series, introduction by Stefan Collini (Cambridge: Cambridge University Press, 1993).

175. Thomas Neville Bonner, *To the Ends of the Earth: Women's Search for Education in Medicine* (Cambridge, Mass.: Harvard University Press, 1992), 48–54, 70–75, 120–137; Yvonne Knibiehler and Catherine Fouquet, *La femme et les médecins: analyse historique* (Paris: Hachette, 1983), chap. 6.

176. Jean Donnison, *Midwives and Medical Men: A History of Inter-professional Rivalries and Women's Rights* (London: Heinemann Educational, 1977).

177. David H. J. Morgan, *Discovering Men* (London and New York: Rout-ledge, 1992), chap. 8. See also Susan Bordo's seminal work in "The Car-tesian Masculinization of Thought," *Signs: A Journal of Women in Culture and Society,* 11 (Spring 1986), 439–456; and Bordo, *The Flight to Objec-tivity: Essays on Cartesianism and Culture* (Albany: State University of New York Press, 1987), chap. 6.

178. See Genevieve Lloyd's study *The Man of Reason: "Male" and "Female" in Western Philosophy* (1984), 2nd ed. (Minneapolis: University of Minne-sota Press, 1993).

179. For the classic statement of this idea, see Evelyn Fox Keller, *Reflections on Gender and Science* (New Haven and London: Yale University Press, 1985), chap. 5, esp. p. 79.

180. Anne K. Mellor, *Romanticism and Gender* (New York and London: Routledge, 1993), Introduction and chap 1.

181. Susan J. Wolfson, "*Lyrical Ballads* and the Language of (Men) Feeling: Writing Women's Voices," in Thais E. Morgan, ed., *Men Writing the Fem-inine: Literature, Theory, and the Question of Genders* (Albany: State Uni-versity of New York Press, 1994), 29–57. See also Alan Richardson, "Romanticism and the Colonization of the Feminine," in Anne K. Mellor, ed., *Romanticism and Feminism* (Bloomington: Indiana Univer-sity Press, 1988), 13–25.

182. Susan J. Wolfson, "Individual in Community: Dorothy Wordsworth in Conversation with William," in Mellor, *Romanticism and Feminism* (1988), 139–166.

183. Quoted in Richardson, "Romanticism and the Colonization of the Feminine," in Mellor, *Romanticism and Feminism* (1988), 20.

184. On androgyny as a creative strategy of European Romanticism, see Mircea Eliade, *Mephistopheles and the Androgyne: Studies in Religious Myth and Symbol,* trans. from the French by J. M. Cohen (New York: Sheed and Ward, 1965), and Diane Long Hoeveler, *Romantic Androgyny—The Woman Within* (University Park and London: Pennsylvania State Uni-versity Press, 1990).

185. Chateaubriand, *Atala/René* (1802), Preface by Pierre Reboul (Paris: Garnier-Flammarion, 1964), 148.

186. Margaret Waller discusses René's "mental femininity" in *The Male Mal-ady: Fictions of Impotence in the French Romantic Novel* (New Brunswick, N.J.: Rutgers University Press, 1993), 39–44.

187. Dr. Henri Albert Potiquet, *Chateaubriand et l'hystérie: Essai de psychologie* (Paris: Laisney, 1911).

188. These are the observations of Glyn Holmes, *The "Adolphe Type" in French Fiction of the First Half of the Nineteenth Century* (Sherbrooke,

Québec: Éditions Naaman, 1977); Michael J. Call, *Back to the Garden: Chateaubriand, Senancour, and Constant* (Saratoga, Calif.: Anma Libri, 1988); and Waller, *Male Malady* (1993).

189. Sally Shuttleworth, "'Preaching to the Nerves': Psychological Disorder in Sensation Fiction," in Marina Benjamin, ed., *A Question of Identity: Women, Science, and Literature* (New Brunswick, N.J.: Rutgers University Press, 1993), 192–222, 242–244; Shuttleworth, "'The Surveillance of a Sleepless Eye': The Constitution of Neurosis in *Villette*," in George Levine, *One Culture: Essays in Science and Literature* (Madison: University of Wisconsin Press, 1987), 313–335; Jane Wood, "'The Disorder of Literary Men': Sensitive Men and Victorian Ideals of Manliness" (typescript), 13; and Wood, *Passion and Pathology in Victorian Fiction* (Oxford and New York: Oxford University Press, 2001), 1–7, 59–77, and 215–218. My thanks to Jane Wood for sharing her work in progress with me.

190. Wood, *Passion and Pathology in Victorian Fiction* (2001), 78–109; Shuttleworth, "'Preaching to the Nerves,'" in *Question of Identity* (1993), 195.

191. The following discussion again draws on Micale, *Approaching Hysteria* (1996), 243–245, 250–252. See also Micale, "Littérature, Médecine, Hystérie: le cas de *Madame Bovary* de Gustave Flaubert," *L'Évolution psychiatrique*, 60 (1995), 901–918.

192. Baudelaire, "*Madame Bovary* par Gustave Flaubert," in Baudelaire, *L'Art romantique, Oeuvres complètes de Charles Baudelaire,* ed. Jacques Crépet, 17 vols. (Paris: Louis Conard, 1925), III: 393–408.

193. See the letter from Flaubert to Baudelaire, dated October 21, 1857, in *Correspondance, 1850–1859,* in *Oeuvres complètes de Flaubert,* 16 vols. (Paris: Club de l'Honnête Homme, 1971), 13: 610.

194. Nancy Rubino explores this same theme in a later Flaubert novel but reaches quite different conclusions in "Impotence and Excess: Male Hysteria and Androgyny in Flaubert's *Salammbô,*" *Nineteenth-Century French Studies,* 29 (Fall-Winter, 2000–2001), 78–99. Also relevant is Flaubert's Middle Eastern travel journal in which the novelist extensively discusses his own volatile mental condition. See *Voyage en Égypte/ Gustave Flaubert,* Édition intégrale du manuscrit original établie et présentée par Pierre-Marc de Biasi (Paris: B. Grasset, 1991).

195. For the passages and some discussion see Micale, *Approaching Hysteria* (1995), 243–245; Jacqueline Carroy-Thirard, "Hystérie, théâtre, littérature au dix-neuvième siècle," *Psychanalyse à l'université,* 7 (March 1982), 299–317; and André Bolzinger, "Bovary, Baudelaire, Briquet: hystérie 1856," *L'Évolution psychiatrique,* 49 (1984), 1165–1172.

196. "Autobiography," *Oxford English Dictionary,* 2nd ed. (Oxford: Claren-

don Press, 1989), I: 801; Robert Folkenflik, "Introduction: The Institution of Autobiography," in *The Culture of Autobiography: Constructions of
Self-Representation* (Stanford: Stanford University Press, 1993), 1–7.

197. See Peter Gay, *The Bourgeois Experience: Victoria to Freud,* vol. 4: *The Naked Heart* (New York: Norton, 1995), chap. 2; Heidi I. Stull, *The Evolution of the Autobiography from 1770–1850: A Comparative Study and Analysis* (New York: Peter Lang, 1985); and Jerome Hamilton Buckley, *The
Turning Key: Autobiography and the Subjective Impulse since 1800* (Cambridge, Mass.: Harvard University Press, 1984).

198. Linda H. Peterson, *Victorian Autobiography: The Tradition of Self-
Interpretation* (1986), 2–3, 21–22; Gay, *Naked Heart* (1995), 106–114.

199. Martin A. Danahay, *A Community of One: Masculine Autobiography and
Autonomy in Nineteenth-Century Britain* (Albany: State University of
New York Press, 1993), chaps. 2, 4–6. David H. J. Morgan makes this
same point in "Masculinity, Autobiography, and History," *Gender and
History,* 2 (1990), 34–39.

200. Nicholas Capaldi, *John Stuart Mill: A Biography* (Cambridge and New
York: Cambridge University Press, 2004), 56–66; Michael St. John
Packe, *The Life of John Stuart Mill* (New York: Macmillan, 1954), 74–86.

201. Citations are from John Stuart Mill, *Autobiography and Other Writings,*
edited and with an introduction by Jack Stillinger (Boston: Houghton
Mifflin, 1969), chap. 5, 80–110.

202. Ibid., 81.

203. Ibid., 84, 88, 89, 80, 81.

204. Ibid., 85.

205. Ibid., 86.

206. John Stuart Mill to John Sterling, letter dated May 24, 1832, in Francis
E. Mineka, ed., *The Early Letters of John Stuart Mill, 1812–1848* (Toronto: University of Toronto Press, 1963), 99.

207. Mill's earlier drafts of his autobiography have been preserved. The most
conspicuous changes involve toning down the emotionally charged
parts of the chronicle. See Jack Stillinger, ed., *The Early Draft of John
Stuart Mill's Autobiography* (Urbana: University of Illinois Press, 1961),
1–33.

208. Jo Ellen Jacobs, *The Voice of Harriet Taylor Mill* (Bloomington: Indiana
University Press, 2002); Jo Ellen Jacobs, ed., *The Complete Works of Har-
riet Taylor Mill* (Bloomington: Indiana University Press, 1998); Ann P.
Robson and John M. Robson, eds., *Sexual Equality: Writings by John
Stuart Mill, Harriet Taylor Mill, and Helen Taylor* (Toronto: University of
Toronto Press, 1994), vii–xxxiv.

209. Stillinger, ed., *Early Draft of John Stuart Mill's Autobiography* (1961), 1–33.
210. Mill, *Autobiography and Other Writings* (1969), 84.
211. Ibid., 81–82. Mill is referring to Act V, Scene III of Shakespeare's play where Macbeth wails: "Canst thou not minister to a mind diseas'd?"
212. Ibid., 89–90. See Stephen Gill, *William Wordsworth: A Life* (Oxford: Clarendon Press, 1989), 354, and St. John Packe, *Life of John Stuart Mill,* 81–82, 107, 131.
213. Mill, *Autobiography,* 80, 84, 88, 89, 90, 82, 87.
214. The Hume/Mill comparison seems not to have occurred to biographers of either figure. The similarities in their stories, however, are so detailed that they raise the question of a direct textual influence. Hume's "Epistle to Dr. Arbuthnot," it turns out, was discovered by John Hill Burton, Hume's early Victorian biographer, who first published the document in 1846 in his *Life and Correspondence of David Hume,* 2 vols. (Edinburgh: W. Tait), 1: 30–47, along with an analysis. It seems likely that Mill would have been familiar with Burton's biography.

## 3. Charcot and *La Grande Hystérie Masculine*

1. The factual material in this chapter draws on several of my previous publications: "The Salpêtrière in the Age of Charcot: An Institutional Perspective on Medical History in Late Nineteenth-Century France," *Journal of Contemporary History,* 20 (October 1985), 703–731; "Diagnostic Discriminations: Jean-Martin Charcot and the Nineteenth-Century Idea of Masculine Hysterical Neurosis," Ph.D. diss., Yale University, 1987; "Charcot and the Idea of Hysteria in the Male: Gender, Mental Science, and Medical Diagnosis in Late Nineteenth-Century France," *Medical History,* 34 (1990), 363–411; "Hysterical Male/Hysterical Female: Reflections on Comparative Gender Construction in Nineteenth-Century Medical Science," in Marina Benjamin, ed., *Science and Sensibility: Essays on Gender and the History of Science in Nineteenth-Century Britain* (London: Basil Blackwell, 1991), 200–239; *Approaching Hysteria* (1995), 88–97, 149–154, 260–284; "Jean-Martin Charcot and *les névroses traumatiques:* From Medicine to Culture in French Trauma Theory of the Late Nineteenth Century," in Mark S. Micale and Paul Lerner, eds., *Traumatic Pasts: History, Psychiatry, and Trauma in the Modern Age, 1870–1930* (Cambridge and New York: Cambridge University Press, 2001), chap. 6; and "Charcot, Jean-Martin," in John Merriman and Jay Winter, eds., *Europe, 1789–1914,* 5 vols. (New York: Thomson/Gale, 2006), vol. 1: 407–411.

2. The three indispensable book-length studies of Charcot are Georges Guillian, *J.-M. Charcot, 1825–1893: His Life—His Work,* ed. and trans. from the French by Pearce Bailey (New York: Hoeber, 1959); Bernard Brais, "The Making of a Famous Nineteenth Century Neurologist: Jean-Martin Charcot (1825–1893)," M. Phil. thesis, University College London, 1990; and Christopher G. Goetz, Michel Bonduelle, and Toby Gelfand, *Charcot: Constructing Neurology* (New York: Oxford University Press, 1995).

3. Goetz, Bonduelle, and Gelfand, *Charcot: Constructing Neurology* (1995), chap. 4.

4. Jack D. Ellis, *The Physician-Legislators of France: Medicine and Politics in the Early Third Republic, 1870–1914* (Cambridge and New York: Cambridge University Press, 1990).

5. Brais, "Making of a Famous Nineteenth Century Neurologist" (1990), chaps. 3–4; Goetz, Bonduelle, and Gelfand, *Charcot: Constructing Neurology* (1995), 222–231.

6. *Oeuvres complètes de J. M. Charcot,* 9 vols. (Paris: Bureaux du Progrès Médical, Delahaye & Lecrosnier, 1886–1893).

7. Goetz, Bonduelle, and Gelfand, *Charcot: Constructing Neurology* (1995), 90–97.

8. Henri Ellenberger, "Charcot and the Salpêtrière School" (1965), reproduced in Mark S. Micale, ed., *Beyond the Unconscious: Essays of Henri F. Ellenberger in the History of Psychiatry* (Princeton: Princeton University Press, 1993), chap. 4; Brais, "Making of a Famous Nineteenth Century Neurologist" (1990), 149–158.

9. "Charcuterie" is the French term for a pork butcher's shop.

10. Ellenberger, "Charcot and the Salpêtrière School" (1993), 142–143, 153; Bertrand Marquer, *Les romans de la Salpêtrière: Réception d'une scénographie clinique: Jean-Martin Charcot dans l'imaginaire fin-de-siècle* (Geneva: Droz, 2008).

11. Brais, "Making of a Famous Nineteenth Century Neurologist" (1990), 116–127; Bernard Brais, "Désiré Magloire Bourneville and French Anticlericalism during the Third Republic," in Dorothy Porter and Roy Porter, eds., *Doctors, Politics and Society: Historical Essays* (Amsterdam and Atlanta: Rodopi, 1993), chap. 4. See also Jan Goldstein, "The Hysteria Diagnosis and the Politics of Anticlericalism in Late Nineteenth-Century France," *Journal of Modern History,* 54 (1982), 209–239.

12. Goetz, Bonduelle, and Gelfand, *Charcot: Constructing Neurology* (1995), chap. 9; Brais, "Making of a Famous Nineteenth Century Neurologist" (1990), chap. 6.

13. The most important of Charcot's writings from this period on female hysteria are the seven lectures in the first volume of the *Leçons sur les maladies du système nerveux* (hereafter cited as *LMSN*), recueillies et publiées par Bourneville (1872–78) in *Oeuvres completes* (1892), 1: 275–405 and 427–448. See also D.-M. Bourneville and P. Régnard, *Iconographie photographique de la Salpêtrière*, 3 vols. (Paris: Bureaux du Progrès Médical, Delahaye & Lecrosnier, 1876–1880).

14. Case of Pierre de Bassonnière, Archives de l'assistance publique. Salpêtrière, *Registre de diagnostics,* 6-R-90 (1880–1883).

15. "De l'hystérie chez les jeunes garçons," *Progrès médical,* 10 (50–51) (December 16–23, 1882), 985–987, 1003–1004, reprinted in *LMSN,* recueillies et publiées par M. M. Babinski, Bernard, Féré, Guinon, Marie, and Gilles de la Tourette, *Oeuvres complètes,* vol. 3 (1890), lecture 6: 79–96.

16. "Le somnambulisme hystérique spontané considéré au point de vue nosographique et médico-légal," *Gazette hebdomadaire de médecine et de chirurgie* 30 (1) (January 7, 1893), 2–7.

17. *LMSN,* vol. 3, lecture 6: 89–91, 92–96; lecture 8: 117–123; lecture 16: 229–237; lecture 17: 238–252; lecture 18: 261–267, 267–271, 272 279; lecture 19: 284, 283–284 n.1, 284–289, 289–298; lecture 20: 300–307; lecture 21: 321–327, 327 334; lecture 22: 344–369; lecture 23: 370–385; lecture 24: 394–398; lecture 25: 399–421; lecture 26: 422–438; Appendix 1: 441–459, 459–462; and Appendix V: 483 512.

18. *Leçons du mardi à la Salpêtrière. Professor Charcot. Policliniques. 1887–1888. Notes de cours de MM. Blin, Charcot, et Colin,* vol. 1 (Paris: Bureaux du Progrès Médical, Delahaye & Lecrosnier, 1887 [*sic*]), lesson 4: 60–62, 62–65; lesson 11: 199–209, 209–213; lesson 12: 227–229; lesson 16: 288–300, 305–309; lesson 18: 338–343, 344–347, 348–353; lesson 19: 357–363, 367–368; lesson 20: 378–384, 386–387, 387–388; *Leçons du mardi à la Salpêtrière Professor Charcot. Policlinique. 1888–1889. Notes de cours de MM. Blin, Charcot, Henri Colin,* vol. 2 (Paris: Bureaux du Progrès Médical, E. Lecrosnier & Babé, 1889), lesson 2: 19–37; lesson 3: 43–53; lesson 5: 83–100; lesson 6: 121–125; lesson 7: 131–139; lesson 9: 189–198; lesson 12: 261–265, 265–269; lesson 13: 285–292, 292–299; lesson 15: 347–353; lesson 17: 393–399, 399–403; lesson 18: 419–433; lesson 19: 436–462; lesson 21: 502–509, 518–523; Appendix I: 528–535; Appendix III: 543–548.

19. *Clinique des maladies du système nerveux. M. le Professeur Charcot. Leçons du Professeur, Mémoires, Notes et Observations, 1889–1890 et 1890–91,* publiés sous la direction de Georges Guinon, 2 vols. (Paris: Bureaux du

Progrès Médical, Babé & Cie, 1892–93), vol. 1: lecture 2: 30–45; lecture 3: 53–61, 61–64, 64–69; lecture 5: 95–116; lecture 14: 292–307; vol. 2, Appendix II: 461–472, 472–474.

20. "Spasme glosso-labié unilatéral des hystériques. Diagnostic entre l'hémiplégie capsulaire et l'hémiplégie hystérique," *Semaine médicale* 7 (1887), 37–38; "Des paralysies hystéro-traumatiques chez l'homme," ibid., 490–491; "Sur un cas de monoplégie brachiale chez l'homme, présentant des difficultés de diagnostic," ibid., 12 (1892), 225–227; "Le somnambulisme hystérique," *Gazette hebdomadaire* (1893), 2–7.

21. Case of "Guénin," Countway Medical Library, Boston, Rare Book Room, Manuscripts Collection, Charcot, Folio C96; Wellcome Institute for the History of Medicine, London, Manuscripts Collection, Charcot.

22. Archives de l'assistance publique, Salpêtrière, *Registre de diagnostics,* 6-R-90.

23. G. Daumezon, "Essai historique et critique de l'appareil d'assistance aux malades mentales dans le département de la Seine depuis le début du XIXè siècle," *L'Information psychiatrique,* 1 (1960), 26; "Hospice de la Vieillesse: Plan Général," in Ludwig Hirt, *Das Hospiz 'La Salpêtrière' in Paris und die Charcot'sche Klinik für Nervenkrankheiten* (Breslau: Grass-Barth, 1883), with annotations by Charcot.

24. Auguste Klein, *De l'hystérie chez l'homme* (Doctoral diss., Paris Medical Faculty, 1880).

25. Micale, "On the 'Disappearance' of Hysteria: A Study in the Clinical Deconstruction of a Diagnosis," *Isis,* 84 (1993), 496–526.

26. On the self-image of the Salpêtrians, see Charles Richet, "Aux temps héroïques de la médecine, 1872–1878," *Progrès medical,* 50 (December 16, 1922), 589ff.

27. See, for example, the opening comments in Léon de Casaubon, *L'hystérie chez les jeunes garçons* (Doctoral diss., Paris Medical Faculty, 1884); Émile Batault, *Contribution à l'étude de l'hystérie chez l'homme* (Doctoral diss., Paris Medical Faculty, 1885); and Paul Michaut, *Contribution à l'étude des manifestations de l'hystérie chez l'homme* (Doctoral diss., Paris Medical Faculty, 1890).

28. Étienne Trillat, *L'Histoire de l'hystérie* (Paris: Seghers, 1986), 121–125.

29. Micale, *Approaching Hysteria* (1995), 138–139; Marcel Gauchet and Gladys Swain, *Le vrai Charcot: Les chemins imprévus de l'inconscient* (Paris: Calmann-Lévy, 1997), 13–95.

30. Lawrence D. Longo, "The Rise and Fall of Battey's Operation: A Fashion in Surgery," *Bulletin of the History of Medicine,* 53 (Summer 1979), 244–267.

31. *LMSN,* vol. 3, lecture 23: 372–373, and *Leçons du mardi,* vol. 1, lesson 4: 63–64; Gilles de la Tourette, "Du traitement chirurgical de l'hystérie," *Archives de tocologie et de gynécologie,* 22 (June 20, 1895), 409–420; Georges Gilles de la Tourette, *Traité clinique et thérapeutique de l'hystérie,* 3 vols. (Paris: E. Plon, Nourrit, et Cie, 1891–1895), III: 529–545.

32. *Leçons du mardi,* vol. 2, lesson 2 (October 30, 1888), 37.

33. "A propos de six cas d'hystérie chez l'homme (1)," *LMSN,* vol. 3, lecture 18: 253; *Leçons du mardi,* vol. 2, lesson 17 (March 12, 1889), 393.

34. These are the cases of the Breton boy "François X," found in *LMSN,* vol. 3, lectures 16 and 17: 229–237, and the factory worker "P...on" in *Leçons du mardi,* vol. 2, lesson 3: 43–53.

35. Briquet, *Traité clinique et thérapeutique de l'hystérie* (Paris: J. B. Bailliere, 1859), 36, and Charcot, *LMSN,* vol. 3, lecture 8: 114.

36. Charcot, *Leçons du mardi,* vol. 2, lesson 12 (January 29, 1889), 256. Later in the lesson Charcot adds: "il est remarquable que chez les sujets rustiques des classes ouvrières, les affections nerveuses sans 'substratum' organique—la neurasthénie, l'hystérie, par exemple—se montrent généralement, toutes choses égales d'ailleurs, plus graves et plus tenances que chez les sujets plus délicats, plus impressionnables des classes lettrées" (p. 261).

37. *LMSN,* vol. 3, lecture 6: 92–96; *Leçons du mardi,* vol. 1, lesson 22: 199–209.

38. Charcot in fact elsewhere refers to the male variant of hysteria as "l'hystérie des artisans" and "l'hystérie du maçon, du serrurier" ("the bricklayer and locksmith's hysteria"), *Leçons du mardi* (January 31, 1888), 2nd ed. (1892), vol. 1, lesson 8: 123; "Des paralysies hystéro-traumatiques chez l'homme," *Semaine médical* (1887), 490.

39. *Leçons sur l'hystérie virile,* Preface by Michèle Ouerd (Paris: Le Sycomore, 1984), Introduction, 21.

40. George Weisz, *The Medical Mandarins: The French Academy of Medicine in the Nineteenth and Early Twentieth Centuries* (New York: Oxford University Press, 1995), 215.

41. These are the cases of the beggar Klein, the circus saltimbanque "Lap...sonne," and the street singer "Ro...eau," all in the second volume of the *Leçons du mardi,* lessons 15 and 17, 347–353, 393–403.

42. Ibid., 393.

43. Ouerd, *Leçons sur l'hystérie virile* (1984), Introduction; Ursula Link-Heer, "'Male Hysteria': A Discourse Analysis," *Cultural Critique,* 15 (Spring 1990), 215–217.

44. Feuchtersleben, *The Principles of Medical Psychology* [1845], trans. from the German by H. Evans Lloyd, rev. and ed. by B. G. Babington (Lon-

don: Sydenham Society, 1847), 228; Reynolds, "Hysteria," in Reynolds, ed., *A System of Medicine,* 5 vols. (London: Macmillan, 1866–1879), vol. 2: 307.

45. "Deux cas de contracture hystérique d'origine traumatique (2)," *LMSN,* vol. 3, lecture 8: 115.

46. Ibid., lecture 18: 256.

47. Ibid., lecture 8: 117.

48. Case of Antoine Charnu, Bibliothèque Charcot.

49. Case of Jean-Pierre Mattivet, Bibliothèque Charcot.

50. Charcot and Valentin Magnan, "Inversion du sens génital et autres perversions sexuelles," *Archives de neurologie,* 2 pts., 3 (January 1882), 53–60; 4 (November 1882), 296–322. For analysis of the case, see G. Bonnet, "Diagnostic et mot d'esprit: À propos de la réédition de 'Inversion du sens génital et autres perversions sexuelles,'" *L'Evolution psychiatrique,* 53 (1988), 395–407.

51. *Leçons du mardi,* vol. 2, lesson 18 (March 19, 1889), 420.

52. Prosper Lucas, *Traité philosophique et physiologique de l'hérédité naturelle dans les états de santé et de maladie du système nerveux,* 2 vols. (Paris: J. B. Baillière, 1847–1850); B. A. Morel, *Traité des dégénérescences physiques, intellectuelles, et morales de l'espèce humaine* (Paris: J. B. Baillière, 1857); J. J. Moreau de Tours, *La psychologie morbide dans ses rapports avec la philosophie de l'histoire* (Paris: Masson, 1859).

53. Ian Dowbiggin, "Degeneration and Hereditarianism in French Mental Medicine, 1840–1890: Psychiatric Theory as Ideological Adaptation," in W. F. Bynum, Roy Porter, and Michael Shepherd, eds., *The Anatomy of Madness,* 3 vols. (London: Tavistock, 1985), I: 188–232; Jean-Christophe Coffin, *La transmission de la folie: 1850–1914* (Paris: L'Harmattan, 2003), chaps. 3, 4.

54. Although the concepts of "functional" and "dynamic" disorders assumed purely psychological significance in the twentieth century, they remained within the organicist paradigm during the late nineteenth century—as Charcot states clearly in "Médecine empirique et médecine scientifique," *Oeuvres complètes,* vol. 7: xxiii–xxiv; and *LMSN,* vol. 3, lecture 1: 12, and lecture 21: 321.

55. Charles Féré, "La famille névropathique," *Archives de neurologie,* 2 pts. (January-March, 1884), 7 (19–20): 1–43, 173–191, with remarks on hysteria on pp. 11ff.

56. *LMSN,* vol. 3, lecture 8: 115. See also Charcot's instructions regarding the separation of hysterical boys from their mothers in *Leçons du mardi,* vol. 1, lesson 11: 208.

57. Guinon, *Les agents provocateurs de l'hystérie* (Paris: Bureaux du Progrès Médical, Delahaye & Lecrosnier, 1889).

58. Ibid., 72–119; Charcot, *Leçons du mardi*, vol. 2, lesson 19: 437.

59. Ibid., lesson 2: 35, and lesson 5: 93–94.

60. *LMSN*, vol. 3, lecture 19: 280–284; *Leçons du mardi*, vol. 2, lesson 12: 261–265; ibid., lesson 19: 436–462, and Appendix III: 543–548.

61. *LMSN*, vol. 3, lecture 23: 370–385; ibid., Appendix I: 458–462; *Leçons du mardi*, vol. 2, lesson 7: 131–139; ibid., Appendix I: 528–535; *Clinique des maladies du système nerveux*, vol. 1, lecture 3: 61–64.

62. *Leçons du mardi*, vol. 2, lesson 3: 43–52; ibid., lesson 6: 121–125; *Clinique des maladies du système nerveux* (1892–93), vol. 2, Appendix II: 461–472. See also Paul Berbez, "L'hystérie toxique," *Gazette des hôpitaux*, 61(6) (January 14, 1888), 45–50.

63. *LMSN*, vol. 3, Appendix I: 443; *Leçons du mardi*, vol. 1, lesson 16: 297; ibid., vol. 2, lesson 7: 134.

64. Mark S. Micale, "Jean-Martin Charcot and *les névroses traumatiques:* From Medicine to Culture in French Trauma Theory," in Micale and Lerner, eds., *Traumatic Pasts* (2001), chap. 6.

65. Patricia E. Prestwich, *Drink and the Politics of Social Reform: Antialcoholism in France since 1870* (Palo Alto, Calif.: Society for the Promotion of Science and Scholarship, 1988), chap. 3; Susanna Barrows, "After the Commune: Alcoholism, Temperance, and Literature in the Early Third Republic," in John M. Merriman, ed., *Consciousness and Class Experience in Nineteenth-Century Europe* (New York: Holmes & Meier, 1979), 205–218.

66. Michael J. Freeman, *Railways and the Victorian Imagination* (New Haven: Yale University Press, 1999), 18–25; Esther Fischer-Homberger, "Die Büchse der Pandora: Der mythische Hintergrund der Eisenbahnkrankheiten des 19ten Jahrhunderts," *Sudhoffs Archiv*, 56 (1971), 297–317.

67. In Britain, Parliament passed the first Employers' Liability Act in 1880, followed in 1897 by the more comprehensive Workmen's Compensation Act. The German Reichstag implemented the Industrial Injury Law in 1885. And in 1891 the first International Congress for Workers' Accidents was held in Amsterdam.

68. V. P. Comiti, "Les maladies et le travail lors de la révolution industrielle française," *History and Philosophy of the Life Sciences*, 1 (1980), 215–239.

69. Léon Chertok, "On Objectivity in the History of Psychotherapy," *Journal of Nervous and Mental Disease*, 153 (1971), 73.

70. "Sur un cas de coxalgie hystérique de cause traumatique chez l'homme (2)," *LMSN*, vol. 3, lecture 24: 388, 390.

71. "A propos d'un cas d'hystérie masculine," *Clinique des maladies du système nerveux* (1892–93), vol. 1, lecture 14: 305.

72. *Leçons du mardi*, vol. 2, lesson 2: 30.

73. Ibid., vol. 1, lesson 18: 348–353.

74. Freud, "Notes upon a Case of Obsessional Neurosis" (1909), in James Strachey and Anna Freud, eds., *The Standard Edition of the Complete Psychological Works of Sigmund Freud*, 24 vols. (London: Hogarth Press, 1955), vol. 10: 157.

75. "Deux nouveaux cas de paralysie hystéro-traumatique chez l'homme," *LMSN*, vol. 3, Appendix I: 441–459.

76. Charcot's "psychological" analysis of "Le Log." appears in "Deux nouveaux cas de paralysie hystéro-traumatique chez l'homme," ibid., Appendix I: 450–456. "Auto-suggestion involontaire" is from *Clinique des maladies du système nerveux* (1892–93), vol. 1, lecture 2: 32.

77. My view that Charcot moves timidly toward psychogenic explanations through his work on select topics while remaining within the reigning neurophysiological paradigm of his time is most in accord with Esther Fischer-Homberger's "Charcot und die Ätiologie der Neurosen," *Gesnerus*, 28 (1971), 35–46.

78. Michel Foucault, *Histoire de la sexualité*, vol. 1: *La volonté de savoir* (Paris: Gallimard, 1976), 74–76; Georges Didi-Huberman, *Invention de l'hystérie: Charcot et l'Iconographie photographique de la Salpêtrière* (Paris: Macula, 1982), passim; Didi-Huberman, *Invention of Hysteria*, trans. from the French by Alisa Hartz (Cambridge, Mass.: MIT Press, 2003), passim.

79. Guinon, *Agents provocateurs de l'hystérie* (1889), 98–119; Georges Gilles de la Tourette, "Hystérie et syphilis," *Progrès Médical,* 2nd series, 6 (December 17, 1887), 511–512.

80. *Leçons du mardi,* vol. 1, lesson 4: 62–65; Charcot and Pierre Marie, "Hysteria, mainly Hystero-epilepsy," in Daniel Hack Tuke, ed., *A Dictionary of Psychological Medicine,* 2 vols. (London: J. & A. Churchill, 1892), vol. 1: 637; *LMSN,* vol. 3, lecture 18: 272, 267.

81. See the case of the 24-year-old "Me...ier" (*Leçons du mardi,* vol. 2, lesson 9: 189–198) in which Charcot states that the onset of the patient's illness coincided with the rejection of an offer of marriage and that one of the symptoms is an intense genital hyperaesthesia, but then hurries to assure readers that the case is not one of "Hysteria virilis amatoria."

82. Bourneville and Régnard, *Iconographie photographique de la Salpêtrière* (1876–1880); Didi-Huberman, *Invention de l'hystérie* (1982), passim.

83. Guinon, *Agents provocateurs de l'hystérie* (1889), 129–133.

84. Freud, *On the History of the Psychoanalytic Movement,* in *Standard Edition,* vol. 14: 13–14.

85. Havelock Ellis, "Hysteria in Relation to the Sexual Emotions," *Alienist and Neurologist,* 19(4) (1898), 599–615, reprinted in *Studies in the Psy-*

*chology of Sex,* 7 vols. (Philadelphia: F. A. Davis, 1901–1928), vol. 1: 139–164.

86. Charles Lasègue, "Les hystériques, leur perversité, leurs mensonges," *Annales médico-psychologiques,* series 6 (1881), 111–118; Henri Huchard, "Caractère, moeurs, état mental des hystériques," *Archives de neurologie,* 3(8) (1882), 187–211.

87. Havelock Ellis, *Man and Woman: A Study of Human Secondary Sexual Characters* (London: Walter Scott, 1894), 283.

88. Freud, "Charcot" (1893), in *Standard Edition,* III: 13.

89. Charcot and Marie, "Hysteria, mainly Hystero-Epilepsy," in Tuke, *Dictionary of Psychological Medicine* (1892), 628.

90. The best overview of the symptomatology of Charcotian hysteria is in ibid., 629–639.

91. Albert Pitres, *Des anesthésies hystériques* (Bordeaux: Davezac, 1887).

92. Henri Parinaud, "The Ocular Manifestations of Hysteria," in William F. Norris and Charles A. Oliver, eds., *System of Diseases of the Eye,* 4 vols. (London: J. B. Lippincott, 1900), vol. 4: 727–769.

93. Paul Richer, *Paralysies et contractures hystériques* (Paris: Octave Doin, 1892).

94. Case of "Guénin," Countway Medical Library, Manuscripts Division, Charcot, Folio C96; Charcot and Marie, "Hysteria, mainly Hystero-Epilepsy," in Tuke, *Dictionary of Psychological Medicine* (1892), 635–636; Gilles de la Tourette, *Traité clinique et thérapeutique de l'hystérie* (1895), III: chap. 14, 159–245.

95. *LMSN,* vol. 3, lecture 26: 422–438; ibid., Appendix V: 483–512; *Leçons du mardi,* vol. 1, lesson 19: 357–363; ibid., vol. 2, lesson 12: 265–269.

96. *Leçons du mardi,* vol. 1, lesson 4: 60–62; ibid., lesson 11: 209–213; ibid., vol. 2, lesson 1: 13–17. See also Charcot, "Des tics et tiqueurs," *Tribune médicale,* 19 (November 25, 1888), 571–573.

97. James Paget, "Nervous Mimicry" (1873), reprinted in Stephen Paget, ed., *Selected Essays and Addresses by Sir James Paget* (London: Longmans, Green, 1902), 73–144.

98. *Leçons du mardi,* vol. 2, lesson 21: 516–523.

99. "Des tremblements hystériques," *Clinique des maladies du système nerveux* (1892–93), vol. 1, lecture 3: 46–69.

100. *Leçons du mardi,* vol. 2, lecture 17: 393–399; ibid., lecture 18: 419–433.

101. Paul Fabre, "De l'hystérie chez l'homme," *Gazette médicale de Paris,* 3(49) (December 3, 1881), 687.

102. Ten of Charcot's male patients, or 16 percent, reported the sensation of the hysterical *boule.*

103. The most detailed portraits of the Salpêtrian attack, including many

cases in men, are in Paul Richer, *Études cliniques sur la grande hystérie ou l'hystéro-épilepsie,* 2nd rev. ed. (Paris: Delahaye & Lecrosnier, 1885). From Charcot's writings, see "Description de la grande attaque hystérique" (1879) in *LMSN,* vol. 1: 435–448, and J. M. Charcot and Paul Richer, *Les démoniaques dans l'art* (Paris: Delahaye & Lecrosnier, 1887), 96–106.

104. *LMSN,* vol. 3, lecture 18: 275.

105. The influences on his formulation of the concept, however, were numerous. They include Catholic demonology, with its notion of sensory stigmata; early French and German sexological literature, which traffics in the notion of the "erotogenic zones"; and the discovery by the neurophysiologist Brown-Séquard of a "zone épileptogène" in laboratory animals.

106. "De l'hystérie chez les jeunes garçons," *LMSN,* vol. 3, lecture 6: 88. See also Charcot, "Des zones hystérogènes," *Progrès médical,* 8(51) (December 18, 1880), 1036–1038.

107. *Leçons du mardi,* vol. 2, lesson 9: 92, 97. See also Raoul Gaube, "Recherches sur les zones hystérogènes" (Doctoral diss., University of Bordeaux, 1882).

108. *LMSN,* vol. 3, lecture 21: 331; *Leçons du mardi,* vol. 2, lecture 2: 33–34; and the case of "Guénin," Countway Medical Library, Manuscripts Collection, Charcot, Folio C96.

109. *Leçons du mardi,* vol. 1, lesson 4: 63.

110. Ibid., vol. 2, lesson 17: 401. See the similar descriptions in *LMSN,* vol. 3, lecture 18: 274–275, and the case of Albert Rose, Bibliothèque Charcot.

111. P. Foet, "Attaque d'hystérie chez un homme, traitée et guérie par la compression des testicules," *Gazette hebdomadaire de médecine et chirurgie,* 11(50) (December 11, 1874), 798; A. Mossé, "Observations de grand hystérie chez l'homme—Crises convulsives arrêtées par la compression du testicule gauche," *Gazette hebdomadaire des sciences médicales de Montpellier,* 9(2) (January 8, 1887), 13–18; P.-J.-E. Bitôt and J. Sabrazès, "Anesthésie testiculaire dans l'hystérie mâle," *Bulletin de la Société d'anatomie et de physiologie de Bordeaux,* 12 (December 14, 1891), 279–281.

112. Foucault, *Histoire de la sexualité* (1976), vol. 1: 75.

113. *Leçons du mardi,* vol. 2, lesson 19: 454, 456; "Des paralysies hystéro-traumatiques chez l'homme," *Semaine médicale,* 7 (1887), 491.

114. Gilles de la Tourette, *Traité clinique et thérapeutique de l'hystérie* (1891), I: 299–300.

115. The second possibility deserves consideration. Included in the nineteenth-century medical literature are a number of cases of pseudo-

cyesis, or hysterical pregnancy, in men. These male Anna O.'s tended to develop their symptoms—faintness, morning nausea, leg cramps, and, in one case, a large tympanitic swelling of the abdomen—during the pregnancies of their wives or mistresses. See Wilhelm Griesinger, *Die Pathologie und Therapie der psychischen Krankheiten,* 2nd ed. (Stuttgart: A. Krabbe, 1861), 186; S. Weir Mitchell, *Lectures on Diseases of the Nervous System, especially in Women,* 2nd rev. and enl. ed. (Philadelphia: Lea Brothers, 1885), 63–64; and Francis W. Clark, "Hysteria in Men," *Journal of Mental Science,* 33 (January 1888), 545–546.

116. Gilles de la Tourette, *Traité clinique et thérapeutique de l'hystérie* (1891), I: 300.

117. M. D'Olier, "De la coexistence de l'hystérie et de l'épilepsie . . . considerée dans des deux sexes et en particulier chez l'homme," *Annales médico-psychologiques,* series 6 (1881), 196. For a British statement of this idea, see Thomas Savill's "Case of Hysteria Minor with 'Ovarian Phenomena' in a Male Subject," *Lancet,* 133 (May 11, 1889), 934–935.

118. *LMSN,* vol. 3, lecture 6: 89; ibid., lecture 18: 253–254; *Leçons du mardi,* vol. 2, lesson 5: 96. Guinon also emphasizes the point in "L'hystérie chez l'homme comparée à l'hystérie chez la femme," *Gazette médicale de Paris,* 56 (May 16, 1885), 231–234.

119. For the exceptions, see *Leçons du mardi,* vol. 1, lesson 4: 62–65; and ibid., vol. 2, lesson 7: 131–139.

120. Ibid., vol. 2, lesson 6: 124–125; ibid., lesson 19: 456–457.

121. Ibid., Appendix I: 533.

122. *Leçons du mardi,* vol. 2, lesson 3: 50.

123. Paul Lucas-Championnière, "Hospice de la Salpêtrière: hystérie chez l'homme," *Journal de médicine et de chirurgie pratique,* 11(56) (1885), 445.

124. Foucault wrote of the "hystérisation du corps de la femme" in the introductory volume of his *Histoire de la sexualité* (1976), 137.

125. On issues of gender in Charcot's overall medical career, see Christopher G. Goetz, "Charcot and the Myth of Misogyny," *Neurology,* 52 (May 1999), 1678–1686.

## 4. Male Hysteria at the Fin de Siècle

1. A. E. Carter, *The Idea of Decadence in French Literature, 1830–1900* (Toronto: University of Toronto Press, 1958), 145–146.

2. Robert A. Nye, *Crime, Madness, and Politics in Modern France: The Medical Concept of National Decline* (Princeton: Princeton University Press, 1984), chap. 5.

3. Susan Kingsley Kent, *Gender and Power in Britain, 1640–1990* (London and New York: Routledge, 1999), chap. 10.

4. Michelle Perrot, "The New Eve and the Old Adam: Changes in French Women's Condition at the Turn of the Century," in Margaret R. Higonnet et al., eds., *Behind the Lines: Gender and the Two World Wars* (New Haven and London: Yale University Press, 1987), chap. 3; Jennifer Waelti-Walters and Steven C. Hause, eds., *Feminisms of the Belle Époque: A Historical and Literary Anthology* (Lincoln and London: University of Nebraska Press, 1994), Appendix I.

5. Thomas Neville Bonner, *To the Ends of the Earth: Women's Search for Education in Medicine* (Cambridge, Mass.: Harvard University Press, 1992), chap. 3.

6. Yvonne Knibiehler and Catherine Fouquet, *La femme et les médecins: analyse historique* (Paris: Hachette, 1983), 193–200.

7. Elaine Showalter, *Sexual Anarchy: Gender and Culture at the Fin de Siècle* (New York: Viking, 1990), chap. 3; Mary Louise Roberts, *Disruptive Acts: The New Woman in Fin-de-Siècle France* (Chicago and London: University of Chicago Press, 2002); Sally Ledger, *The New Woman: Fiction and Feminism at the Fin de Siècle* (Manchester: Manchester University Press, 1997).

8. Peter Gay, "The Powerful, Weaker Sex," in *The Cultivation of Hatred*, vol. 3: *The Bourgeois Experience: Victoria to Freud* (New York and London: W.W. Norton, 1993), chap. 4; Christine Bard, ed., *Un siècle d'antiféminisme* (Paris: Fayard, 1999); Ute Planert, *Antifeminismus im Kaiserreich: Diskurs, soziale Formation und politische Mentalität* (Göttingen: Vandenhoeck & Ruprecht, 1998).

9. Bram Dijkstra, *Idols of Perversity: Fantasies of Feminine Evil in Fin-de-Siècle Culture* (Oxford: Oxford University Press, 1986), passim; Birgit Zilch-Purucker, *Die Darstellung der geisteskranken Frau in der bildenden Kunst des 19. Jahrhunderts am Beispiel der Melancholie und Hysterie* (Aix-la-Chapelle: Verlag Murken-Altrogge, 2001), chaps. 8–9.

10. Jeffrey Weeks, *Sex, Politics, and Society: The Regulation of Sexuality since 1800*, 2nd ed. (London and New York: Longman, 1989), 115; Alan Sinfield, *The Wilde Century: Effeminacy, Oscar Wilde, and the Queer Moment* (London and New York: Cassell, 1994), chap. 1.

11. Matt Cook, *London and the Culture of Homosexuality, 1885–1914* (New York and Cambridge: Cambridge University Press, 2003), 1–6, 22–41; William A. Peniston, *Pederasts and Others: Urban Culture and Sexual Identity in Nineteenth-Century Paris* (New York: Harrington Park Press, 2004), pt. II.

12. Antony R. H. Copley, *Sexual Moralities in France, 1780–1980: New Ideas on the Family, Divorce, and Homosexuality* (London and New York: Routledge, 1989), chap. 6.

13. George Robb and Nancy Erber, eds., *Disorder in the Court: Trials and Sexual Conflict at the Turn of the Century* (New York: New York University Press, 1999), chaps. 2 and 5; Peniston, *Pederasts and Others* (2004), chaps. 1–4; Isabel V. Hull, *The Entourage of Kaiser Wilhelm II, 1888–1918* (Cambridge: Cambridge University Press, 1982), 109–145.

14. Mosse, "Masculinity and the Decadence," in Roy Porter and Milulas Teich, eds., *Sexual Knowledge, Sexual Science* (Cambridge: Cambridge University Press, 1994), chap. 11; Michael S. Foldy, *The Trials of Oscar Wilde: Deviance, Morality, and Late-Victorian Society* (New Haven and London: Yale University Press, 1997), chap. 6.

15. Claude Quétel, *History of Syphilis*, trans. from the French by Judith Braddock and Brian Pike (London: Polity Press, 1990), chap. 6; Erwin H. Ackerknecht, *A Short History of Psychiatry*, trans. from the German by Sulammith Wolff (New York: Hafner, 1959), 66.

16. Flaubert, *Bouvard and Pécuchet*, trans. from the French by A. J. Krailsheimer (Harmondsworth: Penguin, 1976), 327.

17. Judith Surkis, *Sexing the Citizen: Morality and Masculinity in France, 1870–1920* (Ithaca and London: Cornell University Press, 2006), chap. 7; Alain Corbin, "La grande peur de la syphilis," in Jean-Pierre Bardet et al., eds., *Peurs et terreurs face à la contagion: choléra, tuberculose, syphilis, XIXe–XXe siècles* (Paris: Fayard, 1988), 328–348.

18. Andrew R. Aisenberg, *Contagion: Disease, Government, and the "Social Question" in Nineteenth-Century France* (Stanford: Stanford University Press, 1999), chap. 3.

19. Gerald N. Izenberg, *Modernism and Masculinity: Mann, Wedekind, Kandinsky through World War I* (Chicago and London: University of Chicago Press, 2000), Introduction; James Gilbert, *Men in the Middle: Searching for Masculinity in the 1950s* (Chicago and London: University of Chicago Press, 2005), chap. 2.

20. Michael C. C. Adams, *The Great Adventure: Male Desire and the Coming of World War I* (Bloomington: Indiana University Press, 1990), passim.

21. Kent, *Gender and Power in Britain* (1999), chap. 9; Christopher E. Gittings, ed., *Imperialism and Gender: Constructions of Masculinity* (New Lambton, Australia: Dangaroo Press, 1996); Graham Dawson, *Soldier Heroes: British Adventure, Empire, and the Imagining of Masculinity* (London and New York: Routledge, 1994).

22. George L. Mosse, *Nationalism and Sexuality: Respectability and Abnormal Sexuality in Modern Europe* (New York: Howard Fertig, 1985), passim.

23. Nye, *Crime, Madness, and Politics in Modern France* (1984), 141–143, 166–169; Karen Offen, "Depopulation, Nationalism, and Feminism in fin-de-siècle France," *American Historical Review*, 89 (1984), 648–676.

24. Christopher E. Forth, *The Dreyfus Affair and the Crisis of French Manhood* (Baltimore and London: Johns Hopkins University Press, 2004). For the background to French notions of middle-class male honor, see Robert A. Nye, *Masculinity and Male Codes of Honor in Modern France* (New York: Oxford University Press, 1993).

25. Christophe Prochasson, *Paris 1900: Essai d'histoire culturelle* (Paris: Calmamm-Lévy, 1999), chaps. 1–3.

26. Nancy Erber, "The French Trials of Oscar Wilde," *Journal of the History of Sexuality,* 6 (1996), 549–588.

27. Nye, *Crime, Madness, and Politics in Modern France* (1984), 169. My national portrait follows Nye's influential monograph on French degenerationism.

28. Christopher E. Forth, "Moral Contagion and the Will: The Crisis of Masculinity in Fin-de-Siècle France," in Alison Bashford and Claire Hooker, eds., *Contagion: Historical and Cultural Studies* (London and New York: Routledge, 2001), 61–75; Forth, "Neurasthenia and Manhood in *fin-de-siècle* France," in Marijke Gijswijt-Hofstra and Roy Porter, eds., *Cultures of Neurasthenia from Beard to the First World War* (Amsterdam and New York: Rodopi, 2001), chap. 15.

29. Darwin, *The Descent of Man, and Selection in Relation to Sex,* 2 vols. (London: J. Murray, 1871), chaps. 19–20.

30. Cynthia Eagle Russett, *Sexual Science: The Victorian Construction of Womanhood* (Cambridge, Mass: Harvard University Press, 1989), 83–94; Evelleen Richards, "Darwin and the Descent of Woman," in David Oldroyd and Ian Langham, eds., *The Wider Domain of Evolutionary Thought* (Dordrecht: D. Reidel, 1983), 57–111.

31. For two particularly clear examples, the first British and the second American, see Henry Maudsley, "Sex in Mind and in Education," *Fortnightly Review,* 15 (1874), 466–483, and W. K. Brooks, "The Condition of Women from a Zoological Point of View," *Popular Science Monthly,* 15 (1879), 145–155, 347–356.

32. Lombroso and Ferrero, *La donna deliquente, la prostituta e la donna normale* (Turin: L. Roux, 1893); Lombroso and Ferrero, *Criminal Woman, the Prostitute, and the Normal Woman,* trans. from the Italian by Nicole Rafter and Mary Gibson (Durham: Duke University Press, 2004).

33. Chandak Sengoopta, "Transforming the Testicle: Science, Medicine and Masculinity, 1800–1950," *Medicina nei Secoli Arte e Scienza,* 13 (2001), 637–655.

34. Robert A. Nye, "Sex Difference and Male Homosexuality in French Medical Discourse, 1830–1930," *Bulletin of the History of Medicine,* 63 (1989), 32–51.

35. Krafft-Ebing, *Psychopathia Sexualis: mit besonderer Berücksichtigung der conträren Sexualempfindung*, 2nd ed. (Stuttgart: Ferdinand Enke, 1887).

36. Showalter, *Sexual Anarchy* (1990), 4. See also Georges Lanteri-Laura, *Lecture des perversions: Histoire de leur appropriation médicale* (Paris: Masson, 1979).

37. Huxley, *Evolution and Ethics* (London and New York: Macmillan, 1893).

38. Harry Oosterhuis, *Stepchildren of Nature: Krafft-Ebing, Psychiatry, and the Making of Sexual Identity* (Chicago and London: University of Chicago Press, 2000), 275–285.

39. Paul A. Robinson, *The Modernization of Sex: Havelock Ellis, Alfred Kinsey, William Masters and Virginia Johnson* (New York: Harper & Row, 1976), chap. 1.

40. Eugen Steinach, *Sex and Life: Forty Years of Biological and Medical Experiments* (New York: Viking Press, 1940), 20.

41. Anne Fausto-Sterling, *Sexing the Body: Gender Politics and the Construction of Sexuality* (New York: Basic Books, 2000), chaps. 6 and 7; Chandak Sengoopta, "Glandular Politics: Experimental Biology, Clinical Medicine, and Homosexual Emancipation in fin-de-siècle Central Europe," *Isis*, 89 (1998), 445–473.

42. Weininger, *Geschlecht und Charakter; eine prinzipielle Untersuchung* (Vienna: W. Braumüller, 1903).

43. Weininger, *Geschlecht und Charakter* (Munich, 1980), v–xi.

44. Ibid., chap. 6.

45. Jeffrey Herf, *Reactionary Modernism: Technology, Culture, and Politics in Weimar and the Third Reich* (New York and Cambridge: Cambridge University Press, 1984).

46. David S. Luft, *Eros and Inwardness in Vienna: Weininger, Musil, Doderer* (Chicago and London: University of Chicago Press, 2003), chaps. 1–2; Chandak Sengoopta, *Otto Weininger: Sex, Science, and the Self in Imperial Vienna* (Chicago and London: University of Chicago Press, 2000); Jacques Le Rider, *Modernity and Crises of Identity: Culture and Society in Fin-de-Siècle Vienna*, trans. from the French by Rosemary Morris (New York: Continuum, 1993), passim.

47. Weininger, *Sex and Character* (1906), 8.

48. Luft, *Eros and Inwardness* (2003), 3, 54–65.

49. *Table des thèses soutenues devant la Faculté de Médecine de Paris, 1856–1980*, typescript, Bibliothèque de la Faculté de Médecine, Paris.

50. Batault, *Contribution à l'étude de l'hystérie chez l'homme* (Paris: Georges Steinheil, 1885), 145–155.

51. *Index-Catalogue: The Library of the Surgeon-General's Office*, United States Army, First and Second Series (Washington, D.C.: GPO, 1880–1916).

For the first series, see vol. VI (1885): 764–765; for the second series, vol. VII (1902): 798–801.

52. Augustin Berjon, *Une observation de grande hystérie chez l'homme* (Paris, Medical Dissertation, 1886), 3.

53. Marquézy, "L'Homme hystérique," *Bulletin médical*, 69 (August 29, 1888), 1143.

54. Debove, "Hystérie chez les hommes," *Revue médicale française et étrangère*, 65 (December 5, 1885), 918–919.

55. Dr. Olier, "De la coexistence de l'hystérie et de l'épilepsie considérée dans les deux sexes," *Annales médico-psychologiques*, series 6 (September 1881), 194.

56. Marie, "L'Hystérie à la consultation du Bureau Central des Hôpitaux de Paris—Étude statistique," *Progrès médical*, 10 (July 27, 1889), 69.

57. Alexandre Souques, "De l'hystérie mâle dans un service hospitalier," *Archives générales de médecine*, series 7, 16 (August 1890), 169.

58. Paul Michaut, *Contributions à l'étude des manifestations de l'hystérie chez l'homme* (Paris, Medical Dissertation, 1890), 14–17.

59. Émile Bitot, *L'hystérie mâle dans le service de Dr. Pitres à Bordeaux* (Paris: Octave Doin, 1890), 3–4.

60. Bodenstein cited in Gilles de la Tourette, *Traité clinique et thérapeutique de l'hystérie*, 3 vols. (Paris: Plon, Nourrit, 1891–1895), I: 57.

61. André Pitres cited in ibid., I: 66.

62. Ibid.

63. N. M. Popoff, "Un cas singulier de l'hystérie mâle," *Archives de neurologie*, 25 (May 1893), 367–373; Dr. Natier, "Contributions à l'étude du mutisme hystérique," *Revue de laryngoscopie*, 4 (1888), 16–29.

64. Charcot, *Leçons du mardi*, II, lesson 16 (March 12, 1889), 393.

65. Marie, "L'hystérie à la consultation du Bureau Central des Hôpitaux de Paris—Étude statistique," *Progrès médical*, 10 (July 27, 1889), 68–70.

66. Ibid., 68–69.

67. Ibid., 69. Italics in the original.

68. Michaut, *Contributions à l'étude des manifestations de l'hystérie chez l'homme*, (1890), 17; Fulgence Raymond, "Hystérie chez l'homme," *Mémoires de le Société de Biologie* (July 27, 1885), 237–242.

69. Léon Casaubon, *L'Hystérie chez les jeunes garçons* (Paris, Medical Dissertation, 1884).

70. Arthur Clopatt, *Études sur l'hystérie infantile* (Helsinki: J. C. Frenckell, 1888).

71. Mlle. H. Goldspiegel, *Contribution à l'étude de l'hystérie chez les enfants* (Paris, Medical Dissertation, 1888). See also Étienne Burnet, *Contribution à l'étude de l'hystérie infantile* (Paris, Medical Dissertation, 1891).

72. Klein, *De l'hystérie chez l'homme* (1880), 14–15.

73. A. Coustans, "Un cas d'hystérie mâle sans attaque," *Archives de médecine et de pharmacie militaires,* 10 (November 1886), 375–378.

74. Terrien, "De l'hystérie en Vendée," *Archives de neurologie,* 26 (December 1893), 447–475. See also Terrien, "Hystérie infantile en Vendée," *Archives de neurologie,* series 2, 4 (October-November 1897), 299–320, 369–389; and Terrien, *L'Hystérie et la neurasthénie chez le paysan* (Angers, 1906), 10–16, 25–85.

75. Léopold Jannet, *De l'hystérie chez l'homme* (Paris, Medical Dissertation, 1880).

76. Dr. Glorieux, "L'Hystérie chez l'homme," *Archives médicales belges,* series 3, 31 (1887), 234–238.

77. Quinqueton, *De l'hystérie chez l'homme* (Paris, Medical Dissertation, 1885), 13.

78. Émile Duponchel, "L'Hystérie dans l'armée," *Revue de médecine,* 6 (June 1886), 517–542.

79. Ibid., 517, 534, 540.

80. Ibid., 520–540.

81. Ibid., 535.

82. Klein, *De l'hystérie chez l'homme* (1880), 46, 47–62, passim.

83. Moty, "Hystérie chez l'homme," 30 (March 12, 1885), 235.

84. Elisé-Samuel Maricourt, *Contribution à l'étude de l'hystérie chez l'homme* (Paris, Medical Dissertation, 1877), 42.

85. Joseph Grasset, and S. Jeannet, *Quelques cas d'hystérie mâle et de neurasthénie* (1891), 9–11.

86. Ingelrans and Brongniart, "Manifestations urétrales de l'hystérie mâle," *L'Écho médical du Nord,* 3 (February 12, 1899), 78–80.

87. Paul Fabre, "De l'hystérie chez l'homme," series 5, 13 (1875), 357–359.

88. Klein, *De l'hystérie chez l'homme* (1880), 28.

89. For a sampling, see P. Foet, "Attaque d'hystérie chez un homme, traitée et guérie par la compression des testicules," *Gazette hebdomadaire de médecine et de chirurgie,* 2 (December 11, 1874), 798; A. Mossé, "Observation de grande hystérie chez l'homme avec crises convulsives arrêtées par la compression du testicule gauche," *Gazette hebdomadaire de sciences médicales de Montpellier,* 9 (January 8, 1887), 13–18; and P.-J.-E. Bitot and J. Sabrazès, "Anesthésie testiculaire dans l'hystérie," *Bulletin de la Société d'anatomie et physiologie de Bordeaux,* 12 (December 14, 1891), 279–281.

90. M. Sevestre, "Quelques cas d'hystérie chez l'homme," *L'Union médicale,* series 3, 35 (April 29, 1883), 734.

91. Bitot and Sabrazès, "Anesthésie testiculaire dans l'hystérie" (1891), 281.

See also Casaubon, *L'hystérie chez les jeunes garçons* (1884), 36, and Sevestre, "Quelques cas d'hystérie chez l'homme," *L'Union médicale* (1883), 736.

92. Léon Camuset, "Un cas de dédoublement de la personnalité," *Annales médico-psychologiques,* series 6, 7 (January 1882), 75–86; Legrand du Saulle, *Les hystériques—état physique et état mental* (Paris: Baillière, 1883), 279–286; Berjon, *Une observation de grande hystérie chez l'homme* (1886), 7–78; Ribot, *Les maladies de la personnalité* (Paris: Alcan, 1885), 82–85; Jules Voisin, "Note sur un cas de grande hystérie chez l'homme, avec dédoublement de la personnalité," *Archives de neurologie,* 10 (September 1885), 212–225; and Quinqueton, *De l'hystérie chez l'homme* (1885), 41–51.

93. Voisin, "Note sur un cas de grande hystérie chez l'homme avec dédoublement de la personnalité," *Archives de neurologie* (1885), 215.

94. Berjon, *Observation de grande hystérie chez l'homme* (1886), 14; Quinqueton, *De l'hystérie chez l'homme* (1885), 42.

95. Quinqueton, *De l'hystérie chez l'homme* (1885), 49.

96. Berjon, *Observation de grande hystérie chez l'homme* (1886), 14.

97. Ibid., 224.

98. Ibid., 12.

99. Quinqueton, *De l'hystérie chez l'homme* (1885), 47.

100. Ibid., 51.

101. Berjon, *Observation de grande hystérie chez l'homme* (1886), 13.

102. Voisin, "Un cas de grande hystérie chez l'homme," *Archives de neurologie* (1885), 213.

103. See the cases in M. G. Lecoq, "Un cas d'hystérie chez l'homme," *La France médicale,* 1, 60–61 (May 23, 1882), 709–714, 722–726; Sevestre, "Quelques cas d'hystérie," *Union médicale* (1883), 733–737; and J.-M.-L. Lucas-Championnière, "Contribution à l'étude de l'hystérie chez l'homme," *Archives de neurologie,* 14 (July 1887), 15–46.

104. Roubinovitch, *Hystérie mâle et dégénérescence* (Paris, Medical Dissertation, 1890), 9. See also Émile Bitot, "Note sur l'hystérie mâle," *Le Mercredi médical,* 2, no. 3 (January 21, 1891), 25.

105. Charcot, *Notes et observations,* I, lecture 14, 285–286.

106. Briquet, *Traité clinique et thérapeutique de l'hystérie* (1859), 33.

107. Axenfeld and Huchard, *Traité des névroses,* 2nd ed. (Paris, 1883), passim.

108. W. R. Gowers, *A Manual of Diseases of the Nervous System,* 2 vols. (London: J. and A. Churchill, 1888), II: 903–946; 2nd ed. (1893), II: 984–1030. "Some disposition to hysteria is inherent, if not in all women, at least in the vast majority," declares Gowers, who should have known better (p. 985).

109. H. C. Wood, *Nervous Diseases and Their Diagnosis* (Philadelphia: J. B. Lippincott, 1887), 97–102, 120–122, passim; William A. Hammond, *A Treatise on the Diseases of the Nervous System*, 8th ed. (New York: D. Appleton, 1888), 750–765; Charles L. Dana, *Textbook of Nervous Diseases* (New York: William Wood, 1892), 416–431. See also James Ross, *Handbook of the Diseases of the Nervous System* (London, 1885), 336–341.

110. J. A. Ormerod, "Hysteria," in *A System of Medicine*, ed. Sir Thomas Clifford Allbutt, 8 vols. (London and New York: Macmillan, 1898), VIII: [88–127], 90; Christfried Jakob, *Atlas of the Nervous System*, trans. from the German by Edward D. Fisher as *Saunder's Medical Hand Atlas* (Philadelphia and London: W. B. Saunders, 1901), 158–162; Oppenheim, *Lehrbuch der Nervenkrankheiten für Ärzte und Studierende*, 3rd enl. ed. (Berlin: S. Karger, 1901), 900–949.

111. Bernutz, "Hystérie," in S. Jaccoud, ed., *Nouveau dictionnaire de médecine et de chirurgie pratiques*, 40 vols. (Paris: Baillière, 1884), XVIII: 190.

112. Berger, *Principes élémentaires de la neurologie clinique* (Toulouse, 1886), 136. For two exceptions, see Joseph Grasset, "Hystérie," in *Dictionnaire encyclopédique des sciences médicales*, ed. A. Dechambre and L. Lereboullet, 100 vols., series 4 (Paris: G. Masson and Asselin Houzeau, 1889), XV: 252–253, and Ludwig Hirt, *The Diseases of the Nervous System: A Textbook for Physicians and Students*, trans. from the German by August Hoch (New York: D. Appleton, 1896), 519.

113. Legrand du Saulle, *Les Hystériques—état physique et état mental* (Paris, 1883), 14.

114. Jannet, *De l'hystérie chez l'homme* (Paris, Medical Dissertation, 1880), passim.

115. Ibid., 67, 81.

116. Chairou, *Études cliniques sur l'hystérie; nature, lésions anatomiques, traitement* (Paris, 1870); Augustin Fabre, *L'Hystérie viscérale: nouveaux fragments de clinique médicale* (Paris, 1883), 71; Bernard Meurisse, *Syndrome utérin et manifestations hystériques* (Paris, 1895).

117. William S. Playfair, "The Nervous System in Relation to Gynaecology," in Thomas Clifford Allbutt and W. S. Playfair, eds., *A System of Gynaecology by Many Writers* (London: Macmillan, 1897), 220–231; Graily Hewitt, *The Pathology, Diagnosis, and Treatment of the Diseases of Women*, 4th ed. (London: Longmans Green, 1882), 549–563; S. C. Gordon, "Hysteria and Its Relation to Diseases of the Uterine Appendages," *Journal of the American Medical Association*, 6 (1886), 561–567.

118. Lucien Israël, *L'Hystérique, le sexe et le médecin* (Paris, 1979), 60.

119. T[homas]. G. Stewart's *Lectures on Giddiness and on Hysteria in the Male*, 2nd ed. (Edinburgh: Pentland, 1898).

120. A. Stodart Walker, "Some Notes on 'Hysteria' with Special Reference to 'Hysteria' in the Male," *Edinburgh Medical Journal,* 40 (1894), 313.

121. Donkin, "Hysteria," in Daniel Hack Tuke, ed., *A Dictionary of Psychological Medicine,* 2 vols. (London: J. and A. Churchill, 1892), I: 624.

122. Georges Audiffrent, *Des maladies du cerveau et de l'innervation* [1874], 2nd ed. (Paris: Ernest Leroux, 1884), [349–369], 369.

123. Bouchut, "Hystérie," *Dictionnaire de médecine et de thérapeutique médicale et chirurgicale,* ed. E. Bouchut and Armand Després, 5th ed. (Paris: Félix Alcan, 1889), 783.

124. John S. Bristowe, "Hysteria and Its Counterfeit Presentments," *Lancet,* 125 (June 13–20, 1885), 1069–1072, 1113–1117.

125. Paul Fabre, "De l'hystérie chez l'homme," *Gazette médicale de Paris,* series 6, 52 (November 19, 1881), 654.

126. For three examples of this ploy, see Émile Laurent, "De l'hystérie pulmonaire chez l'homme," *L'Encéphale,* 9 (1889), 23–50; Dr. Crésantignes, "Epistaxis et mutisme hystérique chez l'homme," *Bulletin et mémoires de la Société de médecine pratique de Paris* (1888), 681–685; and Benjamin K. Hays, "Phantom Tumors in a Man," *Medical Record: A Weekly Journal of Medicine and Surgery,* 54 (October 8, 1898), 525.

127. A. Stodart Walker, "Some Notes on 'Hysteria' with Special Reference to 'Hysteria' in the Male," *Edinburgh Medical Journal,* 40 (1894), 312–322.

128. Israël, *L'Hystérique, le sexe et le médecin* (1979), 60–62.

129. See August Klein, *De l'hystérie chez l'homme* (1880), 15, and Batault, *Contribution à l'étude de l'hystérie chez l'homme* (1885), 39–41, who observes that the disorder is distributed equally among artisans, farmers, soldiers, priests, and professionals.

130. Marie, "L'Hystérie à la consultation du Bureau Central des hôpitaux de Paris," *Progrès médical* (1889), 69.

131. Souques, "De l'hystérie mâle," *Archives générales de médecine* (1890), 173.

132. Michaut, *Contribution à l'étude des manifestations de l'hystérie chez l'homme* (1890), 3, 81.

133. Klein, *De l'hystérie chez l'homme* (1880), 12.

134. Duponchel, "L'Hystérie dans l'armée," *Revue de médecine* (1886), 532.

135. Jannet, *De l'hystérie chez l'homme* (1880), 16.

136. Bourneville and P. Sollier, "Deux nouvelles observations d'hystérie mâle," *Archives de neurologie,* 22 (October 1891), 380.

137. Roubinovitch, *Hystérie mâle et dégénérescence* (1891), 61.

138. Quinqueton, *De l'hystérie chez l'homme* (1885), 12.

139. Henri Colin, *Essai sur l'état mental des hystériques* (1890), 14.

140. Fabre, "De l'hystérie chez l'homme," *Annales médico-psychologiques,* series 5, 13 (May 1875), 363–365.

141. British medical texts trafficked in the same stereotypes. See J. Russell

Reynolds, "Hysteria," *System of Medicine*, 3 vols. (Philadelphia: Henry C. Lea's Sons & Co., 1880), I: 631–642; Charles Hilton Fagge, *Principles and Practice of Medicine*, 2nd ed., compiled by Philip H. Pye-Smith, 2 vols. (London: J. and A. Churchill, 1888), I: 837; and William R. Gowers, *Epilepsy and Other Chronic Convulsive Disorders*, 2nd ed. (London: J. and A. Churchill, 1901), 187.

142. Marquézy, "L'Homme hystérique," *Bulletin médical* (1888), 1142–1143.

143. Collineau, "L'Hystérique," *Archives d'anthropologie criminelle*, 4 (1889), 331.

144. Bernutz, "Hystérie," *Nouveau dictionnaire de médecine et de chirurgie pratiques* (1884), XVIII: 190.

145. For rebuttals of this charge, see Souques, "De l'hystérie mâle," *Archives générales de médecine* (1890), 168–170, and Bitot, "Note sur l'hystérie mâle," *Mercredi médical*, 2 (1891), 26–27.

146. John B. Tuke and Edwin Bramwell, "Hysteria," *Encyclopaedia Britannica*, 11th ed. (1910), XIV: 211, 212.

147. Preeminently, see Mendel, "Über Hysterie beim männlichen Geschlecht," *Berliner klinische Wochenschrift*, 20–22 (May-June 1884), 314–317, with discussion on 330–331 and 346–348.

148. Hannah S. Decker, *Freud in Germany: Revolution and Reaction in Science, 1893–1907*, published as *Psychological Issues*, 11, 1, monograph 41 (New York, 1977), 78–80.

149. Cited in Charcot, *Notes et observations*, I, lecture 14, 289. Charcot does not reveal the author of this alleged accusation.

150. N. A., "Revue critique: L'Hystérie en Allemagne," *Progrès médical*, 2nd series, 5 (November 19, 1887), 440–442.

151. Ibid., 440. For other French defenses, see Glorieux, "L'Hystérie chez l'homme," *Archives médicales belges* (1887), 234–235, and Souques, "De l'hystérie mâle," *Archives générales de médecine* (1890), 170.

152. N. A., "L'Hystérie en Allemagne," (1887), 441.

153. A. Strümpell, "Antikritische Bemerkungen," *Neurologisches Centralblatt*, 6 (October 15, 1887), 488.

154. Drs. Andrée and Knoblauch, "Über einen Fall von Hystero-Epilepsie bei einem Manne," *Berliner klinische Wochenschrift*, 26 (March 11, 1889), 204–207.

155. Charcot, *Leçons du mardi*, II, lesson 18 (March 19, 1889), 427.

156. Gilles de la Tourette, "L'Hystérie dans l'armée allemande," *Nouvelle iconographie photographique de la Salpêtrière*, 1 (January-February 1889), 317–326. The quotation is on p. 317.

157. Moty, "Hystérie chez l'homme," *Gazette des hôpitaux*, 30 (March 12, 1885), 235–236.

158. Lucas-Championnière, "Contribution à l'étude de l'hystérie chez

l'homme—troubles de la sensibilité chez les orientaux—les aissaoua,"
*Archives de neurologie,* 14 (July 1887), 24.

159. Ibid., 46. See also Gilles de la Tourette's remarks on male hysteria in
Tunisia and Madagascar in *Traité clinique et thérapeutique de l'hystérie*
(1891), I: 121–122.

160. Philip S. Ray, "Hysteria in the Negro," *The Medical Record: A Weekly
Journal of Medicine and Surgery,* 34 (July 14, 1888), 39–40; Ray, "L'Hystérie
chez le nègre," *L'Encéphale,* 8 (1888), 563–566.

161. Cited in Gilles de la Tourette, *Traité clinique et thérapeutique de l'hystérie*
(1891), I: 122.

162. Collineau, "L'Hystérique—point de vue ethnographique," *L'Homme—
journal illustré des sciences anthropologiques,* 22 (November 25, 1887),
674–675.

163. Ibid., 673–687.

164. C. Shah, "An Interesting Case of Hysteria in a Boy," *Indian Medical Re-
cord,* 23 (1888), 302; Joseph Benjamin, "Strange Hysterical Fits in a
Young Man," *Indian Medical Record,* 6 (March 1, 1894), 144; J. R. M.
Thomson, "A Case of Hysteria in a Male," *Intercolonial Medical Journal of
Australasia,* 2 (1897), 660–663.

165. Charcot, *Leçons du mardi,* II, lesson 1 (October 23, 1888), 11–12.

166. Ibid., lesson 15 (February 19, 1889), 353.

167. "L'Hystérie en Allemagne," *Progrès médical* (1887), 440.

168. Raymond, "Résumé des principaux travaux russes concernant la neurologie," *Archives de neurologie,* 17 (May 1889), 472. For context and
commentaries, see Sander Gilman, "Jews and Mental Illness: Medical
Metaphors, Anti-Semitism, and the Jewish Response," *Journal of the History of Behavioral Sciences,* 20 (1984), 150–159, and Jan Goldstein, "The
Wandering Jew and the Problem of Psychiatric Anti-Semitism in Fin-
de-Siècle France," *Journal of Contemporary History,* 20 (1985), 521–552,
as well as Céline Kaiser and Marie-Luise Wünsche, *Die "Nervosität der
Juden" und andere Leiden an der Zivilisation: Konstruktionen des Kollektiven
und Konzepte individueller Krankheit im psychiatrischen Diskurs um 1900*
(Paderborn, Germany: Schöningh, 2003), 23–40, 89–109.

169. Henry Meige, "Le Juif-errant à la Salpêtrière: étude sur certains névropathes voyageurs," *Nouvelle iconographie de la Salpêtrière,* 6 (1893),
191–204, 277–291, 333–358.

170. Ibid., 337.

171. Ibid., 191, 192.

172. One can argue that this historical figure also appears in Anglo-American
medical literature on the related diagnosis of neurasthenia published
during the 1880s and 1890s. I have not, however, included a chapter on

medical neurasthenia—partly because my coverage of the late nineteenth century, encompassing three chapters, is already extensive; partly because the key analytical points about this body of medical writing would duplicate those of Chapter 1 (that is, like the Enlightenment-era nervous distempers, Gilded-Age neurasthenia, as a "new" diagnosis with a flattering etiology, favorable prognosis, and pleasurable therapeutics, was a nonstigmatizing label); and partly because excellent studies of the topic already exist. Among book-length studies, see Francis G. Gosling, *Before Freud: Neurasthenia and the American Medical Community, 1870–1910* (Urbana and Chicago: University of Illinois Press, 1987); Tom Lutz, *American Nervousness, 1903: An Anecdotal History* (Ithaca: Cornell University Press, 1991); Eric Caplan, *Mind Games: American Culture and the Birth of Psychotherapy* (Berkeley: University of California Press, 1998), chap. 3; Joachim Radkau, *Das Zeitalter der Nervosität: Deutschland zwischen Bismarck und Hitler* (Munich: Carl Hanser, 1998); Marijke Gijswijt-Hofstra and Roy Porter, eds., *Cultures of Neurasthenia from Beard to the First World War* (Amsterdam: Rodopi, 2001); Hans-Georg Hofer, *Nervenschwäche und Krieg: Modernitätskritik und Krisenbewältigung in der österreichischen Psychiatrie, 1880–1920* (Vienna: Böhlau, 2004), pt. 1; Andreas Killen, *Berlin Electropolis: Shock, Nerves, and German Modernity* (Berkeley: University of California Press, 2006), chaps. 2 and 3; and Petteri Pietikainen, *Neurosis and Modernity: The Age of Nervousness in Sweden* (Leiden and Boston: Brill, 2007).

173. "The Princess; A Medley" (1847), in *The Poetical Works of Alfred Lord Tennyson* (New York: Thomas Crowell, 1897), pt. V, 423. Tennyson's surrounding lines read: "Man for the field and woman for the hearth/ Man for the sword and for the needle she/ Man with the head and woman with the heart/ Man to command and woman to obey."

174. Sally Ledger, "The New Woman and the Crisis of Victorianism," in Sally Ledger and Scott McCracken, eds., *Cultural Politics at the Fin de Siècle* (Cambridge and New York: Cambridge University Press, 1995), chap. 2.

175. Louis Marquèze-Pouey, *Le mouvement décadent en France* (Paris: Presses universitaires de France, 1986), pt. III.

176. Debora Leah Silverman, *Art Nouveau in Fin-de-Siècle France: Politics, Psychology, and Style* (Berkeley: University of California Press, 1989), 78, 332 n. 15.

177. Barbara Spackman, *Decadent Genealogies. The Rhetoric of Sickness from Baudelaire to D'Annunzio* (Ithaca: Cornell University Press, 1989), viii.

178. Pierre Vareilles, "Le Progrès," in *Le Décadent*, ed. Anatole Baju, 1 (April 10, 1886), n.p.

179. Nordau, *Degeneration* [1892], intro. by George L. Mosse, trans. from the German (New York: Howard Fertig, 1968), 296–337; Émile Laurent, *La poésie décadente devant la science psychiatrique* (Paris: Maloine, 1897).

180. Thaïs Morgan, "Victorian Effeminacies," in Richard Dellamora, ed., *Victorian Sexual Dissidence* (Chicago and London: University of Chicago Press, 1999), chap. 4; Joseph Bristow, *Effeminate England: Homoerotic Writing after 1885* (Buckingham: Open University Press, 1995), 1–15.

181. As Richard Dellamora highlights in *Masculine Desire: The Sexual Politics of Victorian Aestheticism* (Chapel Hill and London: University of North Carolina Press, 1990).

182. Eve Kosofsky Sedgwick, *Between Men: English Literature and Male Homosocial Desire* (New York: Columbia University Press, 1985), passim.

183. Paul A. Robinson, *Gay Lives: Homosexual Autobiography from John Addington Symonds to Paul Monette* (Chicago: University of Chicago Press, 1999); Philippe Lejeune, "Autobiographie et homosexualité en France au XIXe siècle," *Romanticisme/Romanticism,* 56 (1987), 79–100; William A. Peniston and Nancy Erber, eds., *Queer Lives: Men's Autobiographies from Nineteenth-Century France* (Lincoln and London: University of Nebraska Press, 2007).

184. Timothy d'Arch Smith, *Love in Earnest: Some Notes on the Lives and Writings of English "Uranian" Poets from 1889 to 1930* (London: Routledge & Kegan Paul, 1970), 46–106, 235–255; Michel Larivière, ed., *Les amours masculines: Anthologie de l'homosexualité dans la littérature* (Paris: Lieu commun, 1984), 251–283.

185. Jeffrey Meyers, *Homosexuality and Literature, 1890–1930* (London: Athlone Press, 1977); James W. Jones, *"We of the Third Sex": Literary Representations of Homosexuality in Wilhelmine Germany* (New York: Peter Lang, 1990), chap. 10.

186. Janet Oppenheim, *"Shattered Nerves"* (1991), 166–167, 174–179.

187. Frédéric Fladenmuller, "Le nerveux narrateur dans *A la recherche du temps perdu,*" *Bulletin Marcel Proust,* 17 (1986), 35–42; Marie Miguet, "La Neurasthénie entre science et fiction," *Bulletin Marcel Proust* (1990), 28–42.

188. Martha Noel Evans, *Fits and Starts: A Genealogy of Hysteria in Modern France* (Ithaca and London: Cornell University Press, 1991), 64–68; William C. Carter, *Marcel Proust: A Life* (New Haven and London: Yale University Press, 2000), 400–403.

189. Adrien Proust and Gilbert Ballet, *L'Hygiène du neurasthénique* (Paris: Masson, 1897).

190. Michael R. Finn, *Proust, the Body, and Literary Form* (Cambridge and New York: Cambridge University Press, 1999), 34.

191. Michael Finn reads the two texts comparatively in ibid., 56–64.

192. The case of the fin-de-siècle Austrian novelist Arthur Schnitzler, whose father was also a physician, provides in many ways a Viennese counterpart to Proust. See Peter Gay, *Schnitzler's Century: The Making of Middle-Class Culture, 1815–1914* (New York: W. W. Norton, 2002), xxvii–xxix, 35–38, and pt. II, passim.

193. Joseph Bristow, *Empire Boys: Adventures in a Man's World* (London and Boston: Unwin Hyman, 1991).

194. Charcot, *Leçons sur les maladies du système nerveux,* ed. Babinski et al., 3 vols. (Paris: Bureaux du Progrès médical, 1887), III: lecture 18, "A propos de six cas d'hystérie chez l'homme (1)," 249–277. Gui's case appears on 269–277.

195. J. M. Charcot, *Clinical Lectures on Certain Diseases of the Nervous System,* trans. E. P. Hurd (Detroit: George S. Davis, 1888), 123–130. Quotations on pp. 125, 127, and 129.

196. *LMSN,* III, lecture 18, 274–276.

197. Didi-Huberman, *Invention of Hysteria* (2003). Sander Gilman does not reference them either in his "Image of the Hysteric," in Gilman et al., *Hysteria beyond Freud* (Berkeley: University of California Press, 1993), 345–452.

198. For a reproduction of the catalogue, see *Cimaise: Art et architecture actuels,* 31 (November–December 1984), 29–34.

199. Michael Peppiatt, *Francis Bacon: Anatomy of an Enigma* (London: Weidenfeld & Nicolson, 1996), 142–143; Dennis Farr and Massimo Martino, curators, *Francis Bacon: A Retrospective* (New York: Harry N. Abrams, 1999), 36; Michel Frizot, *The New History of Photography,* trans. from the French by Susan Bennett et al. (Cologne: Könemann, 1998), 260.

200. My thanks to Dr. Margarita Cappock and Jessica O'Donnell, archivists at the gallery, for allowing me to consult the source and aiding my investigation.

201. Peppiatt, *Francis Bacon* (1996), chap. 12.

202. On Bacon's interest in photography generally, including medical and scientific images, see Martin Harrison, *In Camera: Francis Bacon—Photography, Film, and the Practice of Painting* (New York: Thames and Hudson, 2005).

203. Clearly, the photographs cry out for theoretical exegesis. Londe's medical collection can be seen as part of a larger photographic archive of marginalized people maintained by European governments in the late nineteenth century, which Allan Sekula explores in "The Body and the Archive," *October,* 39 (Winter 1986), 3–64. For contemporaneous rep-

resentations of the strenuous male nude in Parisian visual culture, see Anthea Callen, "Doubles and Desire: Anatomies of Masculinity in the Later Nineteenth Century," *Art History*, 26 (November 2003), 669–699, and Tamar Garb, "Gustave Caillebotte's Male Figures: Masculinity, Muscularity and Modernity," in *Bodies of Modernity: Figure and Flesh in Fin-de-Siècle France* (London: Thames and Hudson, 1998), chap. 1. On the visual codification of scientific data, refer to Barbara Maria Stafford's "Presuming Images and Consuming Words: The Visualization of Knowledge from the Enlightenment to Postmodernism," in John Brewer and Roy Porter, eds., *Consumption and the World of Goods* (London and New York: Routledge, 1993), chap. 22. And on medical/technological imaging practices and "the neurological gaze," see Lisa Cartwright, *Screening the Body: Tracing Medicine's Visual Culture* (Minneapolis and London: University of Minnesota Press, 1995), chap. 3.

## 5. Freud and the Origins of Psychoanalysis

1. Kenneth Levin, *Freud's Early Psychology of the Neuroses: A Historical Perspective* (Pittsburgh: University of Pittsburgh Press, 1978), 16.

2. Freud, *An Autobiograpical Study* (1925), in *The Standard Edition of the Complete Psychological Works of Sigmund Freud*, trans. from the German under the General Editorship of James Strachey, in collaboration with Anna Freud, assisted by Alix Strachey and Alan Tyson, 24 vols. (London: The Hogarth Press and the Institute of Psycho-analysis, 1966), XX: 11.

3. *Letters of Sigmund Freud,* selected and edited by Ernst L. Freud, trans. from the German by Tania and James Stern (New York: Basic Books, 1960; 2nd ed., 1975), 171–211.

4. Letter from Sigmund Freud to Martha Bernays, dated November 24, 1885, in *Letters of Sigmund Freud* (1960), 184–185; letters from Sigmund Freud to Carl Koller, dated January 1, 1886, and October 13, 1886, reproduced in Hortense Koller Becker, "Carl Koller and Cocaine," *Psychoanalytic Quarterly,* 32 (1963), 356, 357.

5. Freud, "Charcot" (1893), in *Standard Edition, III:* 17.

6. Letter from Sigmund Freud to Martha Bernays, dated November 24, 1885, in *Letters of Sigmund Freud* (1960), 185. Later in his career, Freud hung a signed photograph of Charcot and a black-and-white lithograph of Brouillet's *A Clinical Lesson at the Salpêtrière* in his Vienna office. Andreas Mayer contends that Freud also modeled his library and consulting room in part on Charcot's lavish two-story study. See Mayer, "Objektwelten des Unbewussten: Fakten und Fetische in Charcots Museum und Freuds Behandlungspraxis," in Anke te Heesen and Emma C. Spary, eds., *Sammeln als Wissen: Das Sammeln und seine wissen-*

*schaftsgeschichtliche Bedeutung* (Göttingen: Wallstein Verlag, 2001), 169–198.

7. Freud, *An Autobiographical Study* (1925), in *Standard Edition*, XX: 13.

8. Freud, "Charcot" (1893), in *Standard Edition*, III: 22.

9. Ibid., 11–23, passim; Freud, *Autobiographical Study* (1925), in *Standard Edition*, XX: 13–14.

10. *Gazette des hôpitaux* (1885), passim, esp. 684–685, 1109–1110; *Gazette des hôpitaux* (1886), passim, esp. 157.

11. The *Index-Catalogue of the Library of the U.S. Surgeon General's Office* lists nineteen French publications dedicated to masculine hysteria in the years 1885–1886, including the dissertations of Batault, Quinqueton, and Berjon, and the article series by Émile Duponchel about hysteria in the French army.

12. Freud, "Report on My Studies in Paris and Berlin" (1886), in *Standard Edition*, I: 11.

13. J. M. Charcot, *Neue Vorlesungen über die Krankheiten des Nervensystems, insbesondere über Hysterie,* translated from the French by Sigmund Freud (Leipzig: Toeplitz & Deuticke, 1886).

14. Charcot, "Über einen Fall von hysterischer Coxalgie aus traumatischer Ursache bei einem Manne," *Weiner medizinische Wochenschrift,* 36 (May 15 and 22, 1886), 711–715, 756–759.

15. J.-M. Charcot, *Poliklinische Vorträge, 1887–1888,* trans. into German by Sigmund Freud (Leipzig and Vienna: Deuticke, 1892–1894). See also *Standard Edition*, I: 131–148.

16. Quoted in Becker, "Carl Koller and Cocaine," *Psychoanalytic Quarterly* (1963), 358. The early psychoanalytic historians Siegfried and Suzanne Bernfeld reported anecdotally that one of Freud's first patients was a second-hand bookstore owner who as a boy had been run down by a horse-drawn taxi in the Ringstrasse, had developed hysterical fits from the shock, and was treated, successfully, by Freud with electrotherapy. (Bernfeld and Bernfeld, "Freud's First Year in Practice, 1886–1887," *Bulletin of the Menninger Clinic*, 16 [1952], 39.)

17. Freud, "Report on My Studies in Paris and Berlin," in *Standard Edition*, I: 3–15. Quote on p. 5.

18. Ibid., 12.

19. Ibid., 9, 12.

20. For the organization during this time, see Karl Hermann Spitzy, ed., *Gesellschaft der Ärzte in Wien, 1837–1987* (Vienna and Munich: Edition Christian Brandstätter, 1987), 26–33.

21. Unfortunately, the lecture itself has been lost, and scholars must rely on the Society's official minutes as well as five stenographic accounts of

the meeting's proceedings recorded for several German and Austrian medical weeklies. See *Anzeiger der k. k. Gesellschaft der Aerzte in Wien*, 25 (1896), 149–152; *Allgemeine Wiener medizinische Zeitung*, 31 (1886), 506–507; *Wiener medizinische Presse*, 27 (1886), 1407–1409; *Wiener medizinische Wochenschrift*, 36 (1886), 1444–1447; *Münchener medizinische Wochenschrift*, 33 (1886), 768; and *Wiener medizinische Blätter*, 9 (1886), 1292–1294, all of which have been usefully gathered and reprinted in *Luzifer-Amor: Zeitschrift zur Geschichte der Psychoanalyse*, 1 (1988), 156–175.

22. Freud, *Autobiographical Study* (1925), in *Standard Edition*, XX: 15.

23. Freud, *The Interpretation of Dreams* (1900), in *Standard Edition*, V: 438.

24. Freud, "Beobachtung einer hochgradigen Hemi-anästhesie bei einem hysterischen Manne," *Wiener medizinische Wochenschrift*, 36 (December 1886), 1633–1638, translated in *Standard Edition*, I: 23–31.

25. Ibid., 25.

26. Ibid., 30–31.

27. Freud, *Autobiographical Study* (1925), in *Standard Edition*, XX: 15–16.

28. Henri Ellenberger, "La conférence de Freud sur l'hystérie masculine (15 octobre 1886): Étude critique," *L'Information psychiatrique*, 44 (1968), 921–929, English trans. in Mark S. Micale, ed., *Beyond the Unconscious: Essays of Henri F. Ellenberger in the History of Psychiatry* (Princeton: Princeton University Press, 1993), chap. 3; Frank J. Sulloway, *Freud, Biologist of the Mind: Beyond the Psychoanalytic Legend* (New York: Basic Books, 1979), 35–42; K. Codell Carter, "Germ Theory, Hysteria, and Freud's Early Work in Psychopathology," *Medical History*, 24 (1980), 259–274. I hope to address elsewhere this scholarly tempest in a teapot.

29. See Henri Codet and René Laforgue, "L'Influence de Charcot sur Freud," *Le progrès médical* (1925), 801–802; J.-B. Pontalis, "Freud in Paris," *International Journal of Psycho-Analysis*, 55 (1974), 455–458; Léon Chertok, "Freud à Paris: Étape décisive," *L'Évolution psychiatrique*, 34 (1969), 733–750; Jacques Nassif, *Freud l'Inconscient: Sur les commencements de la psychanalyse* (Paris: Éditions Galilée, 1977), pt. I; Julian A. Miller et al., "Some Aspects of Charcot's Influence on Freud," in *Psychological Issues*, monograph 34/35: *Freud: The Fusion of Science and Humanism* (1976), 115–132; Elisabeth Roudinesco, *La bataille de cent ans: histoire de la psychanalyse en France*, 2 vols. (Paris: Editions Ramsay, 1982, 1986), I: chap. 1; Malcolm Macmillan, "Souvenir de la Salpêtrière: M. le Dr Freud à Paris, 1885," *Australian Psychologist*, 21 (March 1986), 3–29.

30. Ernest Jones, *The Life and Work of Sigmund Freud*, 3 vols. (New York: Basic Books, 1953–1957), I: chap. 11; Peter Gay, *Freud: A Life for Our Time* (New York: W. W. Norton, 1988), 63–69.

31. In chronological order: J.-M. Charcot, *Poliklinische Vorträge* [1887–1888], trans. Sigmund Freud (1892–1894), in *Standard Edition*, I: 131–143; Freud, "Some Points for a Comparative Study of Organic and Hysterical Motor Paralyses" (1893), in *Standard Edition*, I: 155–172; Freud, "On the Psychical Mechanism of Hysterical Phenomena: A Lecture" (1893), in *Standard Edition*, III: 25–39; Breuer and Freud, "On the Psychical Mechanism of Hysterical Phenomena: Preliminary Communication" (1893), in *Standard Edition*, II: 1–17; Freud, "The Neuro-Psychoses of Defence" (1894), in *Standard Edition*, III: 41–61; Breuer and Freud, *Studies on Hysteria* (1895), in *Standard Edition*, II; Freud, "Heredity and the Etiology of the Neuroses" (1896), in *Standard Edition*, III: 141–156; Freud, "The Etiology of Hysteria" (1896), in *Standard Edition*, III: 187–221; Freud, "Further Remarks on the Neuro-Psychoses of Defence" (1896), in *Standard Edition*, III: 159–185, esp. 163–168.

32. Ola Andersson, *Studies in the Prehistory of Psychoanalysis: The Etiology of Psychoneuroses and Some Related Themes in Sigmund Freud's Scientific Writings and Letters, 1886–1896* (Stockholm: Norstedt, 1962); Toby Gelfand, "'Mon Cher Docteur Freud': Charcot's Unpublished Correspondence to Freud, 1888–1893," annotations, translations, and commentary by Toby Gelfand, *Bulletin of the History of Medicine*, 62 (Winter 1988), 563–588; Gelfand, "Charcot's Response to Freud's Rebellion," *Journal of the History of Ideas*, 50 (1989), 293–307; and Gelfand, "Sigmund-sur-Seine: Fathers and Brothers in Charcot's Paris," in Toby Gelfand and John Kerr, eds., *Freud and the History of Psychoanalysis* (Hillsdale, N.J.: Analytic Press, 1992), chap. 2.

33. "Hysteria" (1888), in *Standard Edition*, I: 39–57. The quotations are on p. 56.

34. Alain de Mijolla, "Les lettres de Jean-Martin Charcot à Sigmund Freud (1886–1893): Le crépuscule d'un dieu," *Revue française de psychanalyse*, 52 (1988), 702–725; Gelfand, "Charcot's Response to Freud's Rebellion," *Journal of the History of Ideas* (1989).

35. This point has been explored in depth by Katrien Libbrecht and Julien Quackelbeen in "On the Early History of Male Hysteria and Psychic Trauma: Charcot's Influence on Freudian Thought," *Journal of the History of the Behavioral Sciences*, 31 (October 1995), 370–384.

36. Sander L. Gilman, *Freud, Race, and Gender* (Princeton: Princeton University Press, 1993), 93–113.

37. Freud, "Heredity and the Etiology of the Neuroses" (1896), in *Standard Edition*, III: 143, 151.

38. Ibid., 151

39. Peter W. Halligan, Christopher Bass, and John C. Marshall, eds., *Con-*

*temporary Approaches to the Study of Hysteria* (Oxford and New York: Oxford University Press, 2001), passim.

40. *Studies on Hysteria,* in *Standard Edition,* II: 21–181.

41. Sara van den Berg, "Textual Bodies: Narratives of Denial and Desire in *Studies on Hysteria,*" in Mary G. Winkler and Letha B. Cole, eds., *The Good Body: Asceticism in Contemporary Culture* (New Haven and London: Yale University Press, 1994), chap. 9.

42. *Studies on Hysteria,* in *Standard Edition,* II: 160–161.

43. Lisa Appignanesi and John Forrester, *Freud's Women* (London: Basic Books, 1992), 63–116.

44. *Studies on Hysteria* (1895), in *Standard Edition,* II: 100–101, 163–164, 169–170, 175–176, 180–181.

45. Freud, "Etiology of Hysteria" (1896), in *Standard Edition,* III: 207–208; Freud, "Further Remarks on the Neuro-Psychoses of Defence" (1896), in *Standard Edition,* III: 163.

46. Ilse Grubrich-Simitis, *Early Freud and Late Freud,* trans. from the German by Philip Slotkin (London and New York: Routledge, 1997), 18.

47. Freud and Breuer, *Studies on Hysteria,* Introduction by Rachel Bowlby, trans. Nicola Luckhurst (London and New York: Penguin Books, 2004), xix.

48. Freud, "On the Psychical Mechanism of Hysterical Phenomenon" (1893), in *Standard Edition,* III: 27.

49. Freud, "Quelques considérations pour une étude comparative des paralysies motrices organiques et hystériques," *Archives de neurologie,* 26 (July 1893), 29–43; Freud, "L'Hérédité et l'étiologie des névroses," *Revue neurologique,* 4 (March 1896), 161–169.

50. Jean Garrabé and R. Rechtman, "Les écrits français (1893–1896) de Freud," paper delivered on May 13, 1995, at the conference on "Freud's Pre-Analytical Writings (1877–1900)" in Gent, Belgium; Nicole Edelman, "Freud, les hystériques et les Français," in Edelman, *Les métamorphoses de l'hystérique: Du début du XIXe siècle à la Grande Guerre* (Paris: Éditions La Découverte, 2003), 297–306.

51. "Preliminary Communication" (1893), in *Standard Edition,* II: 17.

52. Franziska Lamott, *Die vermessene Frau: Hysterien um 1900* (Munich: Wilhelm Fink Verlag, 2001).

53. Breuer and Freud, *Studies on Hysteria* (1895), in *Standard Edition,* II: xxxi.

54. The exception is "Sexuality in the Etiology of the Neuroses" (1898), in *Standard Edition,* III: 259–285.

55. Ernst Kris, "Wilhelm Fliess's Scientific Interests," in *Origins of Psycho-Analysis* (1954), 3–14; Sulloway, *Freud, Biologist of the Mind* (1979), chaps. 5 and 6.

56. Sigmund Freud, *Aus den Anfängen der Psychoanalyse: Briefe an Wilhelm Fliess* (London: Imago, 1950); *The Origins of Psycho-Analysis: Letters to Wilhelm Fliess, Drafts and Notes: 1887–1902, by Sigmund Freud,* ed. Marie Bonaparte, Anna Freud, and Ernst Kris, trans. from the German by Eric Mosbacher and James Strachey (New York: Basic Books, 1954); *The Complete Letters of Sigmund Freud to Wilhelm Fliess, 1887–1904,* trans. and ed. Jeffrey Moussaieff Masson (Cambridge, Mass.: Harvard University Press, 1985); *Sigmund Freud Briefe an Wilhelm Fliess, 1887–1904,* Herausgegeben von Jeffrey Moussaieff Masson, Bearbeitung der deutschen Fassung von Michael Schröter, Transkription von Gerhard Fichtner (Frankfurt am Main: S. Fischer, 1986).

57. Letter from Sigmund Freud to Wilhelm Fliess, dated May 2, 1897, in *Complete Letters,* 240; *Sigmund Freud Briefe an Wilhelm Fliess,* 255.

58. *Origins of Psychoanalysis,* 126; *Sigmund Freud Briefe an Wilhelm Fliess,* 146.

59. Gay, *Freud: A Life for Our Time* (1988), 96; letter from Freud to Fliess, dated February 9, 1898, in *Complete Letters,* 299; *Sigmund Freud Briefe an Wilhelm Fliess,* 326.

60. Max Schur, *Freud: Living and Dying* (New York: International Universities Press, 1972), chap. 4; Mark Kanzer and Jules Glenn, eds., *Freud and His Self-Analysis* (New York: J. Aronson, 1983); Gay, *Freud: A Life for Our Time* (1988), 96–99.

61. Freud to Fliess, *Origins of Psychoanalysis,* 234; *Sigmund Freud Briefe an Wilhelm Fliess,* 305.

62. *Studies on Hysteria,* in *Standard Edition,* II: 117. See also Heinz Schott, "Elemente der Selbstanalyse in den '*Studien über Hysterie*': Erlauterungen zum Ursprung der psychoanalytischen Technik," *Gesnerus,* 37 (1980), 235–256, and Siegfried Bernfeld, "An Unknown Autobiographical Fragment by Freud," *American Imago,* 4 (1946), 3–19.

63. Didier Anzieu, *Freud's Self-Analysis* [1959], trans. from the French by Peter Graham (Madison, Conn.: International Universities Press, 1986). See also Heinz Schott, "Elemente der Selbstanalyse in den *Studien über Hysterie*: Erlauterungen zum Ursprung der psychoanalytischen Technik," *Gesnerus,* 37 (1980), 235–256, and Siegfried Bernfeld, "An Unknown Autobiographical Fragment by Freud," *American Imago,* 4 (1946), 3–19.

64. Freud, *Interpretation of Dreams* (1900), in *Standard Edition,* IV: xxvi.

65. Michel Serres, *Hermes—Literature, Science, Philosophy* (Baltimore: Johns Hopkins University Press, 1982), chap. 2.

66. Letters dated May 6, 1894, and September 29, 1896, in *Complete Letters,* 70, 198; *Sigmund Freud Briefe an Wilhelm Fliess,* 65, 209.

67. Freud to Fliess, *Complete Letters,* letters dated August 14, 1897, and Oc-

tober 3, 1897, 261 and 269; *Sigmund Freud Briefe an Wilhelm Fliess,* 280, 289.

68. Freud to Fliess, *Complete Letters,* 254; *Sigmund Freud Briefe an Wilhelm Fliess,* 271.

69. Freud to Fliess, *Complete Letters,* letter dated July 7, 1897, 255; *Sigmund Freud Briefe an Wilhelm Fliess,* 272.

70. Letters from Freud to Fliess, dated October 31, 1897, and January 4, 1898, *Complete Letters,* 275–276, 291–293.

71. Freud to Fliess, *Complete Letters,* 261; *Sigmund Freud Briefe an Wilhelm Fliess,* 281.

72. *Complete Letters,* letter dated October 3, 1897, 269; *Sigmund Freud Briefe an Wilhelm Fliess,* 289.

73. *Complete Letters,* letter dated August 31, 1898, 325; *Sigmund Freud Briefe an Wilhelm Fliess,* 355.

74. Max Schur, who later was Freud's physician, discusses Freud's "hysterical tachycardia" in *Living and Dying* (1972), chap. 2. After first reading the Fliess letters in 1950, James Strachey characterized Freud as Fliess's "hysterical partner." (Quoted in Riccardo Steiner, "'Et in Arcadia Ego . . . ?' Some Notes on Methodological Issues in the Use of Psychoanalytic Documents and Archives," *International Journal of Psychoanalysis,* 76 [August 1995], 752.) Even Ernest Jones ruefully admitted that "however unpalatable the idea may be to hero-worshippers, the truth has to be stated that Freud did not always possess the serenity and inner sureness so characteristic of him in the years when he was well known. . . . There is ample evidence that for ten years or so—roughly comprising the nineties—he suffered from a very considerable psychoneurosis" (Jones, *Life and Work of Sigmund Freud,* 1: 304).

75. William J. McGrath, *Freud's Discovery of Psychoanalysis: The Politics of Hysteria* (Ithaca and London: Cornell University Press, 1986), esp. chap. 4; Marianne Krüll, *Freud and His Father,* trans. from the German by Arnold J. Pomerans (New York: W. W. Norton, 1986); John E. Toews, "Historicizing Psychoanalysis: Freud in His Time and for Our Time," *Journal of Modern History,* 63 (September 1991), 516–524.

76. Freud's letters of August 23, 1894, August 16, 1895, October 13, 1895, November 2, 1896, and January 11, 1897, in *Complete Letters,* 92–94, 135, 148, 202, and 222, all discuss male patients.

77. As best I can tell, the thin line of scholarship on the case goes as follows: *Origins of Psychoanalysis* (1954), 131 n. 1; Anzieu, *Freud's Self-Analysis* (1986), 161, 190, 521–525; Eva Rosenblum, "Le premier parcours psychanalytique d'un homme relaté par Freud," *Études psychothérapeutiques,* 4 (1973), 51–58; Peter L. Rudnytsky, *Freud and Oedipus* (New York:

Columbia University Press, 1987), 56–62; Douglas A. Davis, "Freud's Unwritten Case," *Psychoanalytic Psychology,* 7 (1990), 185–209; Juliet Mitchell, *Mad Men and Medusas: Reclaiming Hysteria* (New York: Basic Books, 2000), 64–71; and Douglas A. Davis, "Freud's Unwritten Case: The Patient 'E.,'" at *www.haverford.edu/psych/ddavis/freud_e.html.*

78. The psychoanalytic sleuth Peter Swales claims that the patient's real name was Oscar Fellner. Communication from Peter Swales to the author, August 10, 2006; my thanks to Mr. Swales for kindly sharing this information with me.

79. Letter from Freud to Fliess, dated October 31, 1895, *Complete Letters,* 148; *Sigmund Freud Briefe an Wilhelm Fliess,* 153.

80. *Complete Letters,* letter dated November 2, 1895, 149; *Sigmund Freud Briefe an Wilhelm Fliess,* 153. (Freud's italics.)

81. Draft L: "Architecture of Hysteria," *Complete Letters,* 242.

82. Ibid., letters dated December 29, 1897, and February 19, 1899, 290, 345–346.

83. Ibid., letter dated December 29, 1897, 290.

84. Ibid., letters dated December 21, 1899, 391–392 (Freud's italics) and January 8, 1900, 395; *Sigmund Freud Briefe an Wilhelm Fliess,* 430, 434. Heinrich Schliemann was the nineteenth-century German archaeologist who excavated many ancient sites in Greece and Turkey, including, he believed, the Homeric city of Troy.

85. Rosenblum, "Le premier parcours psychanalytique," *Études psycho-thérapeutiques* (1973), 56; Rudnytsky, *Freud and Oedipus* (1987), 56; Davis, "Freud's Unwritten Case," *Psychoanalytic Psychology* (1990), 191–195.

86. Letter dated December 21, 1899, *Complete Letters,* 392.

87. Letter from Freud to Fliess, dated December 21, 1899, *Complete Letters,* 391; *Sigmund Freud Briefe an Wilhelm Fliess,* 430. See also Anzieu, *Freud's Self-Analysis* (1986), 161, 523.

88. Letter dated April 16, 1900, *Complete Letters,* 409; *Sigmund Freud Briefe an Wilhelm Fliess,* 448–449. (Freud's italics.)

89. I might have added a fourth figure, namely Shakespeare. For Freud's observations on "Hamlet the hysteric," see his letters to Fliess dated September 21, October 15, and November 5 of 1897, in *Complete Letters,* 265, 272–273, 277.

90. For the fullest analyses, written respectively from the perspectives of feminist and gay studies, see Shirley Nelson Garner, "Freud and Fliess: Homophobia and Seduction," in Dianne Hunter, ed., *Seduction and Theory: Readings of Gender, Representation, and Rhetoric* (Urbana and Chicago: University of Illinois Press, 1989), chap. 5, and Wayne Koesten-

baum, *Double Talk: The Erotics of Male Literary Collaboration* (New York and London: Routledge, 1989), chap. 1. See also Gay, *Freud, A Life for Our Time* (1988), 86–87, 275–277.

91. Jones, *Life and Work of Sigmund Freud* (1953), I: 287n.

92. Letters from Freud to Fliess, dated June 22, 1894, August 7, 1894, and May 18, 1898, in *Complete Letters*, 84, 89, 313; *Sigmund Freud Briefe an Wilhelm Fliess*, 77, 83, 342.

93. Letters dated August 16, 1895, and January 4, 1898, *Complete Letters*, 135, 292.

94. Jones, *Life and Work of Sigmund Freud* (1953), I: 287.

95. On the breakup, see *Complete Letters*, 459–468; Sulloway, *Freud, Biologist of the Mind* (1979), 223–235; and Peter Heller, "A Quarrel over Bisexuality," in Gerald Chapple and Hans H. Schulte, eds., *The Turn of the Century: German Literature and Art, 1890–1915* (Bonn: Bouvier Verlag, 1983), 87–115.

96. Letter from Freud to Fliess, dated May 7, 1900, *Complete Letters*, 412; *Sigmund Freud Briefe an Wilhelm Fliess*, 452.

97. Letter dated August 7, 1901, *Complete Letters*, 447; *Sigmund Freud Briefe an Wilhelm Fliess*, 492.

98. Letters from Freud to Ferenczi, dated October 6 and October 17, 1910, in *The Correspondence of Sigmund Freud and Sándor Ferenczi*, ed. Eva Brabant, Ernst Falzeder, and Patrizia Giampieri-Deutsch, trans. from the German by Peter T. Hoffer, 3 vols. (Cambridge, Mass.: Belknap Press of Harvard University Press, 1993–2000), vol. 1: 221, 227.

99. Letter from Freud to Ernest Jones, dated December 8, 1912, cited in Jones, *Life and Work of Sigmund Freud* (1953), I: 317.

100. Douglas Davis in "Freud's Unwritten Case," *Psychoanalytic Psychology* (1990), 194–195, also emphasizes this point.

101. For related interpretations of this period in Freud's career, see John E. Toews, "Fashioning the Self in the Story of the 'Other': The Transformation of Freud's Masculine Identity between 'Elisabeth von R.' and 'Dora,'" in Suzanne L. Marchand and Elizabeth Lunbeck, eds., *Proof and Persuasion: Essays on Authority, Objectivity, and Evidence* (Amsterdam: Brepols Press, 1996), chap. 10, and Liliane Weissberg, "Was will der Mann? Gedanken zum Briefwechsel von Sigmund Freud und Wilhelm Fliess," in Claudia Benthien and Inge Stephan, eds., *Männlichkeit als Maskerade: Kulturelle Inszenierungen vom Mittelalter bis zur Gegenwart* (Cologne: Böhlau, 2003), 81–99.

102. As Juliet Mitchell has also argued in her important study *Mad Men and Medusas* (2000), Preface and chap. 2. See as well Tamar Garb and Mignon Nixon, "A Conversation with Juliet Mitchell," *October*, 113 (Summer 2005), 9–26.

103. See Jones, *Life and Work of Sigmund Freud* (1953), I: 287–289; and Masson, ed., *Complete Letters* (1985), Introduction, 1–13.

104. Jones, *Life and Work of Sigmund Freud,* I: 288.

105. Strictly speaking, this is not true: in *From the History of an Infantile Neurosis* (1918) Freud locates hysterical components in the Wolf Man's obsessional personality, and in "Dostoevsky and Parricide" (1928) the Russian novelist suffers hystero-epileptic fits.

106. Freud, *Three Essays on the Theory of Sexuality* (1905), in *Standard Edition,* VII: 123–245.

107. Ibid., 220.

108. Sulloway, *Freud, Biologist of the Mind* (1979), chap. 8; Jacques Le Rider, *Modernity and Crises of Identity: Culture and Society in Fin-de-Siècle Vienna* [1990], trans. from the French by Rosemary Morris (New York: Continuum, 1993), 77–79, 101–107, 171–173.

109. Freud, "Hysterical Phantasies and Their Relation to Bisexuality" (1908), in *Standard Edition,* IX: 157–166; see especially the closing paragraphs of the essay. For an intelligent discussion of Freud's thinking on this theme, see Elisabeth Young-Bruehl, ed., *Freud on Women: A Reader* (New York: W. W. Norton, 1990), Introduction. And on the implicit lines of gender analysis in early psychoanalytic theory that Freud chose *not* to explore, see John Brenkman, "Freud the Modernist," in Mark S. Micale, ed., *The Mind of Modernism: Medicine, Psychology, and the Cultural Arts in Europe and America, 1880–1940* (Stanford: Stanford University Press, 2004), 190–196.

110. Scholars occasionally contrast "Freud's women of the 1890s" and "Freud's men of the 1900s." To restate their point interrogatively, how did a theory and therapy of female hysteria yield a psychology of universal psychological processes that takes male experience as its prototype? My answer is that the theorization of male neurosis, although hidden from the printed record, was present in Freud's life and thought all along the way.

111. Carolyn G. Heilbrun, *Toward a Recognition of Androgyny* (New York: Knopf, 1973), ix.

## Conclusion

1. "Wir sind uns unbekannt, wir Erkennenden, wir selbst uns selbst: das hat seinen guten Grund. Wir haben nie nach uns gesucht—wie sollte es geschehn, dass wir eines Tages uns *fanden?* . . . Für uns sind wir keine 'Erkennenden.'" In *Zur Genealogie der Moral,* ed. W. D. Williams (Oxford: Basil Blackwell, 1972), 3; *On the Genealogy of Morals,* trans. from the German by Walter Kaufmann and R. J. Hollingdale (New York: Vintage Books, 1967), 15.

2.  This pattern is borne out in one historical setting after another. Illustratively, see James Gilbert, *Men in the Middle: Searching for Masculinity in the 1950s* (Chicago and London: University of Chicago Press, 2005); Kristin L. Hoganson, *Fighting for American Manhood: How Gender Politics Provoked the Spanish-American and Philippine-American Wars* (New Haven and London: Yale University Press, 1998); Mary Louise Roberts, *Civilization Without Sexes: Reconstructing Gender in Postwar France, 1917–1927* (Chicago and London: University of Chicago Press, 1994); Clare A. Lees, ed., *Medieval Masculinities: Regarding Men in the Middle Ages* (Minneapolis: University of Minnesota Press, 1994); and André Rauche, *Le premier sexe: mutations et crise de l'identité masculine* (Paris: Hachette, 2000).

3.  See Camille Paglia, *Sexual Personae: Art and Decadence from Nefertiti to Emily Dickinson* (New York: Vintage, 1991), passim; Lisa Appignanesi, *Femininity and the Creative Imagination: A Study of Henry James, Robert Musil, and Marcel Proust* (London: Vision Press, 1973), 1–19, 217–223.

4.  This is the memorable phrase of Peter Middleton in *The Inward Gaze: Masculinity and Subjectivity in Modern Culture* (London and New York: Routledge, 1992), chap. 1. See also Kaja Silverman, *Male Subjectivity at the Margins* (New York and London: Routledge, 1992), 15–51, and E. Ann Kaplan, "Is the Gaze Male?" in Ann Snitow, Christine Stansell, and Sharon Thompson, eds., *Powers of Desire: The Politics of Sexuality* (New York: Monthly Review Press, 1983), 309–327.

5.  To date, psychoanalytic psychology provides the most compelling explanation of the possible psychodynamics at work: males entering adulthood, unlike teenage females, must decisively separate themselves from their nurturing mothers in order to achieve independent gender identity as men. The critical threat to masculinity in the boy is not, as Freud maintained obsessively, castration by the father but engulfment by the mother. The psychological imperative to free oneself from infant maternal identification, therefore, requires a continual censuring of the eternal "feminine within"; hence the more difficult passage from adolescence to manhood than to womanhood. See C. G. Jung, *Aspects of the Masculine*, trans. from the German by R. F. C. Hull (Princeton: Princeton University Press, 1989), 9–23; Ralph R. Greenson, "The Struggle against Identification," *Journal of the American Psychoanalytic Association*, 2 (1954), 200–217; Nancy J. Chodorow, *The Reproduction of Mothering: Psychoanalysis and the Sociology of Gender* (Berkeley: University of California Press, 1978); Chodorow, *Femininities, Masculinities, Sexualities: Freud and Beyond* (Lexington, Ky.: University Press of Kentucky, 1994), chap. 3; and Elisabeth Badinter, *XY: De l'identité masculine* (Paris: Éditions Odile Jacob, 1992).

6. Jonathan Rutherford, *Men's Silences: Predicaments in Masculinity* (London: Routledge, 1992).
7. Elaine Showalter, *Sexual Anarchy: Gender and Culture at the Fin de Siècle* (New York: Vintage, 1990), 133–134. See also Stephen M. Whitehead, "Man: The Invisible Gendered Subject?" in Stephen M. Whitehead and Frank J. Barrrett, eds., *The Masculinities Reader* (Cambridge: Polity Press, 2001), chap. 20, and the essays by Claudia Benthien and Walter Erhart in Claudia Benthien and Inge Stephan, eds., *Männlichkeit als Maskerade: Kulturelle Inszenierungen vom Mittelalter bis zur Gegenwart* (Cologne and Weimar: Böhlau Verlag, 2003).
8. Private communication from Robert Nye to the author, August 30, 2001.
9. Among the book-length studies, see Eric J. Leed, *No Man's Land: Combat and Identity in World War I* (Cambridge and New York: Cambridge University Press, 1979); Elaine Showalter, *The Female Malady: Women, Madness, and English Culture, 1830–1980* (New York: Pantheon, 1985), chap. 7; Marc Roudebush, "A Battle of Nerves: Hysteria and Its Treatment in France during World War I," Ph.D. diss., University of California, Berkeley, 1995; Ben Shephard, *A War of Nerves: Soldiers and Psychiatrists in the Twentieth Century* (Cambridge, Mass.: Harvard University Press, 2001), chaps. 1–10; Mark S. Micale and Paul Lerner, eds., *Traumatic Pasts: History, Psychiatry, and Trauma in the Modern Age, 1870–1930* (New York: Cambridge University Press, 2001); Peter Leese, *Shell Shock: Traumatic Neurosis and the British Soldiers of the First World War* (New York: Palgrave, 2002); Paul Lerner, *Hysterical Men: War, Psychiatry, and the Politics of Trauma in Germany, 1890–1930* (Ithaca: Cornell University Press, 2003); and Hans-Georg Hofer, *Nervenschwäche und Krieg: Modernitätskritik und Krisenbewältigung in der österreichischen Psychiatrie (1880–1920)* (Vienna: Böhlau, 2004).
10. The quotation is from Isaiah Berlin, in Michael Ignatieff, *Isaiah Berlin: A Life* (New York: Metropolitan Books, 1998), 301.
11. Davis S. Gutterman, "Postmodernism and the Interrogation of Masculinity," in Harry Brod and Michael Kaufman, eds., *Theorizing Masculinities* (Thousand Oaks, Calif.: Sage Publications, 1994), 219–238.

# Index

workers, 138, 154, 155, 158, 239,
  316n67. *See also* artisans; class
workers' accident legislation, 140
World War One. *See* First World War

York (city of), 91
Young-Bruehl, Elisabeth, xii, 345n109.

*See also* bisexuality; Freud, Sigmund;
psychoanalysis

Zola, Émile, 167, 169, 186, 211, 232,
  255